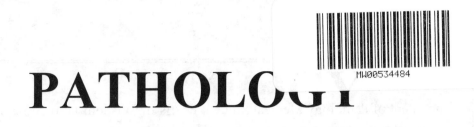

# PATHOLOGY

# MEDICAL STUDENT

## USMLE BOARD PART I

## PEARLS OF WISDOM

**Cory A. Roberts**

## NOTE

The intent of Pathology Medical Student Pearls of Wisdom is to serve as a study aid to improve performance on a standardized examination. It is not intended to be a source text of the knowledge base of medicine or to serve as a reference in any way for the practice of clinical medicine. Neither Boston Medical Publishing Corporation nor the editors warrant that the information in this text is complete or accurate. The reader is encouraged to verify each answer in several references. All drug use indications and dosages must be verified by the reader before administration of any compound.

The editors would like to extend thanks to Terri Lair for her excellent managing and editorial support.

This book was produced using Times and Symbols fonts and computer based graphics with Macintosh® computers

ISBN: 1-58409-018-9

# DEDICATION

*When I decided to undertake writing this book, I did so with every intention to make it a valuable aid in studying for the USMLE Board examination.  I wanted to make certain that it was of the quality that I would have wanted, used and benefited from as a medical student.  Thus, my goal was to make a high quality text that I would be extremely proud to have my name upon as the sole author.  Suffice it to say that the book would not be on the shelf now if I did not feel that I held up my end of my self imposed guidelines.  However, I leave it to you, the reader, as the sole judge as to whether you feel that I have succeeded or not.*

*While my goals for this text were lofty, I owe a mountain of gratitude to a number of people who inspired me throughout my career.  Several of the people who trained me taught me that the phrase "lofty goals" is, in fact, redundant.  They taught me to aim for goals that others have not deemed possible or, better yet, have not even thought of.  This project was initially offered to me by way of James R. Newland, MD here at the University of Nebraska who himself is a dedicated teacher who has taught me the importance of investing one's energy in a tireless manner in order to train future physicians.  He is a man for whom I have great respect.  Samuel M. Cohen, MD, PhD and Rodney S. Markin, MD, PhD, serve as Chair and Vice Chair of the Department of Pathology at the University of Nebraska.  They have created an atmosphere in which pursuit of scholarly activities is expected and fostered. Dr. James Linder exemplified thinking beyond the normal boundaries.  Drs. Julie Breiner, Cary Buresh and Stan Radio offered me some of the images used in this text.  In addition, Drs. Buresh and Breiner taught me a great deal of pathology during our years of training together.  They forced me to work hard so as to not be left behind as they grew into outstanding pathologists.*

*The work that went into this book was tremendous.  My sons, Nathan and Nolan, served as the energy source from which I was rejuvenated when the late nights took their toll.  They are the best things I have on this earth.  Of course, my wife, Tiffany Roberts, MD, made the entire project a reality by allowing me to spend an inordinate amount of time away from many duties usually assigned to me and she did so without complaint.  She is a better wife than I deserve and makes my boys the most blessed children anywhere.  My own mother worked harder than I ever will to make sure that my brothers and I had everything that everyone else had.  I can assure you that I would not be in my current position without her.  Again, another example of someone who gave me more than I could have ever earned.*

*For you, Mom.  A drop in the bucket compared to what you gave me.*

*....CAR*

Cory A. Roberts, MD
Assistant Professor
Department of Pathology and
Microbiology
University of Nebraska Medical Center
Omaha, Nebraska

## WE APPRECIATE YOUR COMMENTS!

We appreciate your opinion and encourage you to send us any suggestions or recommendations. Please let us know if you discover any errors, or if there is any way we can make Pearls of Wisdom more helpful to you. We are also interested in recruiting new authors and editors. Please call, write, fax, or e-mail. We look forward to hearing from you.

## Return to:

**Boston Medical Publishing Corporation**
**237 S. 70th Street, Suite 206, Lincoln, NE, 68510**

**888-MBOARDS (626-2737)**
**402-484-6118**
**Fax: 402-484-6552**
**E-mail: bmp@emedicine.com**
**www.emedicine.com**

# INTRODUCTION

Congratulations! Pathology Medical Student Pearls of Wisdom will help you learn about pathology as well as prepare for the pathology USMLE board examination. This book is structured in a question and answer format. This permits the reader to concentrate on areas of interest or weakness. Some readers will find answering questions the preferred way to study for a board exam. After completing a Pearls chapter, these readers are encouraged to examine the corresponding textbook chapter entirely, for comprehensiveness.

Most readers will probably use this book in a post-textbook review mode. One such method involves reading a chapter in a textbook then proceeding to answer the questions posed in this book. Other readers will prefer to comprehensively study the contents of a pathology text entirely and use this book afterwards. The purpose of the last two methods is to permit the reader to uncover areas of weakness and to become familiarized with the process of answering questions. Answering questions during a board exam is a cognitive task that is optimized by preparing a specific set of cognitive skills.

It must be emphasized that a question and answer book is most useful as a learning tool when used in conjunction with a textbook of pathology. This is because the question/answer format is an active learning process that is at its best when the questioning process continues farther along than ending with answering the Pearls question. The more active the learning process, the better the understanding. When the reader approaches a question that he/she cannot recall the answer to or uncovers a topic of interest, he/she is encouraged to read in the textbook at hand.

Most of the questions are short with short answers. This facilitates moving through a large body of knowledge. Some of the questions have longer answers. In these situations, the questions were not altered because of the clinically interesting question posed.

Certain topics have been repeated in a single chapter and across chapters. This was intentional. Some topics are so important to a practitioner that repetition was utilized as a learning tool.

Each question is preceded by two boxes, to permit the reader to check off areas of interest, weakness or simply noting that it had been read. This allows for re-reading without having uncertainty of what was reviewed earlier.

Great effort has been made to verify that the questions and answers are accurate. Some answers may not be the answer you would prefer. Most often this is attributable to variance between original sources. Please make us aware of any errors you find. We hope to make continuous improvements and would greatly appreciate any input with regard to format, organization, content, presentation or about specific questions. We also are interested in recruiting new contributing authors and publishing new textbooks. Contact our manager at Boston Medical Publishing, Terri Lair, at (toll free) 1-888-MBOARDS. We look forward to hearing form you!

Study hard and good luck!

C. A. R.

# TABLE OF CONTENTS

# THE CELL

❏❏ **What is the basic structure of the cytoplasmic membrane?**

Lipid bilayer.

❏❏ **What cellular components are responsible for protein production and processing?**

Rough and smooth endoplasmic reticulum.

❏❏ **What cellular component is responsible for energy production?**

Mitochondria.

❏❏ **Name the cellular component responsible for enzymatic degradation of intracellular debris.**

Lysosomes.  Primary lysosomes contain enzymes and become secondary lysosomes upon ingestion and phagocytosis of intracellular debris.

❏❏ **What is the cellular adaptation whereby a cell increases in size?**

Hypertrophy.  Remember, hyperplasia refers to an increase in number of cells while hypertrophy refers to an increase in size of a cell.

❏❏ **What is the nuclear chromatin composed of?**

DNA (deoxyribonucleic acid).

❏❏ **What is the nucleolus, located within the nucleus, composed of?**

RNA (ribonucleic acid).

❏❏ **What is the primary energy source for the cell?**

ATP (adenosine triphosphate).

❏❏ **What type of necrosis would one expect following an ischemic injury?**

Coagulative necrosis. This is the most common type of necrosis and follows ischemia.  Chemical injury is marked by cell swelling with subsequent rupture and coagulation of cytoplasmic proteins.  Histologically, it is composed of bland, eosinophilic material without cellular nuclei.

❏❏ **What type of cell death is regulated or programmed?**

Apoptosis.  In apoptosis, the cells shrink resulting in condensation of chromatin and fragmentation of DNA and the nucleus.  This stands in contrast to the cell swelling seen in coagulative necrosis.

❏❏ **What is the term used to describe fragmentation of a nucleus in cell death?**

Karyorrhexis.

❏❏ **What is the term used to describe condensation of a nucleus, resulting in nuclear hyperchromasia on its way to death?**

Pyknosis.

❑❑  **What type of necrosis consists of amorphic eosinophilic material with cellular debris, and is associated with lesions seen in tuberculosis?**

Caseous necrosis.

❑❑  **What is autolysis?**

Autolysis is self-digestion or necrosis due to release of a cell's own hydrolytic enzymes.  The pancreas is particularly susceptible to autolysis due to its high content of digestive enzymes.

❑❑  **Hypoxia results in decreased cellular energy (ATP) production by what mechanism?**

Aerobic respiration or mitochondrial oxidative phosphorylation is decreased or discontinued due to the lack of oxygen.  Subsequently, the cell attempts to maintain energy by producing ATP from glycogen via anaerobic glycolysis.

❑❑  **What type of cellular damage is largely responsible for progression from reversible to irreversible cellular injury?**

Damage to the cell membrane which results in loss of intracellular components necessary for ATP production and influx of other components.  For instance, reperfusion of an area following hypoxia can result in a massive influx of calcium into the cell.  Understanding the process of cell membrane permeability following injury is critical in laboratory detection of such injury in certain organs.  For example, cardiac muscle contains lactate dehydrogenase (LDH) and creatine kinase (CK) which are elevated following myocardial infarction.

❑❑  **What is a free radical?**

Free radicals are chemical compounds which contain an unpaired electron in an outer orbital.  They are largely responsible for the injury seen following reperfusion of an ischemic site.

❑❑  **What are the two mechanisms whereby chemicals induce cell injury?**

Either by direct combination with an organelle or vital component of the cell or by conversion to a toxic metabolite which then acts on the cell.  Direct action by a chemical is typically seen in those that are water soluble (example, mercuric chloride poisoning) while the remaining chemicals are not toxic as parent compounds and are generally lipid soluble (example, carbon tetrachloride).

❑❑  **What enzyme is of critical importance in metabolism of toxic chemicals?**

The P-450 mixed function oxidases which are found predominantly in the liver as well as other organs.

❑❑  **Alcohol causes an accumulation of what substance within the hepatocytes?**

Fat or lipids.  This histologic finding is called steatosis.  Persistent and chronic abuse of alcohol results in further damage in the liver including Mallory bodies, neutrophilic infiltration, individual hepatocyte necrosis, and ultimately cirrhosis.

❑❑  **What is lipofuscin?**

Lipofuscin is a pigment often referred to as the "wear-and-tear" pigment. It is yellow-brown and finely granular.  It is a sign of previous free radical injury and lipid peroxidation.

❑❑  **What is the most common exogenous pigment seen in cells?**

Carbon. This is often seen in the lung and hilar lymph nodes where it is referred to as anthracosis. This is not necessarily an indication of occupational exposure, rather this is seen in virtually anybody living in an urban area due to air pollution.

❏❏ **What are the other major examples of intracellular pigments?**

Besides carbon and lipofuscin mentioned above, melanin, hemosiderin (a hemoglobin-derived iron pigment), and bilirubin.

❏❏ **What is the structure of the protein called amyloid?**

Amyloid contains a beta-pleated sheet structure and is deposited in various tissues and organs in the condition of amyloidosis. Remember, patients with multiple myeloma can develop amyloidosis as a result of production by the abnormal plasma cells.

❏❏ **What are the phases of mitosis?**

Prophase, metaphase, anaphase, and telophase. During cell regeneration, the G1 phase results in production of mRNA, the S phase results in the synthesis of DNA, the G2 phase results in mRNA synthesis for use during mitosis, and the M phase consists of the mitotic phases described above.

❏❏ **Radiation, either intended or unintended, causes damage to cells via what mechanism?**

Free radical formation.

❏❏ **What is dystrophic calcification?**

The deposition of calcium in dead or dying tissue.

❏❏ **What is metastatic calcification?**

This is the deposition of calcium in normal or living tissue. In contrast to dystrophic calcification, this nearly always occurs in the setting of a calcium metabolic disturbance and hypercalcemia.

❏❏ **List some sites where one would expect to find dystrophic calcification.**

Atherosclerotic plaques, old granulomas, scars, damaged heart valves and cusps, and occasionally in tumors. Certain tumors contain characteristic calcifications consisting of round, lamellated calcifications called psammoma bodies. These are often seen in papillary carcinomas of the thyroid, papillary cystadenocarcinomas of the ovary and in certain meningiomas.

❏❏ **Briefly describe the pathogenesis of dystrophic calcification.**

Dystrophic calcification can occur intracellularly, extracellularly or both. Ultimately, the process is composed of two phases, initiation and propagation. Initiation occurs in mitochondria of dead or dying cells when the process is intracellular and in membrane-bound vesicles when the process is extracellular. Propagation of crystal formation follows initiation in either case and depends on calcium and phosphate.

❏❏ **Given that metastatic calcification occurs in a setting of disturbed calcium metabolism, give several clinical settings in which one might expect metastatic calcification.**

Hyperparathyroidism, vitamin D intoxication, hyperthyroidism, adrenocortical insufficiency (Addison's disease), sarcoidosis, chronic renal failure, milk-alkali syndrome, widespread bony metastases, multiple myeloma, and in certain tumors presenting with a paraneoplastic syndrome (example, small cell carcinoma of the lung).

❏❏ **What is the word used to describe the process of a particular cell type being replaced by another cell type due to a particular stimulus?**

Metaplasia. An example is squamous metaplasia of bronchial epithelium in the lungs secondary to cigarette smoking.

❑❑ **What type of metaplasia can one see in the lower esophagus in response to gastroesophageal reflux disease?**

Glandular metaplasia (Barrett's esophagus). The acidic gastric contents can result in metaplasia of the lower esophagus whereby the normal stratified squamous epithelium is replaced by glandular (either gastric or small intestinal) epithelium. Remember, intestinal metaplasia of the lower esophagus is associated with an increased risk of development of adenocarcinoma.

❑❑ **List some of the theories regarding the process of cell aging.**

There are numerous theories regarding the process of cellular aging including: telomeric shortening (results in DNA loss from chromosome ends), free radical damage (see an earlier question), post translational modifications of proteins (an example is glycosylation of proteins in the lens of the eye in cataract formation), presence of "clock genes" that determine rate of aging, and disruption of heat-shock proteins (a cellular adaptive defense mechanism).

❑❑ **What is the term used to describe abnormal maturation or development of tissue which is often a precursor lesion leading to frank malignancy?**

Dysplasia. A prominent example is dysplasia seen in cervicovaginal cytology (Pap smear).

❑❑ **What is the name of the originating cell whose progeny go on to form specific cells of various types?**

Stem cells.

❑❑ **Name the oncogene which inhibits apoptosis resulting in increased cell survival.**

bcl-2 (chromosome 18q21).

❑❑ **What is the gene which is stimulatory for apoptosis and has been shown frequently to be abnormal or completely absent in many malignancies?**

p53

❑❑ **What is the oncogene which can be stimulatory for either apoptosis or cell growth, depending on the presence or absence of other factors such as bcl-2?**

The c-myc oncogene.

❑❑ **Compare and contrast the histologic findings in necrosis versus apoptosis.**

Necrosis features ballooning or swelling of cells, ghost outlines of necrotic cells, and often associated inflammation. Apoptosis, on the other hand, features individual cell death with condensation of chromatin and fragmentation of nuclei and phagocytosis of the individual cells in the absence of other inflammation.

❑❑ **What is the term used to describe an increase in cell mass seen following a regular weightlifting regimen?**

Hypertrophy. Hyperplasia refers to an increase in the number of cells while hypertrophy refers to the size of the cells. Atrophy is the opposite of hypertrophy.

❑❑ **Divide the cells comprising the tissues into three subsets according to their individual ability to replicate.**

1. Labile cells - these are cells which continually replicate and are found in tissues which undergo high turnover (example, gastrointestinal tract).
2. Quiescent or stable cells - these cells replicate slowly, however can undergo rapid proliferation if stressed (example, hepatocytes).
3. Non dividing or permanent cells - these cells are unable to mitotically divide in life and are not part of the cell cycle (example, central nervous system neurons).

❑❑ **Name the two structural components of various epithelia which are necessary for appropriate growth and differentiation.**

Basement membrane and extracellular matrix.

❑❑ **Describe the role of ubiquitin.**

This is a readily available protein which is part of the heat-shock protein family and binds to damaged proteins such that they can be removed.

❑❑ **When a growth factor binds to a particular cell receptor, what is the effect?**

This binding translates into propagation of protein phosphorylation causing a stable or quiescent cell to replicate.

❑❑ **Name one of the signaling proteins which serve to take the extracellular signal for self-proliferation to the cell nucleus for DNA synthesis and replication.**

Phospholipase C-gamma, GTP-binding proteins (including the ras family of proteins) and raf-1.

❑❑ **Name the enzyme which is often activated by binding the growth factors to the receptor in the process of signal transduction in the cell.**

Tyrosine kinase.

❑❑ **Name two mechanisms of inhibition of cell growth.**

Contact inhibition and certain polypeptide factors including transforming growth factor - beta (TGF-b), interferon-beta (IFN-b), and tumor necrosis factor (TNF).

❑❑ **Describe growth factors and name three examples.**

Growth factors are polypeptides which serve to stimulate growth differentiation and even function of cells by various mechanisms. There are numerous growth factors including epidermal growth factors, transforming growth factor-alpha, platelet-derived growth factor, macrophage-derived growth factor, fibroblast growth factor, insulin-like growth factors, hepatocyte growth factor, colony stimulating factors, vasopermeability factor, erythropoietin, various cytokines, nerve growth factor, and others.

❑❑ **What are cytokines?**

Cytokines are a broad group of soluble substances with varied effects on cells including growth stimulation and inhibition. They are released by other cells such as macrophages.

❑❑ **Given that cardiac myocytes do not divide or replicate, what is the cellular response to hypertension resulting in increased heart weight and wall thickness?**

Hypertrophy. In the case of hypertension, left ventricular hypertrophy is the specific result. Histologically, the cells get larger and the nuclei are darker and pleomorphic, often featuring a "boxcar" appearance.

❑❑ **Define the term atrophy.**

This refers to a decreased cell size which can result in decreased organ size. Some common causes of atrophy include aging, poor diet, denervation, decreased vascular supply, and diminished or complete lack of use.

❏❏ **Is metaplastic epithelium capable of undergoing malignant transformation?**

Yes!

❏❏ **What are some causes of metaplasia?**

This is a cellular and subsequently tissue adaptive response. Some common causes include cigarette smoking (respiratory epithelium to squamous epithelium), some vitamin imbalances (vitamin A deficiency or excess), gastroesophageal reflux (Barrett's esophagus), physical injury, chemical exposure, and trauma due to the presence of calculi.

❏❏ **Name the organelle responsible for protein production.**

Rough endoplasmic reticulum.

❏❏ **What organelle is responsible for the paranuclear negative image characteristic of plasma cells?**

Golgi apparatus.

❏❏ **What are the three components of the extracellular matrix?**

Structural proteins (collagen), adhesive glycoproteins (fibronectin and laminin), and proteoglycans.

❏❏ **There are several types of collagens, which type is found as a major component of the basement membrane?**

Type IV.

❏❏ **What is the function of adhesive glycoproteins in the extracellular matrix?**

These proteins (including fibronectin, laminin, thrombospondin, and tenascin) link other constituents of the extracellular matrix and proteins of the cell membrane.

❏❏ **What cellular organelle serves to "package" proteins?**

The Golgi apparatus.

❏❏ **What is the cellular component which functions in the breakdown of glycogen and the synthesis of lipids and carbohydrates?**

The smooth endoplasmic reticulum.

❏❏ **What name is given to the process by which a cell ingests extracellular material?**

Phagocytosis.

❏❏ **Define pinocytosis.**

This is the process by which a cell brings liquid (sometimes containing a solute) into the cell. This is accomplished by forming a vesicle at the cell membrane.

❏❏ **If atrophy is a decrease in cell size, what is involution?**

Involution is a reduction of the number of cells due to a variety of causes. This process involves apoptosis and results in atrophy of a particular organ.

❑❑ **If one removes a stimulus causing hyperplasia, what is the result?**

The affected cells and tissues return to their normal state. Continued stimulation increases the risk of neoplasia.

❑❑ **What type of necrosis does one see following a cerebral infarction?**

Liquefactive or colliquative. This type of necrosis is also often seen in bacterial infections.

❑❑ **What are two ways in which ATP is produced in the cells?**

Oxidative phosphorylation of ADP and glycolysis.

❑❑ **What is the early alteration in intracellular calcium as a result of ischemia or toxic injury?**

Intracellular calcium levels increase secondary to influx and mitochondrial release of calcium.

❑❑ **What happens to membrane permeability in cell injury?**

It is increased, that is, the cell loses its selective permeability.

❑❑ **What is the prognosis of a cell with irreparable mitochondrial damage?**

The cell will die.

❑❑ **In ischemic cell injury, what happens to the intracellular sodium and potassium?**

The sodium increases and potassium decreases secondary to reduced action of the sodium-potassium pump.

❑❑ **What are some of the mechanisms which play a role in membrane damage and irreversible cellular injury?**

Mitochondrial dysfunction, reduction in membrane phospholipids, damage to the cytoskeleton, free radicals, accumulation of lipid breakdown products, and loss of intracellular amino acids.

❑❑ **What are some of the enzymes which act as free radical scavengers by inactivating them?**

Catalase, superoxide dismutase, and glutathione peroxidase.

❑❑ **Are the formation of ultrastructural cellular membrane blebs, myelin figures, and alteration of intercellular adhesions reversible or irreversible cell injuries?**

Reversible.

❑❑ **What effect does apoptosis have on caspases?**

Apoptosis activates several of the cysteine proteases called caspases which result in protein hydrolysis.

❑❑ **What effect does apoptosis have on transglutaminase?**

Apoptosis activates transglutaminase resulting in protein cross-linking.

❑❑ **What effect does chloroquine have on lysosomes?**

Chloroquine serves to increase the pH of lysosomes thereby inactivating their enzymes.

❐❑ **What is the common name of the keratin intermediate filaments which accumulate in some hepatocytes in alcoholic liver disease?**

Mallory bodies or Mallory's hyaline.

❐❑ **What are some common general etiologies of atrophy?**

Disuse, denervation, ischemia, poor nutrition, endocrine hypofunction, natural aging, and physical pressure.

❐❑ **What intercellular pigment is a sign of lipid peroxidation and injury due to free radical formation?**

Lipofuscin.

❐❑ **What is the term used to describe the pigmentation seen in patients with alkaptonuria?**

Ochronosis.

# REPAIR AND INFLAMMATION

❏❏ **What is the definition of the term "inflammation"?**

Inflammation is the tissue response to various injuries.

❏❏ **What are some of the agents which can elicit the inflammatory response?**

Toxic chemicals, infection by microorganisms, immune response (normal or abnormal), heat or cold, trauma, and radiation.

❏❏ **What is the goal of the inflammatory response?**

Inflammation is the cell and tissue response to a harmful insult in an attempt to destroy the harmful agent or prevent further damage. This response can be harmful as well as protective to the tissue.

❏❏ **What are the four classic, historical signs of tissue inflammation?**

Tumor (swelling), calor (warmth), dolor (pain), and rubor (erythema).

❏❏ **What is the term used to describe the replacement of injured tissue during the process of repair?**

Regeneration.

❏❏ **What is the term used to describe a fibroblastic proliferation with subsequent deposition of collagen at the site of previous tissue damage?**

Scar.

❏❏ **What is a keloid?**

This is a hypertrophic scar characterized histologically by dense bundles of collagen arranged in a haphazard fashion. Remember, this occurs in African-Americans more frequently.

❏❏ **List several of the cells which take part in the inflammatory response.**

Polymorphonuclear leukocytes (PMNs or neutrophils), lymphocytes, monocytes, eosinophils, basophils, plasma cells, mast cells, macrophages, and fibroblasts.

❏❏ **What are the two major types of inflammation?**

Acute and chronic.

❏❏ **List the cells predominantly involved in an acute inflammatory response.**

Neutrophils, eosinophils (involved in both acute and chronic), and monocytes/macrophages.

❏❏ **What are three factors which will greatly influence the histologic appearance of inflammation?**

The precise source which is eliciting the inflammatory response (radiation, microorganisms, chemical injury, etc.), the time lapse following the injury (acute, subacute, or chronic), and the immunocompetence of the host.

❑❑ **In general estimates, what are the time frames of the terms acute, subacute, and chronic?**

Acute typically refers to the response which occurs within minutes or hours, subacute refers to days or weeks, and chronic generally means weeks to months. The term subacute is not always used in all tissues; therefore, acute will sometimes refer to inflammation occurring minutes to days following insult.

❑❑ **What are some common examples of the harmful effects of the body's normal inflammatory response?**

The development of adhesions following abdominal surgery, development of contractures due to exuberant scar formation, a ruptured appendix, and fistula formation from the breakdown of tissue. There are many other examples of the potentially harmful effects of normal tissue response.

❑❑ **What are the cells involved in chronic inflammatory response?**

Lymphocytes, macrophages, monocytes, and fibroblasts.

❑❑ **Is acute inflammation always followed by chronic inflammation?**

No. Following insult, the acute inflammatory response can lead to complete resolution of the process, formation of an abscess, a healing phase marked by either regeneration or scar formation, or a chronic inflammatory response if the noxious stimulus persists.

❑❑ **Is chronic inflammation always preceded by acute inflammation?**

No. Chronic inflammation frequently arises without a preceding acute inflammatory response. Examples include chronic lung disease, autoimmune diseases such as rheumatoid arthritis, and granulomatous inflammation as seen in tuberculosis.

❑❑ **What stimulates and orchestrates the inflammatory response?**

Various chemical mediators are produced and released by various cells during inflammation. These mediators then serve to ultimately control the inflammatory response and are responsible for classical signs of inflammation (tumor, rubor, calor, and dolor).

❑❑ **Briefly describe the basic function and properties of the neutrophil (PMN).**

Neutrophils are the initial respondent to an acute insult. They act via phagocytosis and contain various digestive enzymes (oxidase and protease). Histologically, the nucleus normally contains three to five lobes connected by a thin band of chromatin (a segmented neutrophil); however, a young or earlier form of neutrophil has a single lobed, long, drawn out nucleus (a band form). An increase in the band forms has classically been used as an indicator of an infectious process although interobserver reproducibility of identifying band forms is poor.

❑❑ **What is the term used to describe the movement of neutrophils from the blood vessels to the site of tissue injury?**

Diapedesis.

❑❑ **What is the term used to describe the movement of leukocytes within the vascular lumen to the endothelium?**

Margination. The leukocytes marginate, roll along the endothelium, adhere to the endothelium, and eventually transmigrate across the endothelium into the tissue (diapedesis).

❑❑ **What is the predominant enzyme found within neutrophils?**

Myeloperoxidase.

❐❐  **What structure contains the enzymes found within the neutrophils?**

Lysosomes.

❐❐  **What are the three main components of acute inflammation?**

1. Vascular dilatation resulting in increased blood flow.
2. Leakage of plasma from vessels into the tissue.
3. Migration of leukocytes from vessels into the tissue.

❐❐  **What is an exudate?**

Fluid with an increased protein content including most plasma proteins (>3 g/ml and specific gravity > 1.015).

❐❐  **What is a transudate?**

Fluid with a low protein content, predominantly albumin (protein < 3 g/ml and specific gravity less than 1.015).

❐❐  **What is a purulent exudate?**

A purulent exudate or pus is an inflammatory host response. It is simply an exudate which contains many neutrophils, cell debris, and often fibrin.

❐❐  **What is an abscess?**

An abscess is a fibrinopurulent exudate which is localized and "walled-off" with surrounding macrophages, lymphocytes, monocytes, and fibrovascular tissue.

❐❐  **What is edema?**

Edema is an increased amount of extravascular fluid. It is the end result of the increased vascular permeability seen in the acute inflammatory response. The proteins and fluid from the plasma enter the tissue resulting in a decreased intravascular osmotic pressure. At the same time, the hydrostatic pressure is increased secondary to the vascular dilatation which then leads to fluid escaping the intravascular space into the tissue (edema).

❐❐  **What is a macrophage?**

This is a phagocytic cell which is derived from monocytes which have left the intravascular space and entered the tissue.

❐❐  **Where can one find macrophages?**

In the lung (pulmonary alveolar macrophages), the liver (Kupffer cells), lymph nodes (dendritic reticulum cells), and connective tissue histiocytes.

❐❐  **What is the term used to describe phagocytosis of various microorganisms which are coated with either IgG or the complement factor C3b?**

Opsonization. Macrophages have receptors for the Fc fragment of both IgG and C3b which then promotes the phagocytosis of microorganisms which are coated with IgG or C3b.

❐❐  **What is the term used to describe the attraction of leukocytes in the inflammatory process to the site of injury?**

Chemotaxis. Chemotaxis is mediated by a large number of chemical mediators.

❑❑  **What is the most common mechanism of vascular leakage in acute inflammation which occurs very rapidly (in less than half an hour) following injury?**

Endothelial cell contraction. This leads to a gap between endothelial cells (intercellular gap) and typically affects venules and not arterioles.

❑❑  **Name several potential mechanisms which result in vascular leakage during the acute inflammatory response.**

1.  Endothelial cell contraction (rapid, reversible, venules, short-lived)
2.  Endothelial retraction (reversible, long-lived, delayed)
3.  Endothelial injury (effects venules, capillaries, and arterioles, immediate, sustained for several hours, associated with platelet adhesion)
4.  Delayed prolonged leakage (delayed, lasts hours to days, venules and capillaries)
5.  Leukocyte mediated endothelial cell injury (early response, leukocyte products cause endothelial injury)
6.  Leakage from angiogenesis (due to young endothelial cells and capillaries)
7.  Increased transcytosis across endothelial cytoplasm (transports across interconnected vesicles or vacuoles).

❑❑  **What is the term used to describe transient adherence by the leukocytes to the endothelial cell surface?**

Rolling. Eventually the leukocytes become firmly attached to the endothelium creating a lining often referred to as "pavementing".

❑❑  **Compared to neutrophils, how do monocytes go from the bloodstream into the tissue during the acute inflammatory reaction?**

They follow the same process (margination, rolling, adhesion, diapedesis, and tissue migration) that all white cells follow!

❑❑  **How do leukocytes become adherent to and eventually cross between endothelial cells?**

They bind to the endothelial cells via various adhesion molecules.  This process is mediated by various chemoattractants and cytokines.

❑❑  **Name several adhesion molecules which are predominantly present on endothelial cells.**

E-selectin (ELAM-1 or CD62E), P-selectin (GMP-140 or CD62P), ICAM-1, VCAM-1, and LAM-1 (now called CD62L) ligands.

❑❑  **Name several adhesion molecules present on leukocytes (leukocyte receptors).**

Sialyl-Le glycoprotein, LFA-1, Mac-1, VLA-4, and L-selectin (LAM-1).

❑❑  **What type of conditions are classically known to elicit an eosinophilic response?**

Allergic reactions and parasitic infections.

❑❑  **What are the actions of eosinophils?**

Eosinophils have a phagocytic function.  Importantly, they also contain numerous hydrolytic enzymes within the cytoplasmic granules such as histaminase which serves an important antihistamine function at the site of injury.  Remember, eosinophils can be seen in both acute and chronic inflammatory responses.

❑❑  **What is the function of macrophages?**

Macrophages are important phagocytic cells. They engulf foreign material and cellular debris and also have an important antigen processing function. They also release several cytokines such as interleukin-1 (IL-1).

❏❏  **What are the two most characteristic cells of chronic inflammation?**

 Lymphocytes and plasma cells.

❏❏  **What are the two major types of lymphocytes?**

T-cells and B-cells. Among the T-cells there are both helper/inducer (T4) and suppressor/cytotoxic (T8) cells. These cells are important in a variety of responses in the body, for example, acute or cellular rejection (T-cells) and humoral rejection (B-cells). There is a third type of lymphocytes which do not possess the surface antigens which distinguish T-cells from one another (CD4 and CD8) and are referred to as natural killer cells or large granular lymphocytes.

 ❏❏  **What general tissue site contains a significant number of plasma cells?**

The submucosa, particularly of the respiratory and gastrointestinal tracts, contains large numbers of plasma cells. This is likely secondary to the nearly constant antigen exposure which takes place at these sites.

❏❏  **What non-neoplastic (inflammatory/infectious) condition is classically dominated by the presence of plasma cells?**

 Syphilis!

❏❏  **What is the major basic protein (MBP) and what is its function?**

MBP is one of the proteins found in the cytoplasmic granules of eosinophils. When released or degranulated, it serves to kill bacteria and certain parasites. In addition, it induces mast cell degranulation which can then serve to continue the inflammatory process.

❏❏  **Define a granuloma.**

A granuloma is a specific inflammatory response (chronic inflammation) which is composed of a collection of histiocytes, often in a spherical shape, which frequently have a surrounding rim of lymphocytes. Multinucleated giant cells, a specialized type of histiocyte, may or may not be present. Granulomas are a response to a variety of conditions including foreign bodies (such as suture), fungal infection, certain bacterial infections (classically Mycobacterium tuberculosis), cat scratch disease, sarcoidosis, and many other conditions.

❏❏  **What disease is classically characterized by non-necrotizing granulomas in the lungs and/or mediastinum?**

 Sarcoidosis.

❏❏  **Name a classic example of a fibrinous inflammatory response?**

 Fibrinous pericarditis. One may see fibrinous pericarditis in the setting of uremia. Grossly, the surface of the heart has a "bread and butter" appearance which is due to the presence of the bridging fibrin strands.

❏❏  **What is a serous exudate and where is it often seen?**

This is a nearly clear fluid (often straw-colored) which can contain a mild inflammatory cell content. Overall, the protein content is less than that seen in purulent exudate. This is a common fluid found in pleural, pericardial, and peritoneal effusions.

❏❏  **What is the term used to describe a serous exudate with admixed blood?**

Serosanguinous.

**❑❑  What is the common term used to describe a serous peritoneal effusion which is often found in patients with cirrhosis?**

Serous ascites.

**❑❑  What is a catarrhal exudate?**

This is a watery fluid which contains mucus.  This is typically found on mucous membranes.  One example is bronchitis.

**❑❑  What is a Langhans giant cell?**

This is a type of multinucleated giant cell (fused macrophages) in which the nuclei are arranged around the periphery of the cell.  These cells are not specific; however, they are often seen in tuberculosis.

**❑❑  What is granulation tissue?**

This is a part of the inflammatory and subsequent reparative or regenerative tissue response.  It is marked by the presence of acute and chronic inflammatory cells (more of the latter) in the midst of edematous interstitium.  Fibroblasts and myofibroblasts migrate into the area with endothelial cell proliferation and formation of new, small blood vessels (angiogenesis).

**❑❑  What are some of the substances which are released by macrophages?**

Colony-stimulating factor, tumor necrosis factor, alpha-interferon, IL-1, IL-8, IL-10, and IL-12.

**❑❑  Basophils and mast cells, like eosinophils, contain numerous cytoplasmic granules.  In each of these three cells, how do the chemical mediators found within their granules arrive at their target sites?**

In each case, they arrive via degranulation, NOT by phagocytosis.

**❑❑  These three cells (basophil, eosinophil, mast cell) are similar in another way.  Which immunoglobulin class receptor is found on each of these cell surfaces?**

Each of these cell types contains IgE receptors and will degranulate when the IgE is cross-linked by an antigen.

**❑❑  Can mast cells degranulate and thereby participate in an inflammatory response without IgE activation?**

Yes, or I would not have asked the question.  Complement (C5a), some bacteria, eosinophil-derived cationic protein, platelet factor IV, and monocyte chemotactic protein can all cause mast cell degranulation and/or release of histamine.

**❑❑  Where are plasma cells derived from?**

Plasma cells are differentiated B-cells.  Each plasma cell produces one type of immunoglobulin (IgG, IgM, IgA, IgD, or IgE).

**❑❑  Of the circulating lymphocytes, how many are T-cells and how many are B-cells?**

The vast majority are T-cells (70-80%).

**❑❑  What is the role of the coagulation cascade and its components with regard to vasopermeability?**

Fibrinopeptides A and B, which are cleaved from fibrinogen by thrombin, increase vasopermeability and are chemotactic resulting in buildup of fluid and a cellular response. In addition, the D-dimer and E fragments which are cleaved from polymerized fibrin by plasmin during clot dissolution also increase vasopermeability.

❑❑ **What are several chemical substances which are produced during the inflammatory response and cause the clinical signs and symptoms of inflammation?**

Vasoactive amines (histamine and serotonin), bradykinin, the complement system (both classical and alternate pathways), arachidonic acid metabolites (prostaglandins, leukotrienes), leukocyte enzymes and proteins (myeloperoxidase, etc.), lymphokines (interleukin 2, interferons, etc.).

❑❑ **Briefly, how is bradykinin formed?**

Bradykinin is formed from high molecular weight kininogen by the contact activation system. The system is activated when the Hageman factor (factor XII) is exposed to a negatively charged surface (collagen or basement membrane proteins). The activated factor XII then acts on factor XI and prekallikrein to form a kallikrein-activated factor XI complex. This complex then cleaves high molecular weight kininogen to release bradykinin.

❑❑ **What is the action of bradykinin?**

It results in increased vascular permeability, vascular dilatation, smooth muscle contraction, and elicits pain. Bradykinin's life is brief due to the action of kininase.

❑❑ **Can bradykinin be freed from high molecular weight kininogen without initiation of the complete contact activation system?**

Of course, why else would I ask this question?! Neutrophilic enzymes can release bradykinin from HMWK and kallikrein, in and of itself, can activate factor XII thereby jump-starting the contact activation system.

❑❑ **What are the three main mediators of increased vascular permeability?**

Bradykinin, C3a, and C5a.

❑❑ **What is the main mediator of chemotaxis?**

C5a.

❑❑ **Name several chemical mediators which result in vasodilatation during acute inflammation.**

Histamine, serotonin, bradykinin, and prostaglandins.

❑❑ **What are several chemical mediators which result in increased vascular permeability?**

Histamine, serotonin, bradykinin, complement 3a, complement 5a, prostaglandins and leukotrienes.

❑❑ **Name the acute inflammatory chemical mediator which is the only one which serves to vasodilate, induce vasopermeability, and act as a chemical attractant (chemotactic agent).**

Prostaglandins.

❑❑ **Name several chemical mediators of chronic inflammation.**

Migration inhibition factor, macrophage activation factor, complement 5a (remember, this functions as a chemotactic agent and increases vascular permeability in acute inflammation as well), and eosinophil chemotactic factor of anaphylaxis (ECF-A).

❏❏ **Name several chemical mediators which can directly result in the production of fever during an inflammatory response.**

Interleukin-1, interleukin-6, tumor necrosis factor (TNF) alpha, and interferons.

❏❏ **What is the most likely cause of the tissue destruction seen in acute inflammation?**

Oxygen-derived metabolites, nitric oxide (NO), and the enzymes released from leukocyte lysozymes. Remember, nitric oxide also has a direct vasodilatory effect.

❏❏ **How do oxygen-derived free radicals cause tissue damage?**

They are directly cytotoxic; oppose antiproteases which results in enzymatic activity and destruction of the extracellular matrix; and increase vascular permeability by damaging endothelial cells.

❏❏ **What cells produce histamine and serotonin?**

Mast cells and platelets.

❏❏ **Interleukin-1 (IL-1), interleukin-8 (IL-8), and TNF share a common cellular source, what is it?**

Macrophages. In addition, IL-8 is also produced from endothelial cells.

❏❏ **Name several actions of platelet activating factor (PAF) in the inflammatory response.**

Platelet activation (that's the easy one!), leukocyte aggregation (adhesion), and chemotaxis, in addition to increased vascular permeability.

❏❏ **Does platelet activating factor (PAF) cause vasoconstriction or vasodilatation?**

Yes. That is, PAF causes both bronchoconstriction and vasoconstriction; however, it causes vasodilatation in very low concentrations. In fact, it is many times more potent than histamine in this regard.

❏❏ **What are three different cells which can produce platelet activating factor?**

Neutrophils, macrophages, endothelial cells, platelets, and mast cells or basophils.

❏❏ **What are the functions of the body's inflammatory response?**

The inflammatory attack is designed to isolate and kill or inactivate the agent eliciting the response, "detoxify" any toxins, and, if necessary, "clean up" necrotic cells and tissue.

❏❏ **What is the main phagocytic cell in bacterial infections?**

Neutrophils. Remember, neutrophils are the first inflammatory cell to arrive at the site of damage. Also, since they contain cytoplasmic granules filled with various enzymes, the neutrophils themselves can cause significant damage to the host tissue.

❏❏ **What are some mechanisms by which various cellular adhesion molecules result in leukocyte adhesion and ultimately transmigration?**

Adhesion molecules are redistributed from the cytoplasm to the surface of cells. Secondly, certain cytokines actually promote production and subsequent surface expression of adhesion molecules on endothelial cells. Thirdly, with the appropriate stimulus, certain adhesion molecules present on both leukocytes and endothelial cells develop an increased affinity for one another due to a structural change in the molecules.

❏❏  **Briefly discuss the pathway of arachidonic acid metabolism.**

The arachidonic acid is cleaved from the cell membrane following stimulation and activation of phospholipase A2. Arachidonic acid can be acted upon by either cyclooxygenase or lipoxygenase. Cyclooxygenase results in the formation of prostaglandins E2, F2a, prostacyclin (PGI2), and thromboxane A2. Lipoxygenase action results in production of leukotriene B4, C4, D4, E4, and HETE. E prostaglandins cause vasodilatation, regulate pain, and help induce vascular permeability. Thromboxane A2 promotes aggregation of platelets, and PGI2 and prostacyclin inhibit platelet aggregation. The cyclooxygenase enzyme is present in many tissues while leukocytes are the source of lipoxygenase. Leukotriene B4 is a very strong chemotactic agent for leukocytes. In addition, the other leukotrienes cause contraction of bronchial smooth muscle, increase vascular permeability, and mucous production.

❏❏  **What is the source and action of migration inhibition factor (MIF)?**

This lymphokine inhibits macrophage mobility thereby causing them to collect at the site of tissue injury. This mediator is derived from activated T lymphocytes as is macrophage activation factor (MAF). MAF promotes the phagocytic function of macrophages.

❏❏  **Which single cytokine is most directly responsible for the production of fever?**

Interleukin-1.

❏❏  **What are the two forms of the cytokine tumor necrosis factor (TNF)?**

There is an alpha and a beta form which are similar in molecular weight. They both are toxic to certain tumor cells. In addition, they cause fever, cachexia, and production of acute phase proteins. The alpha form is produced predominantly in macrophages while the beta form is produced in lymphocytes.

❏❏  **What are some signals which cause "activation" of macrophages (increased metabolism, increased phagocytosis)?**

Numerous cytokines (interferon-gamma), bacterial endotoxins, and some extracellular matrix proteins (fibronectin).

❏❏  **Briefly discuss the action of phagocytosis.**

First, the desired particle attaches to the surface of the cell. Remember, the process of opsonization (IgG and C3b) greatly promotes this process. The phagocytic cell then engulfs the particle by surrounding it with pseudopods. This engulfed area pinches off from the cell membrane to create an intracellular phagosome then intracellular lysosomes fuse with the engulfed particle releasing their destructive enzymes. This process requires energy. The enzymes now within the phagosome cause destruction of the particle (such as the bacterium).

❏❏  **List several substances which are produced by the activated macrophage.**

Numerous enzymes, oxygen free radicals, growth factors, fibrogenic and angiogenic factors, coagulation factors and numerous other factors listed previously.

❏❏  **At what point in the arachidonic acid pathway does aspirin cause a blockade?**

Aspirin inhibits cyclooxygenase. Therefore, prostaglandin production is inhibited.

❏❏  **Where in the pathway of production and degradation of arachidonic acid do steroids inhibit?**

Steroids inhibit the phospholipases which are responsible for the release of arachidonic acid from the cell membrane. That is, they act before arachidonic acid as compared to nonsteroidal drugs (aspirin and indomethacin) which act after formation of arachidonic acid on the cyclooxygenase pathway.

❑❑  **Following the action of lipoxygenase on arachidonic acid, what is produced prior to the leukotrienes?**

5-HPETE is produced, which is the 5-hydroperoxy derivative of arachidonic acid.  The 5-HPETE is quickly converted either to 5-HETE (which is a chemotactic agent for neutrophils) or it proceeds on to the family of leukotrienes.  Leukotriene A4 is converted either to leukotriene B4 (a potent chemotactic agent) or the other leukotrienes which, as discussed above, cause vasoconstriction, vascular permeability, and bronchoconstriction.

❑❑  **What are the acute phase proteins?**

These are a group of proteins which show characteristic changes in quantity in response to inflammation and tissue injury.  Most of them are produced in the liver.  Interleukins appear to be key mediators in this process.  Others include alpha-1-antitrypsin, haptoglobin, fibrinogen, C-reactive protein, complement factor 3, ceruloplasmin, and hemopexin among others.

❑❑  **What is the function of alpha-1-antitrypsin?**

Alpha-1-antitrypsin is an antiprotease.  Remember, in alpha-1-antitrypsin deficiency people develop severe liver disease and lung disease even with spontaneous pneumothoraces.

❑❑  **If one sees red streaks extending along the entire length of an extremity, what is occurring?**

The lymphatics are most likely secondarily inflamed as they drain an infectious site (lymphangitis).  The red streaking is highlighting the course of the lymphatic channels.  Most likely, the originating node will be swollen and tender as well.

❑❑  **Describe some acute phase reactions.**

Fever is the first and foremost, others include anorexia, hypertension and tachycardia, protein degradation, and increased slow wave sleep.

❑❑  **What is a leukemoid reaction?**

This refers to a marked leukocytosis with white blood cell counts of 40 to even 100,000.  This is due to both an increased release of cells from the bone marrow (triggered by IL-1 and TNF) and increased bone marrow production due to stimulation by colony stimulating factors.

❑❑  **When does repair and regeneration occur following injury?**

Simultaneously.  Once the body begins responding to the injury, it also begins the process of repairing the damage.

❑❑  **Define labile, stable, and permanent cells.**

Remember this from chapter 1?  Labile cells have a short life span and rapidly regenerate (mucosa of the GI tract).  Stable cells have the ability to regenerate, however, have a slower mitotic rate and a longer overall life (kidney).  Permanent cells do not have mitotic activity and therefore cannot replicate or regenerate (cardiac myocytes and neurons).

❑❑  **What is healing by first intention or primary union?**

This is the process by which a wound is repaired following surgical approximation of the wound edges (staples or sutures).

❑❑  **In primary union, what happens immediately?**

Clotted blood fills the gap between the epithelial edges of the wound.  Subsequently, this forms a "scab".

❑❑  **How long does it take to form an apposed, continuous epithelial surface in healing by first intention?**

Within 48 hours the epithelial cells have regenerated from the edges of the wound toward the middle to the extent that they join in the middle of the wound beneath the overlying scab.  The basement membrane is also in place and, although the epithelium is thin, it is also intact.  Within 24 hours, neutrophils appear at the edge of the wound and begin migration toward the center of the blood clot.

❑❑  **72 hours following primary union, what would one expect to see histologically?**

By this time, the wound is now filled largely with macrophages which have gradually replaced the neutrophils.  In addition, fibroblasts, fibrocytes, and myofibroblasts have begun to appear laying down collagen and forming new blood vessels (granulation tissue).  During this time, the epithelium continues to regenerate and repair gradually.

❑❑  **When would one expect to see bridging of the wound by collagen during primary union?**

At approximately day 5 the wound defect is filled with granulation tissue and collagen has begun to bridge the entire gap of the wound. Gradually, the swelling, granulation tissue, and leukocytes recede over the course of the next seven days.

❑❑  **How long does it take to recover the tensile strength at the site of the wound during primary union?**

Several months.

❑❑  **Histologically, how would one know the site of a previous wound in the skin?**

The conspicuous absence of dermal appendages at the site of the wound, increased dermal collagen and perhaps, if you're lucky, a foreign body reaction to retained suture material.

❑❑  **What is secondary union or healing by second intention?**

This simply refers to the fact that the wound edges cannot be directly apposed to help in the repair process.  The process is very similar to that of healing by first intention except that the process is prolonged and the granulation tissue component in secondary union is much more exuberant.

❑❑  **What cell is responsible for the process of contraction in wound healing?**

The myofibroblast.  This is a fibroblast which has smooth muscle cell properties as well.  The wound contraction is much more pronounced in primary union.

❑❑  **Define a basement membrane.**

This is an extracellular matrix which is found at the junction between the cells and the adjacent or subjacent stroma.  It can surround both individual cells and groups of cells.

❑❑  **Define the lamina rara (or lamina lucida) and lamina densa of the basement membrane.**

The lamina rara portion of the basement membrane is electron lucent and found adjacent to the surface cell membrane.  In contrast, the area adjacent to the interstitium is electron dense and is referred to as the lamina densa.

❑❑  **What are some of the components of the basement membrane?**

Collagen type IV, laminin, entactin, and heparin sulfate proteoglycan.

❐❐ **What are several factors which greatly influence the body's ability to formulate an appropriate inflammatory/reparative response?**

Nutrition, glucocorticoids, infection, age, mechanical factors (location of a wound or tension on wound due to body habitus), vascular supply, presence of foreign bodies, malignancy, superimposed infections, certain diseases (diabetics), and immunosuppression.

❐❐ **What substance provides the tensile strength one finds in healing wounds?**

Collagen.

❐❐ **What type of collagen is found within basement membranes?**

Type IV.

❐❐ **Briefly, what is the process of synthesis of collagen?**

Collagen is synthesized in the endoplasmic reticulum in the form of procollagen. During synthesis in the endoplasmic reticulum, it undergoes numerous enzymatic reactions, particularly hydroxylation of prolene. Remember, collagen has approximately 10% hydroxyprolene content and this process is dependent on vitamin C. Following excretion from the cell, the procollagen is converted to collagen by enzymatic cleavage of the terminal peptide chains and lysylhydroxylysyl oxidation which results in cross linkages imparting the tensile strength and stability of collagen.

❐❐ **What enzymatic family is responsible for the degradation of collagen and other extracellular matrix proteins during remodeling?**

The metalloproteinases.

❐❐ **What are some examples of metalloproteinases?**

Interstitial collagenases, gelatinases, and stromelysins.

❐❐ **What percentage of the original tensile strength is present in a healing wound after seven days?**

Approximately 10%.

❐❐ **What does the phrase "wound dehiscence" mean?**

This is the breakdown of a wound manifested by separation of the edges due to inefficient or inadequate wound healing with subsequent scar formation.

❐❐ **What are two complications which can occur during inflammation and repair involving the viscera?**

Excessive adhesions in the abdomen can result in bowel obstruction, fistulous tracts can develop, and perforation of the viscous can occur (e.g., ruptured appendix).

❐❐ **What are some structural differences seen in elastin compared to collagen?**

Elastin has a very small amount of hydroxyprolene and hydroxylysine and random distribution of glycine residues.

❐❐ **Given the name and function of the myofibroblast, what would one expect to find ultrastructurally?**

There is abundant Golgi apparatus material, extensive endoplasmic reticulum, and contractile filaments in the cytoplasm. Often, they are surrounded by an incomplete basement membrane.

❑❑ **What is the adhesion molecule which is responsible for the attachment and subsequent migration of neutrophils to a site of entry?**

ICAM-1.

❑❑ **What adhesion molecule performs a similar role for leukocytes?**

VCAM-1.

❑❑ **During the repair process, platelets are attracted to the site of blood clot in a wound, and they then release what two important cytokines?**

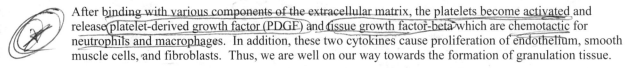

After binding with various components of the extracellular matrix, the platelets become activated and release platelet-derived growth factor (PDGF) and tissue growth factor-beta which are chemotactic for neutrophils and macrophages. In addition, these two cytokines cause proliferation of endothelium, smooth muscle cells, and fibroblasts. Thus, we are well on our way towards the formation of granulation tissue.

❑❑ **What is cicatrization?**

This is a contracture which forms following overly exuberant wound contraction. Classically, one sees this in burned skin.

❑❑ **What are some substances which can induce endothelial retraction and increased vascular permeability in acute inflammation?**

IL-1, TNF, IFN-gamma, and other cytokines.

❑❑ **What is delayed prolonged leakage?**

This is a form of increased vascular permeability seen in acute inflammation that does not begin until 2-12 hours following the insult. It involves venules and capillaries.

❑❑ **What are the substances found on leukocytes that react with endothelial adhesion molecules (ICAM-1 and VCAM-1)?**

Integrins. These are glycoproteins composed of alpha and beta chains and include LFA-1 and MAC-1 (for ICAM-1) and VLA-4 (for VCAM-1).

❑❑ **What receptor is important in "nonopsonic phagocytosis" and is identical to CD11b?**

CR3 which recognizes the stable form of C3b.

❑❑ **What effect does bactericidal permeability increasing protein (BPI) have on microorganisms?**

It results in activation of phospholipase, phospholipid degradation, and ultimately increased permeability of the organism's outer wall.

❑❑ **What are the vascular effects of histamine?**

It dilates arterioles, constricts large arteries, and increases permeability of venules (venular gaps).

❑❑ **What is the most crucial step in the production of the effects of the complement cascade (classic pathway)?**

C3 cleavage following fixation of C1 to an antigen-antibody complex.

❏❏  What parts of the complement cascade comprise the membrane attack complex (MAC)?

C5-9.

❏❏  Which four general systems involved in the inflammatory response can be initiated by activated factor XII (Hageman factor)?

1. Kinin system
2. Clotting system
3. Fibrinolytic system
4. Complement system

❏❏  What two enzymes act on arachidonic acid in the cyclooxygenase pathway?

COX1 and COX2.

❏❏  What effect do lipoxins have on chemotaxis?

They block neutrophil chemotaxis/adhesion and enhance monocyte adhesion.

❏❏  How are lipoxins A4 and B4 generated?

These are produced following the action of platelet 12-lipoxygenase on neutrophilic leukotriene A4 (LTA4).

❏❏  What are some of the actions of platelet-activating factor (PAF)?

Vasoconstriction and bronchoconstriction, vasodilatation, and increased venular permeability (very low concentrations), increased leukocyte adhesion, chemotaxis, degranulation, oxidative burst, and enhanced production of eicosanoids.

❏❏  What happens to the serum levels of C-reactive protein, serum amyloid A, and serum amyloid P during an acute phase reaction?

They are all elevated.  In fact, each may act as an opsonin on bacteria and fix complement.

❏❏  What are the definitions of the three types of intercellular signaling - autocrine, paracrine, and endocrine?

1. Autocrine - secrete and respond to own signals
2. Paracrine - secretory molecules act on cells in close proximity
3. Endocrine - signal produced by one cell and acts on a distant cell

❏❏  What inositol substance binds to receptors on the endoplasmic reticulum within the cell to cause release of calcium when activated?

Inositol 1,4,5-triphosphate (IP3).

❏❏  In particular, which two growth factors are intimately involved in new blood vessel formation (angiogenesis)?

Fibroblast growth factor (FGF), particularly the basic form and vascular endothelial growth factor (VEGF).

❏❏  What are some stimulatory factors for VEGF?

TGF-beta, platelet-derived growth factor (PDGF), TGF-alpha, and tissue hypoxia.

# RBCs, BLEEDING, AND CLOTTING

☐☐ **What is a stem cell?**

Stem cells are progenitor cells that have the unique ability to both replicate themselves and proliferate as well as produce more differentiated cells of various types. In the bone marrow, there are pluripotential stem cells which are able to give rise to both lymphoid and myeloid hematopoietic cells.

☐☐ **What is the term used to describe the production of the cellular components of blood within the bone marrow?**

Hematopoiesis.

☐☐ **What is the name of the factor which is often used clinically to help the bone marrow to increase its production of cells, such as following bone marrow transplantation?**

Colony stimulating factor (CSF). Production of CSF can be increased in certain conditions such as in response to infection.

☐☐ **While still an embryo, what is the site of the first production of blood tissue?**

The yolk sac. There, very primitive cells called mesoblasts will differentiate into primitive erythroblasts and primitive endothelial cells.

☐☐ **At what stage of development does the liver become the predominant site of hematopoiesis?**

The liver assumes the responsibility of being the primary site of hematopoiesis at approximately week 6. At that time, definitive erythroblasts are formed. In addition, myeloid cells and megakaryocytes are also present, although less in number than the erythroid cells.

☐☐ **What is the major organ of hematopoiesis in mid fetal development?**

The liver.

☐☐ **When does the spleen begin to take part in hematopoiesis?**

Toward the middle part of fetal life. The spleen and even lymph nodes produce blood cells; however, the liver remains the dominant organ of production.

☐☐ **Does fetal bone marrow take part in hematopoiesis?**

Of course. Its role becomes increasingly important later and, of course, the bone marrow is the primary site for hematopoiesis during adult life. As the bone marrow becomes more productive, the liver's production recedes.

☐☐ **How is hematopoiesis in fetal bone marrow different from hematopoiesis in other organs?**

There are a greater number of myeloid cells produced in fetal bone marrow hematopoiesis compared to the liver, spleen, or other organs.

❏❏   Besides those listed above, what are other sites of hematopoiesis?

The thymus does produce both erythroid and myeloid cells, however production of leukocytes is its main role, particularly the T lymphocyte subset.

❏❏   What is the term given to describe the presence of islands of erythroid and myeloid precursors within the liver or other organs during adult life?

Extramedullary hematopoiesis (EMH).

❏❏   What happens to the cellularity of the bone marrow as one ages?

A newborn's bone marrow is nearly 100% cellular.  As one ages, more of the bone marrow spaces are occupied by fat leaving fewer islands of hematopoietic cells.  Normal adult bone marrow would be roughly 60% cellular.  A crude estimate of expected normal adult bone marrow cellularity can be arrived at by subtracting the patient's age from 100.

❏❏   In an adult, which bones serve as the primary repositories of hematopoiesis?

The pelvis, sternum, ribs, and vertebrae.  Thus, if one were to sample the bone marrow in diagnostic evaluation, the most accessible sites are the pelvis and sternum.

❏❏   What pathologic condition causes increased erythropoiesis with subsequent expansion of marrow spaces including bones not normally involved in adult hematopoiesis (cranium and long bones) and produces a "hair-on-end" appearance of the calvarium on x-ray, and even malocclusion due to hyperplasia of the maxilla?

Thalassemia major.

❏❏   During normal hematopoiesis, what growth factors are produced and by whom?

Interleukin-6, granulocyte-macrophage colony-stimulating factor (GM-CSF), and stem cell factor (SCF) are produced by stromal cells within the bone marrow.

❏❏   Now suppose there is a stress (such as a viral infection), what is the milieu which stimulates increased hematopoiesis?

The activated monocytes secrete interleukin-1, tumor necrosis factor, macrophage colony stimulating factor (a little selfish, eh?), and granulocyte colony stimulating factor.  The IL-1 serves to excite T cells which then secrete GM-CSF and IL-3.  Finally, the IL-1 and TNF-a result in secretion of IL-6 and GM-CSF from the bone marrow stroma.  All of this results in increased production of granulocytes and lymphoid cells.

❏❏   What is the function of the erythrocyte?

It serves to carry hemoglobin and thus regulate oxygen exchange.

❏❏   What is the function of hemoglobin?

It serves to carry oxygen and carbon dioxide.  Don't forget the carbon dioxide.

❏❏   What is the glycoprotein produced in the liver (fetus) and kidney (adult) in an attempt to compensate for tissue hypoxia?

Erythropoietin.

❏❏   During erythroid differentiation from stem cell to erythrocyte, in which part of that process does erythropoietin carry its heaviest influence?

The last half. The earlier stages of erythrocyte development are controlled partially by GM-CSF, SCF, and IL-3.

❑❑ **In a patient with anemia and chronic renal failure, how might one treat him or her?**

Erythropoietin can be used clinically to prevent multiple transfusions in renal failure patients. Other chronic, debilitating illnesses like malignancy and AIDS can benefit from erythropoietin therapy as well.

❑❑ **While treating a woman with breast cancer who has developed chemotherapy-induced neutropenia, she develops bone pain. Which growth factor are you likely treating her with?**

Granulocyte colony stimulating factor can cause bone pain in approximately 50% of patients.

❑❑ **If you were to desire a rapid increase of panhematopoiesis such as following bone marrow transplantation, which growth factor would you most likely use?**

Granulocyte-macrophage colony-stimulating factor (GM-CSF).

❑❑ **What are the major growth factors involved in eosinophil production?**

IL-3, IL-5 and GM-CSF. Basophils and mast cells are stimulated by stem cell factor and IL-3.

❑❑ **What are the stages of erythrocyte maturation from stem cell to erythrocyte?**

Pronormoblast, basophilic normoblast, polychromatophilic normoblast, orthochromatic normoblast, reticulocyte, and finally erythrocyte.

❑❑ **What are the various stages in progression from myeloblast to a mature myeloid cell (eosinophil, neutrophil, etc.)?**

Myeloblast, promyelocyte, myelocyte, metamyelocyte, band form, and finally the mature myeloid cell, like a segmented neutrophil.

❑❑ **What is the normal life span of an erythrocyte?**

Just making sure you are awake - 120 days.

❑❑ **What is the normal size of an erythrocyte?**

About 5 microns.

❑❑ **Name some conditions in which erythrocyte production increases.**

Anemia, cardiopulmonary dysfunction resulting in hypoxia, and high altitudes.

❑❑ **The compound 2,3-diphosphoglycerate (2,3-DPG) within red cells helps regulate oxygen affinity. What happens to your oxygen affinity if you are standing on top of Mount Everest?**

Oxygen affinity to hemoglobin is decreased in an attempt to combat the hypoxia of that low oxygen tension environment. Thus, the 2,3-DPG increases in concentration resulting in increased delivery of oxygen to tissue (decreased oxygen affinity). That shifts the oxygen dissociation curve to the right.

❑❑ **What other things shift the oxygen dissociation curve to the right (increased oxygen delivery to tissue)?**

Decreased pH, increased concentration of 2,3-DPG and increased temperature.

❑❑ **What is the structure of the hemoglobin molecule?**

Hemoglobin is a tetramer composed of two pairs of polypeptide chains, alpha or alpha-like chains, and beta or beta-like chains. This is in conjunction with a heme portion found in each of the chains between two histadine residues. Each heme portion can bind a molecule of oxygen - four total molecules of oxygen can be bound.

❑❑ **What portion of a normal adult's hemoglobin is normally type A2?**

3% is A2 and the remaining portion is essentially hemoglobin A with a fraction of fetal hemoglobin.

❑❑ **What percentage of hemoglobin F (fetal hemoglobin) is found in a typical neonate?**

About three fourths of the hemoglobin is F type and the vast majority of the remaining portion is composed of adult type hemoglobin (hemoglobin A).

❑❑ **What is anemia?**

Anemia refers to a decrease in the red cell blood cell mass or hemoglobin.

❑❑ **What are the red cell indices and how are they used in evaluating anemia?**

The indices are the parameters used to describe the red cells themselves and include the mean corpuscular volume (MCV), mean corpuscular hemoglobin (MCH), and mean corpuscular hemoglobin concentration (MCHC). These indices then allow one to classify the type of anemia present.

❑❑ **What is a microcytic anemia?**

This represents an anemia in which the MCV is less than 80. If the MCV value is within normal range, it is referred to as normocytic, and if the MCV is greater than the upper limits of normal (100) then one would refer to it as a macrocytic anemia.

❑❑ **What is a hypochromic anemia?**

This refers to the MCHC value. As with the MCV, one can subclassify the anemia as either hypochromic, normochromic, or hyperchromic based on where the MCHC value falls.

❑❑ **What are several causes of a microcytic anemia?**

TAILS. This mnemonic refers to thalassemia, anemia of chronic disease (usually a normocytic anemia but can be microcytic), iron deficiency anemia, lead poisoning, loss of blood, and sideroblastic anemia.

❑❑ **What is the differential diagnosis for normocytic anemias?**

HARAM. That is, hemolysis (and some hemoglobinopathies), anemia of chronic disease, renal failure, aplastic anemia, and myelophthisic processes. The most common cause, far and away, is chronic disease.

❑❑ **What are some causes of macrocytic anemia?**

I don't have an acronym or terribly easy way to remember these. They include vitamin B12 deficiency, aplastic anemia (again), thyroid dysfunction (both hypo and hyperthyroidism), myelodysplastic syndromes, chronic liver disease, dilantin or phenytoin therapy, and even some hemolytic conditions. Look for hypersegmentation of neutrophils (greater than five lobes of the nucleus) in megaloblastic anemias.

❑❑ **If a patient has anemia, what signs and symptoms would you expect clinically?**

Dyspnea, palpitations, fatigue with minimal exertion, tachycardia, and even chest pain. Don't forget, most anemia occurs gradually and thus the symptoms may be less noticeable.

❏❏ **In an anemia which is due to blood loss (such as a chronic gastrointestinal hemorrhage), what would you expect to find in the peripheral smear and bone marrow microscopically?**

The bone marrow would likely demonstrate hyperplasia of the erythroid cells (decreased myeloid to erythroid ratio). A peripheral smear would likely show an increase in circulating reticulocytes. Remember, they are a younger form of the erythrocyte and this would be viewed as an appropriate response of the marrow to the anemia.

❏❏ **If one desired to determine if acute hemolysis had taken place, what plasma protein can be measured?**

The most common determinant is serum haptoglobin. Following hemolysis, the serum haptoglobin would markedly decrease as it is bound by the circulating free hemoglobin. Remember, patients with chronic liver disease may have a low serum haptoglobin in their normal state, thus one may wish to measure a serum haptoglobin on a serum sample which was drawn prior to the bleeding.

❏❏ **Compare the oxygen affinity of fetal hemoglobin (HbF) and adult hemoglobin (HbA).**

Fetal hemoglobin has greater oxygen affinity, predominantly because hemoglobin A has much more 2,3-DPG.

❏❏ **What is the formula which defines mean corpuscular hemoglobin (MCH)?**

MCH = hemoglobin (in grams per liter) / red blood cell count (in millions per microliter)

❏❏ **What is the formula which defines the mean corpuscular hemoglobin concentration (MCHC)?**

MCHC = hemoglobin (grams per deciliter) / hematocrit

❏❏ **What is poikilocytosis?**

This is a general term referring to abnormal erythrocytes.

❏❏ **What is a Howell-Jolly body?**

This is a basophilic cytoplasmic inclusion in red blood cells which represents a remnant of the nucleus which has been extruded and thus is composed of DNA.

❏❏ **What is a Pappenheimer body?**

These are small basophilic granules (more than one, compared to a Howell-Jolly) which represent iron, often in a mitochondrial remnant. One might see these following splenectomy or in sideroblastic anemia.

❏❏ **What is a stomatocyte?**

This is a red cell abnormality in which the cell has a mouth-like appearance. This is due to abnormal membrane permeability.

❏❏ **What is a dacrocyte?**

This is a distorted red blood cell which looks like a tear drop. One often sees these in myelofibrosis as the red cells are distorted in their attempt to traverse the fibrotic bone marrow.

❏❏ **What is a target cell?**

Also known as a codocyte, these red cells simply have a target-like appearance with a "bullseye" in the middle. One should think of thalassemia, hemoglobin C, or liver disease when one sees these cells.

❑❑   **What is an acanthocyte?**

These are also referred to as spur cells and have spicules projecting from the edge of the cell circumferentially.  This is due to an abnormal cell membrane lipid content.

❑❑   **Where would one expect to see acanthocytes?**

Think of abetalipoproteinemia, liver disease, or patients who have had a splenectomy.

❑❑   **What is basophilic stippling?**

This refers to numerous, small basophilic cytoplasmic bodies in red cells. These are composed of ribosomes (RNA).

❑❑   **If one sees coarse basophilic stippling in the peripheral blood smear of an underprivileged child, what is a possible diagnosis that needs to be ruled out?**

Lead poisoning.  Thalassemia also can produce coarse basophilic stippling.

❑❑   **Contrast a spur cell (acanthocyte) with a burr cell (echinocyte).**

The cellular projections on a spur cell are of varying lengths, whereas in burr cells the spicules are short and typically have even spacing.  In addition, spur cells have a dense center while burr cells have more central pallor.  Burr cells are an artifact and can be seen in many conditions such as uremia.

❑❑   **What is rouleaux?**

These are red blood cells which are arranged in a stack simulating a "stack of coins".  This change can be seen in paraproteinemia.  In an exam situation such as the  boards, think of multiple myeloma.

❑❑   **What would you expect the iron stores in the bone marrow to show in a case of chronic hemorrhage (such as a gastrointestinal hemorrhage)?**

One would see decreased iron stores in the marrow and serum in this case. In contrast, "internal blood loss", such as hemolysis, or anemia due to any other disease should show an increase in bone marrow iron stores.

❑❑   **When would one see the maximum number of reticulocytes following acute blood loss?**

10 days after the episode one would find the maximum number of reticulocytes or young red blood cells. Therefore, the MCV may be increased.

❑❑   **What are the polypeptide globin chains that make up hemoglobin A2?**

Two alpha and two delta chains.

❑❑   **What are the polypeptide globin chains which make up hemoglobin F?**

Two alpha and two gamma chains.

❑❑   **Which polypeptide globin chain has an abnormality in sickle cell anemia?**

The beta chain in sickle cell anemia shows a single amino acid substitution (valine for glutamic acid at the 6th position).  The resultant hemoglobin is called hemoglobin S.

❑❑   **Regarding sickle cell anemia, what is the prevalence of both sickle cell trait and sickle cell disease?**

The heterozygote (sickle cell trait) occurs in up to 10% of African-Americans. The homozygote state (sickle cell disease) occurs in approximately 0.2% of African-Americans in the United States. This is an autosomal dominant process.

❑❑  **What causes the sickling of the red blood cells seen in sickle cell disease?**

The amino acid substitution in the beta chain changes the solubility of the resultant hemoglobin. Therefore, at an acidic pH and decreased oxygen tension, the hemoglobin S precipitates in the red cells causing the sickling of the cells. Thus, the abnormally shaped cells cannot traverse the small blood vessels as they normally would causing vascular occlusion, hemolysis, and the clinical signs and symptoms one would expect.

❑❑  **What are the signs and symptoms typically seen in sickle cell anemia?**

Microscopic infarcts of bone with subsequent pain, infarctions of the spleen and kidney, hematuria secondary to papillary necrosis, hepatomegaly, hepatic dysfunction, pulmonary thromboemboli, stroke, and numerous infections.

❑❑  **What is the otherwise somewhat unusual organism that can classically cause osteomyelitis in sickle cell anemia?**

Salmonella.                    (asplenic)

❑❑  **What is the name of the clinical signs and symptoms that one sees as a result of a vascular occlusion from the sickled red blood cells?**

This is referred to as sickle cell crisis. Low flow systems, such as the portal systems, are at particular risk for a vascular occlusion.

❑❑  **In hereditary abnormalities of red blood cell shape, what is the usual cause?**

Typically, the abnormal shape is due to inheritance of abnormal integral proteins which are found in the red cell membrane and charged with maintaining the normal red cell shape and stability.

❑❑  **Within the red cell membrane, name some of the important structural proteins.**

Spectrin, actin, ankyrin, and band 4.1.

❑❑  **In hereditary spherocytosis, what is the membrane defect?**

There is a decreased amount of spectrin in these patients. Sometimes, the spectrin itself may also be qualitatively abnormal.

❑❑  **What typically happens to the red blood cells in a patient with hereditary spherocytosis?**

There is increased splenic sequestration secondary to the abnormal and diminished red blood cell membrane flexibility.

❑❑  **How common is hereditary spherocytosis?**

1 in 5,000 within the United States. It is the most common inherited hemolytic anemia in northern Europeans.

❑❑  **What is the pattern of inheritance of hereditary spherocytosis?**

Autosomal dominant.

❑❑  **What is an important laboratory test used to detect the presence of spherocytes?**

The osmotic fragility test. This is a test used to help determine the competence, or lack thereof, of the red cell membrane. Normal red blood cells can swell to nearly two times the resting volume before hemolyzing. Thus, spherocytes have a much lower threshold and when placed in a hypotonic solution and will burst or hemolyze.

❏❏ **What is another condition which can give similar increased osmotic fragility test values?**

Any condition with spherocytes will show increased values. Thus, autoimmune hemolytic anemia with spherocytosis can show increased values, although not typically to the degree of hereditary spherocytosis.

❏❏ **Name some conditions which can give decreased values in the osmotic fragility test.**

Conditions such as thalassemia, chronic liver disease, and iron deficiency anemia can all cause a decreased degree of hemolysis during the test.

❏❏ **What are the red blood cell indices like in the case of hereditary spherocytosis?**

The MCV, MCH, and MCHC are usually normal.

❏❏ **In questioning other family members regarding the possibility of hereditary spherocytosis, what are some findings one might elicit in their history?**

Documented anemia, "bouts" of jaundice, and cholelithiasis.

❏❏ **How might you surgically treat somebody with hereditary spherocytosis?**

Splenectomy.

❏❏ **What is the typical mode of inheritance of hereditary elliptocytosis?**

Also autosomal dominant.

❏❏ **Would you more likely expect hemolysis in a patient with elliptocytosis or spherocytosis?**

Spherocytosis is more likely to have clinically significant hemolysis.

❏❏ **Is there a specific membrane protein abnormality in elliptocytosis?**

No. A number of abnormalities have been seen including qualitative and quantitative defects in band 4.1 and spectrin.

❏❏ **What is the mode of inheritance of glucose-6-phosphate dehydrogenase deficiency (G6PD)?**

This is an X-linked trait. It is incompletely dominant and occurs in 10% of African-Americans.

❏❏ **What is the function of G6PD?**

It serves to help prevent oxidative injury and hemolysis in red blood cells by maintaining glutathione in a reduced form.

❏❏ **What is a common precipitating event resulting in hemolysis in patients with G6PD deficiency?**

Infections may be the most common cause. In addition, patients who ingest substances with oxidative activity can also elicit hemolytic episodes (such as antimalarial drugs, fava beans, and certain antibiotics like sulfonamides and furantoins).

❏❏  **Does one see increased or decreased numbers of Heinz bodies in patients with G6PD deficiency?**

Increased, or I would not have asked.  The Heinz body test is based on the presumed abnormality of the oxidative pathway of glycolytic red blood cell enzymes in patients with G6PD deficiency.  Thus, blood is collected and methyl violet or neutral red is added to identify the presence or absence of Heinz bodies.  At times, phenylhydrazine can be added to increase the numbers of Heinz bodies present.

❏❏  **What is another condition associated with abnormal red blood cell metabolism?**

Pyruvate kinase deficiency is probably the second most common enzyme deficiency in red blood cell metabolism.

❏❏  **What is beta-thalassemia?**

This is an anemia which is due to a decreased or complete lack of production of the beta chain in hemoglobin.  Thalassemia causes a microcytic and hypochromic anemia.

❏❏  **What ethnicity is commonly associated with thalassemia?**

Mediterranean peoples.

❏❏  **What are the two main types of beta-thalassemia?**

Thalassemia major and thalassemia minor.  As you might guess, major is associated with marked hypochromic, microcytic anemia while minor may have very mild anemia.

❏❏  **What is another name for thalassemia major?**

Cooley's anemia.  Remember, thalassemia major is the homozygote in beta-thalassemia and thalassemia minor patients are heterozygotes.

❏❏  **What about red blood cell (RBC) survival in beta-thalassemia?**

Thalassemia major patients have a diminished RBC life span whereas thalassemia minor patients may have a normal RBC survival.

❏❏  **What is alpha-thalassemia?**

You should get this one.  This is a patient with deficient alpha-globin production in his/her red blood cells.  Again, he/she may be a homozygote or a heterozygote.  The anemia may be mild or nonexistent in the heterozygote form.

❏❏  **What is the direct Coomb's test?**

Also called the direct antiglobulin test (DAT), this test is used to detect the presence of immunoglobulin on a patient's red blood cells.  Thus, rabbit antihuman immunoglobulin is added to a patient's washed red blood cells and agglutination is then evaluated.  Agglutination can vary from absent to 4+ positivity.

❏❏  **In macrocytic anemia, what is the most common cause of megaloblastic macrocytic anemia?**

Deficiencies of folic acid and/or vitamin B12.  Remember, megaloblastic refers to an increase in the physical size of red blood cell precursors within the bone marrow.

❏❏  **What do the neutrophils often look like in patients with megaloblastic macrocytic anemia?**

They are often hypersegmented, which means > 5 nuclear lobes.

❏❏  **In what type of patient does one classically see folic acid deficiency?**

Remember that folic acid is found in vegetables and a deficiency is typically secondary to dietary inadequacy.  The classic test question regarding folic acid deficiency revolves around an alcoholic patient.  Alcoholics often suffer from poor nutrition secondary to their excessive ethanol use.  Certain folic acid antagonists used as chemotherapeutic agents may also result in a similar picture.

❏❏  **What is pernicious anemia?**

This is a type of vitamin B12 deficiency which is due to a lack of intrinsic factor.

❏❏  **What is intrinsic factor?**

This is a substance which is secreted by the parietal cells in the fundus of the stomach.  Intrinsic factor binds vitamin B12 and transports it to the ileum where intrinsic factor receptors bind the complex.  B12 is then absorbed across the mucosa.  In patients with pernicious anemia, they lack this intrinsic factor and subsequently develop vitamin B12 deficiency and megaloblastic anemia.

❏❏  **Given that the intrinsic factor is produced by parietal cells in the stomach, what other symptoms and findings would you expect in a patient with pernicious anemia?**

They lack the parietal cells in the fundus and so one would expect gastric atrophy.  In addition, the parietal cells are responsible for the secretion of hydrochloric acid and these patients will then have achlorhydria.  Remember, pernicious anemia is an autoimmune disorder and these patients have circulating antibodies to the parietal cells.  They are at an increased risk for gastric carcinoma and often have other autoimmune disorders.

❏❏  **Name a common worldwide infection which can cause anemia and massive splenomegaly.**

Malaria.

❏❏  **Name other clinical signs and symptoms associated with folic acid and vitamin B12 deficiency with megaloblastic anemia.**

Atrophic glossitis, lingual atrophy, intestinal metaplasia of the stomach, chronic atrophic gastritis, and neurologic abnormalities.

❏❏  **What happens to the white blood cells in megaloblastic anemia?**

There is generalized leukopenia in addition to thrombocytopenia.

❏❏  **Does one see the same neurologic abnormalities in folate deficiency compared to B12 deficiency?**

No.  Although both feature a megaloblastic anemia, the neurologic findings are restricted to the vitamin B12 deficiency.

❏❏  **What is Blackfan-Diamond syndrome?**

This is an inherited disorder with erythroid hypoplasia.  Obviously, this can cause anemia.

❏❏  **What are other causes of bone marrow aplasia and subsequent anemia?**

Previous radiation, certain drugs (chloramphenicol and benzene derivatives), and viruses.

❏❏  **Name a tumor which can be associated with red cell aplasia.**

Thymoma.

□□  **Name some causes of macrocytic anemia not associated with megaloblastic differentiation.**

Thyroid disease (both hypo- and hyperthyroidism), phenytoin therapy, and chronic liver disease.

□□  **What does the term myelophthisic anemia refer to?**

This refers to replacement of the bone marrow by some process.  This includes metastatic tumors, leukemia, inflammatory processes such as granulomatous disease, and myelofibrosis.

□□  **What is hemoglobin C disease?**

This is a hemoglobinopathy associated with an amino acid substitution of lysine for glutamine in the sixth position of the beta chain.  It is found in 3% of African-Americans.

□□  **How are hemoglobin E and hemoglobin C disease similar?**

Hemoglobin E disease also has a lysine for glutamine substitution in the beta chain; however, this occurs at the number 26 position as opposed to the 6th position in hemoglobin C disease.

□□  **What red cell shape abnormality would you expect in a patient who has suffered from significant burn injury?**

These patients exhibit a marked degree of poikilocytosis with microcytosis and schistocytes.

□□  **What is the condition which is associated with increased red cell susceptibility to lysis by complement and hemoglobinuria at night?**

Paroxysmal nocturnal hemoglobinuria (PNH).

□□  **What are some important laboratory tests used to diagnose PNH?**

These patients have positive Ham's and sucrose hemolysis tests.

□□  **What are some common disease states associated with spherocytosis?**

Hereditary spherocytosis, immune hemolytic anemia, and red cell transfusion.

□□  **What are some common conditions associated with elliptocytosis?**

Hereditary elliptocytosis, iron deficiency, and myeloproliferative/myelodysplastic disorders.

□□  **What are some conditions that are associated with acanthocytosis?**

Severe hepatic disease, abetalipoproteinemia, splenectomy, and McCleod phenotype.

□□  **What is the mechanism of paroxysmal cold hemoglobinuria (PCH)?**

In PCH, one develops IgG antibodies (Donath-Landsteiner antibodies) usually in the setting of a viral infection.  These antibodies activate complement after binding erythrocytes at cold temperatures.  Thus, intravascular hemolysis develops upon warming.

□□  **What is microangiopathic hemolytic anemia?**

This is a result of breaking up of the red blood cells due to trauma as they pass through the vasculature. This is often seen as red cells pass through fibrin and/or platelet strands in a low flow or low pressure situation. Included among the causes of microangiopathic hemolytic anemia are: thrombotic thrombocytopenic purpura (TTP), hemolytic uremic syndrome, disseminated intravascular coagulation, heart valve prostheses, vasculitis, certain drugs,  hypertension, and in congenital vascular malformations.

❑❑  **In blood coagulation, how do platelets become involved?**

When there is injury to the vascular endothelium, the underlying collagen is exposed and the platelets adhere to this exposed collagen. The platelets then release arachidonic acid which causes platelet activation and vasoconstriction. Prostacyclin is released from the endothelium which causes the opposite effects hopefully balancing the tissue reaction.

❑❑  **In addition to the aforementioned endothelial injury, what are the two remaining factors important in maintaining hemostasis (Virchow's triad)?**

Virchow's triad is composed of endothelial injury, alterations in normal blood flow and hypercoagulability. Endothelial injury in and of itself can cause hemostasis; however, alterations in normal blood flow and hypercoagulability in the absence of endothelial injury are sufficient to cause hemostasis.

❑❑  **What are some causes of hypercoagulability?**

Antithrombin III deficiency, protein C deficiency, protein S deficiency, disseminated malignancy, nephrotic syndrome, oral contraceptive use, trauma, pregnancy, smoking, homocystinuria, presence of a Lupus anticoagulant, thrombocytosis, and many others.

❑❑  **What other factors are released by platelets during the process of hemostasis?**

Adenosine diphosphate (ADP), thromboxane A2, and serotonin.

❑❑  **What are some factors which inhibit platelet aggregation?**

PGI2, nitric oxide, and ADPase.

❑❑  **What are two factors which stimulate platelet aggregation and adhesion?**

von Willebrand's factor and platelet-activating factor.

❑❑  **What are the two major arms of the coagulation cascade?**

The intrinsic and extrinsic pathways.

❑❑  **In general, where do the intrinsic and extrinsic arms of the coagulation cascade converge?**

At factor X. The activated factor IX and activated IX in the presence of an activated VIII from the intrinsic pathway activates factor X in the common pathway. From the extrinsic pathway, an activated factor VII aids in the activation of factor IX in the intrinsic pathway and factor X in the common pathway.

❑❑  **What are the initial factors in the intrinsic and extrinsic pathways?**

Factor XII and factor VII, respectively.

❑❑  **What are the activating factors of the intrinsic and extrinsic pathways?**

The Hageman factor (factor XII) activates the intrinsic pathway while the extrinsic pathway is activated by tissue factor.

❑❑  **What are the vitamin K dependent clotting factors and proteins?**

Factors II, VII, IX, and X. In addition, proteins C and S.

❑❑  **Following formation of a fibrin clot, how does the body lyse the clot?**

The fibrinolytic system balances the clotting system. Fibrinolysis is achieved via the activation and conversion of plasminogen to plasmin by plasminogen activator, urokinase and activated factor XII. In addition to lysis of the fibrin clot, plasmin can also cause inactivation of factors V and VIII, and cleave fibrinogen.

## ▢▢  What is disseminated intravascular coagulation (DIC)?

DIC is a consumptive coagulopathy which is seen in a number of clinical scenarios. It is characterized by microthrombi in the small vessel circulation and is often followed by active fibrinolysis and a bleeding diathesis. It can occur in the setting of shock, transfusion reactions, metastatic malignancies, certain leukemias (classically AML FAB M3), and other cases. Clinically, one sees hypofibrinogenemia and an increased level of fibrin split products. Importantly, there is an associated marked thrombocytopenia.

## ▢▢  What is an embolus?

An embolus is a thrombus that has been released from its site of origin and traveled through the bloodstream (example: pulmonary embolus).

## ▢▢  What is idiopathic thrombocytopenia purpura?

This is a cause of thrombocytopenia in which patients develop petechiae. In children, it is often subsequent to a viral infection and the patients bleed into a petechia. In adults, the disorder is characterized by chronicity (years) and it tends to wax and wane. Treatment is immunosuppression, including steroids sometimes leading to splenectomy.

## ▢▢  What are some causes of thrombocytopenia when the origin is found in the bone marrow?

Aplastic anemia causes thrombocytopenia in a setting of marked overall hypocellularity affecting all cell lines. Myelofibrosis and marrow replacement or infiltration by malignancy also can cause a diminished platelet production. Toxic effects of some drugs can preferentially cause a diminished number of megakaryocytes and subsequently thrombocytopenia.

## ▢▢  What is hypersplenism?

This is a cause of thrombocytopenia whereby the spleen sequesters platelets often causing subsequent splenomegaly.

## ▢▢  What is Bernard-Soulier syndrome?

This is an uncommon disorder whereby patients have low platelets, prolonged bleeding time, and qualitatively large platelets in circulation. It is inherited in an autosomal recessive pattern.

## ▢▢  What are the deficiencies that are the cause of Bernard-Soulier syndrome and Glanzman's thrombosthenia?

In Bernard-Soulier, there is a deficiency of the platelet membrane glycoprotein complex (GpIb/IX) which is the platelet receptor for von Willebrand's factor. In Glanzman's thrombosthenia, there is a deficiency of platelet membrane glycoproteins (GpIIb and GpIIIa) which are involved in fibrinogen binding.

## ▢▢  What is the deficiency in hemophilia A (classic hemophilia)?

Factor VIII. Remember, von Willebrand's factor (vWF) acts like a carrier for factor VIII and vWF is thought to bridge collagen and platelets via the GpIb receptor.

## ▢▢  What is von Willebrand's disease?

This is composed of a number of variants and is most commonly inherited in an autosomal dominant pattern. This results in a bleeding diathesis and the variants range from quantitative to qualitative deficiencies of vWF. Also, factor VIII may be reduced in circulation as the vWF stabilizes factor VIII.

❑❑  **What is the inheritance of hemophilia A?**

X-linked recessive.

❑❑  **What is hemophilia B?**

This is factor IX deficiency and is also known as Christmas disease. It is also X-linked recessive.

❑❑  **Briefly outline porphyrin metabolism.**

The porphyrins are ring structures that bind the metal ions found in hemoglobin and myoglobin. Due to various enzyme defects in the various types of porphyrias, various clinical manifestations are seen. The cutaneous manifestations are exacerbated by exposure to the sun. Glycine plus succinyl coenzyme A is converted to aminolevulinic acid (ALA) in the presence of ALA synthetase. ALA dehydrase converts the ALA to porphorbilinogen (PBG). Subsequently, PBG is converted to uroporphyrin, coproporphyrin, and protoporphyrin before the final synthesis of heme in the presence of iron and ferrochelatase.

# WBCs, LYMPH NODES, AND SPLEEN

☐☐ **What is the definition of neutropenia?**

An absolute neutrophil count less than 500 per microliter.

☐☐ **What is the definition of lymphocytopenia?**

An absolute lymphocyte count below 1500 per microliter.

☐☐ **What is the most likely explanation of hypersegmentation of neutrophils?**

A normal neutrophil contains 2-5 lobes. One that contains more than 5 lobes is hypersegmented and generally indicates megaloblastic anemia, most likely secondary to deficiency of vitamin B12, folate or both.

☐☐ **Without therapeutic intervention, which is more likely to follow a rapid and fatal course, acute or chronic leukemia?**

Acute leukemia is characterized by a proliferation of blast cells and is likely to be rapidly fatal without intervention. In contrast, chronic leukemia is characterized by proliferation of mature cells and, although not rapidly fatal, is less likely to be cured than acute leukemia.

☐☐ **What is a leukemoid reaction?**

A leukemoid reaction can be confused with true leukemia. Leukemoid reaction is seen in inflammatory states (often coexisting infection) and results in the presence of immature white blood cells in the peripheral blood. In general terms, leukemoid reactions do not have excessively high blast counts nor is the white blood cell count as elevated as it is in leukemia.

☐☐ **What are some causes of an increased number of peripheral blood eosinophils (eosinophilic leukocytosis)?**

Eosinophils are seen in reaction to asthma, so-called hay fever, some immune related skin diseases, an allergic reaction to medication, and parasitic infections.

☐☐ **In a patient with bacterial infection, one notes numerous large, dark granules in the neutrophils. What are these called?**

Toxic granules which most likely represent atypical azurophilic granules and are reactive and not neoplastic in nature.

☐☐ **What are some causes of an absolute monocytosis?**

While nonspecific, a monocytosis can be seen in systemic lupus erythematosus (SLE), rheumatoid arthritis, inflammatory bowel disease, and chronic infectious states such as tuberculosis, malaria and brucellosis.

☐☐ **What is a Pelger-Huet cell?**

A Pelger-Huet cell is a bi-lobed neutrophil that is inherited in an autosomal dominant fashion. One can see, Pelgeroid cells in patients who do not have the Pelger-Huet anomaly. Occasionally Pelgeroid cells are seen in association with myelodysplasia.

❑❑ **What is chronic granulomatous disease?**

This is a disorder in which neutrophils are able to phagocytose bacteria appropriately; however, there is a metabolic defect in which hydrogen peroxide and hydroxyl radicals are not produced and certain bacteria then are not killed (Staphylococcus aureus most commonly).

❑❑ **What are some laboratory methods by which one can screen for chronic granulomatous disease?**

Measurement of superoxide production chemiluminescence is one screening test. Another, more simple method is one that tests for the reduction of nitroblue tetrazolium to insoluble formazan which is simply called the formazan test.

❑❑ **What are the two basic categories of acute leukemias?**

Acute lymphocytic leukemia and acute myelogenous leukemia.

❑❑ **What is the effect of the accumulation of leukemic blasts on the other bone marrow constituents?**

The immature cells (blasts) have an increased survival time and they suppress the uninvolved hematopoietic stem cells. Thus, the clinical presentation of a patient with acute leukemia is typically related to anemia, thrombocytopenia, and leukopenia.

❑❑ **What is the Chediak-Higashi syndrome?**

This is an autosomal recessive disorder characterized by giant granules in neutrophils and lymphocytes. These patients have neutropenia, delayed microbial killing, and inadequate degranulation making them susceptible to bacterial infections.

❑❑ **What syndrome is characterized by partial albinism, lymphadenopathy, hepatosplenomegaly, pancytopenia, photophobia, and frequent bacterial infections?**

The Chediak-Higashi syndrome.

❑❑ **Describe the inclusion seen in Dohle bodies and the May-Hegglin anomaly.**

It is a pale blue peripheral cytoplasmic inclusion seen in neutrophils.

❑❑ **How is the May-Hegglin anomaly inherited?**

It is autosomal dominant and rare.

❑❑ **Although the inclusions in Dohle bodies and May-Hegglin anomaly are similar by light microscopy, how are they different ultrastructurally?**

Dohle bodies are remnants of the rough endoplasmic reticulum or free ribosomes while the inclusion in the May-Hegglin anomaly is made of RNA and can be removed by treatment with ribonuclease.

❑❑ **What condition contains large purple granules in neutrophilic cytoplasm that may resemble toxic granulation but occurs in the absence of infection?**

The Alder-Reilly syndrome. This is not transient and similar appearing inclusions can be seen in monocytes and lymphocytes in the mucopolysaccharidoses.

□□  In the peripheral blood, are there more circulating T or B lymphocytes?

T lymphocytes outnumber B-cells approximately 2:1.

□□  List some congenital types of absolute neutropenia.

Chronic benign neutropenia, familial severe neutropenia, congenital hypoplastic neutropenia (Kostmann's syndrome), and cyclic neutropenia. Familial severe neutropenia is autosomal dominant while Kostmann's syndrome is autosomal recessive.

□□  What is the syndrome characterized by neutropenia, rheumatoid arthritis, and splenomegaly?

Felty's syndrome.

□□  What is the most common kind of acute leukemia in children?

Acute lymphoblastic leukemia (ALL).  Over 80% of all cases are classified as FAB-L1.

□□  The blasts of an acute leukemia feature basophilic cytoplasm with prominent cytoplasmic vacuoles.  Myeloperoxidase and Sudan black b are negative and oil red O stain is positive within the vacuoles.  What type of acute leukemia is this?

ALL-FAB L3.  The primary differential rests with an acute myelogenous leukemia (FAB-M6).  Of course, AML is typically myeloperoxidase and Sudan black b positive.

□□  In pre B-cell ALL, where is immunoglobulin detected in the blast cells?

Cytoplasm.  Surface immunoglobulin is negative.

□□  In B-cell ALL (L3), what is the TdT and immunoglobulin status?

TdT is negative and immunoglobulin is detectable on the surface.

□□  How does a patient with T-cell ALL compare to B-cell ALL?

Typically older age, earlier relapse, chromosome rearrangements involving the long arm of chromosome 14 (14q11), shorter survival, and 50% have a mediastinal mass.

□□  Which type of ALL is notable for chromosomal translocations involving 8q24?

B-cell ALL (surface immunoglobulin positive).  This type also has a high incidence of an abdominal mass.

□□  The presence of the translocation t(9;22)(q34;q11) in ALL is associated with what type of prognosis?

Unfavorable, both for children and adults.  This is the Philadelphia chromosome ususally seen in chronic myelogenous leukemia (CML).  It is rare in children (approximately 2%) and seen in nearly a quarter of adult cases.

□□  A patient with Burkitt's lymphoma who presents with an acute lymphoblastic leukemia has which FAB subtype?

FAB L3.

□□  Hyperdiploidy (> 50 chromosomes) in ALL is associated with what clinical features?

Lower leukocyte count, age 2-10 years, Caucasian race, and pre B or early pre B-cell phenotype; all of which are favorable prognostic indicators.

❑❑  **How common are chromosomal abnormalities in acute lymphoblastic leukemia?**

Very, 90% of ALL will have some type of cytogenetic abnormality.

❑❑  **How does age at diagnosis play a role in ALL?**

Very young children, less than 2 years old, and adults fare less well than children diagnosed between the ages of 2 and 10.

❑❑  **What leukemia is classically characterized by a B-cell phenotype and often exists with pancytopenia and massive splenomegaly?**

Hairy cell leukemia.

❑❑  **What cytochemical stain has been classically used in the past to diagnose hairy cell leukemia?**

The hairy cells are tartrate resistant acid phosphatase positive (TRAP). Flow cytometry and immunohistochemical stains have greatly decreased reliance on this stain.

❑❑  **The presence of numerous Auer rods, disseminated intravascular coagulation and "faggot" cells are associated with which type of acute leukemia?**

Acute promyelocytic leukemia (FAB M3).

❑❑  **What cytogenetic findings would you expect with FAB M3?**

Translocation between chromosomes 15 and 17, t(15;17).

❑❑  **What is the number one cause of massive splenomegaly worldwide?**

Malaria. Other causes of massive splenomegaly include chronic myelogenous leukemia, myeloid metaplasia with myelofibrosis, and hairy cell leukemia.

❑❑  **Given the appearance of this lesion of the spleen, what is your diagnosis?**

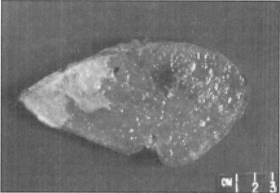

*(Photo courtesy of Julie Breiner, MD - University of Nebraska Medical Center)*

Splenic infarct. It is subcapsular and wedge-shaped.

❑❑  **In a patient with sickle cell disease, what would you expect the spleen to look like?**

These patients undergo "autosplenectomy" as they suffer from multiple splenic infarcts and subsequent fibrosis. Thus, their spleens become quite small.

❑❑  **What is one risk that patients who have undergone surgical or autosplenectomy face?**

They are particularly susceptible to infection with encapsulated organisms such as Streptococci, Klebsiella, and Haemophilus and thus should be given the pneumovax vaccine.

**❏❏  How would the alkaline phosphatase level differ in the leukocytes in chronic myelogenous leukemia compared to a leukemoid reaction?**

The alkaline phosphatase level is low in CML.

**❏❏  What is the classic translocation seen in approximately 90% of patients with CML?**

The Philadelphia chromosome consisting of a reciprocal translocation between chromosomes 9 and 22, t(9;22)(q34;q11).  This results in a bcr-c-abl fusion gene.  This gene then encodes for a protein with tyrosine kinase activity.

**❏❏  Name some drugs that have been reported to cause eosinophilia.**

Pilocarpine, physostigmine, digitalis, para-aminosalicylic acid, and sulfonamides.

**❏❏  Regarding infectious mononucleosis, what is the causal virus and how does it gain entry into the lymphocytes?**

The Epstein-Barr virus is the cause and it is absorbed into B lymphocytes via the C3d complement receptor (CD21).

**❏❏  What is the earliest detectable antibody and the antibody detected in late convalescence and throughout life in patients with infection by the Epstein-Barr virus?**

The IgM antibody to the viral capsid antigen (VCA) is the first detected and the antibody to the nuclear antigen (anti-EBNA) is detected in late convalescence and throughout life.

**❏❏  What is the likelihood of progression to leukemia in a patient with human T-cell leukemia virus-type 1 (HTLV-1)?**

Some 90% of patients with HTLV-1 antibodies are without symptoms at all. Those that do have symptoms will range from a nonspecific viral illness to adult T-cell leukemia.

**❏❏  What is the most common causative agent for a heterophil-negative mononucleosis?**

Cytomegalovirus.  Other causes would include an EBV infection that is heterophil-negative, toxoplasmosis, certain drugs and hepatitis.

**❏❏  What is the neutrophil alkaline phosphatase level in polycythemia vera?**

It is greatly elevated, again in contrast to CML where it is absent or markedly decreased.

**❏❏  What are the myelodysplastic syndromes (MDS)?**

This is a group of stem cell disorders which feature varying degrees of disordered hematopoiesis; however, all fall short of criteria necessary for the diagnosis of acute myelogenous leukemia (AML).

**❏❏  What is the classification of primary MDS?**

Refractory anemia (RA), refractory anemia with ringed sideroblasts (RARS), refractory anemia with excess blasts (RAEB), refractory anemia with excess blasts in transformation (RAEB-T), chronic myelomonocytic leukemia (CMML), chronic myelomonocytic leukemia in transformation (CMML-T), and myelodysplastic syndrome unclassified (MDS-U).

**❏❏  What are the typical patient demographics in someone with MDS?**

There is a slight male predominance and MDS occurs most commonly in patients older than 50 years. It is rare but reported in children. Many cases occur 2-8 years following chemotherapy.

❑❑  **What specific therapies are most commonly related to secondary MDS (therapy related)?**

Alkylating chemotherapeutic agents and radiotherapy.

❑❑  **What percentage of patients with CMML will have hypergammaglobulinemia?**

50%, typically polyclonal.

❑❑  **What three criteria are used to distinguish RAEB from RAEB-T and CMML from CMML-T?**

One or more of these three criteria must be present in addition to the criteria for RAEB or CMML to designate RAEB-T or CMML-T.
1.  5-29% peripheral blood myeloblasts
2.  20-29% bone marrow myeloblasts
3.  The presence of Auer rods

❑❑  **How long after initiation of chemotherapy with alkylating agents does secondary or therapy related MDS typically occur?**

About five years. It is approximately half that in the case of chemotherapy with epipodophyllotoxins.

❑❑  **Of the categories of MDS, which is the most likely to evolve into acute leukemia and thus has the poorest median survival?**

RAEB-T has a median survival of five months and 60% of cases evolve into acute leukemia. In contrast, RARS has the lowest leukemic evolution (8%) and the highest median survival (51 months).

❑❑  **What are some of the cytogenic abnormalities found in MDS?**

5q- is the most common abnormality seen in all classes of MDS. In addition, complete or partial loss of chromosome 8, trisomy 8, deletion or translocation of 11q and/or 12p in addition to many other complex chromosomal abnormalities are seen.

❑❑  **Which type of MDS is most likely to have a cytogenetic abnormality?**

Nearly all cases of therapy-related MDS have cytogenetic abnormalities, whereas less than 40% of primary MDS cases have chromosomal alterations.

❑❑  **Describe the 5q- syndrome.**

Patients have 5q- as the sole cytogenetic abnormality, a stable clinical course, thrombocytosis, refractory anemia subclass of MDS, and abnormal megakaryocytes.

❑❑  **List some factors that are good prognostic indicators in MDS.**

Young age, lack of pancytopenia, lack of peripheral blood myeloblasts and relatively low myeloblasts in the bone marrow, absence of complex chromosomal alterations, presence of ringed sideroblasts, and absence of Auer rods.

❑❑  **Which chromosomes are frequently abnormal in patients treated with alkylating agents and radiotherapy?**

Chromosomes 5 and 8.

❑❑  **What chromosomal abnormalities are associated with an unfavorable prognosis in MDS?**

Monosomy 7 or 7q- and generally complex chromosomal abnormalities.

## ☐☐ Describe the typical patient of monosomy 7 syndrome in childhood.

There is a male predominance and a median age of 10 months. Clinically, they report problems with recurrent infections, hepatosplenomegaly and occasional lymphadenopathy. They typically present with anemia, leukocytosis, and often thrombocytopenia.

## ☐☐ What other disease or condition has been reported in association with monosomy 7 syndrome?

Neurofibromatosis.

## ☐☐ In monosomy 7 syndrome, what is the status of the patient's neutrophils?

The neutrophils have abnormal chemotaxis and dysplastic changes may be present in the peripheral blood granulocytes and monocytes.

## ☐☐ In ringed sideroblasts, where is the iron located that one sees with an iron stain?

The iron is found in mitochondria which ring the nucleus.

## ☐☐ With regard to acute lymphoblastic leukemia, what is the significance of the presence of the following translocation: t(8;14)(q24;q32)?

This translocation is found in 1-3% of all ALL and approximately 90% of FAB L3 (surface immunoglobulin positive mature B-cell ALL) and is associated with a poor prognosis.

## ☐☐ Which subtype of ALL is associated with the presence of the Philadelphia chromosome (t(9;22)(q34;q11))?

That's a trick question. The Philadelphia chromosome is not associated with any specific subtype of ALL; however, it is found in more adults with ALL than children, and patients often have CNS involvement and elevated white counts. It portends a poor prognosis.

## ☐☐ If one were to have a bone marrow aspirate smear featuring relatively undifferentiated blast cells, how would one determine whether they were myeloid or lymphoid in origin?

Cytochemical stains would aid in making this distinction in that myeloid cells would be expected to be myeloperoxidase and Sudan black B positive, while lymphoblasts would be negative for these stains. In addition, the lymphoblasts in T-cell, early pre B-cell, and pre B-cell ALL would be expected to be terminal deoxynucleotidyl transferase (TdT) positive. B-cell ALL is TdT negative.

## ☐☐ In ALL, which subtype features the largest blast cells which also typically have abundant cytoplasmic vacuoles?

FAB-L3.

## ☐☐ What type of ALL is depicted by the following phenotype: DR+, surface Ig-, cytoplasmic mu chain-, CD19+ (a B cell marker), CD10 (CALLA)+?

Early pre-B-cell ALL having either L1 or L2 blast morphology.

## ☐☐ Which type of ALL is both the least frequent (thankfully) and carries the worst prognosis?

Mature B-cell ALL (FAB-L3) which is characterized by the following phenotype: DR+, sIg+, Cmu-, CD19+, and CD10+.

❏❏ **As opposed to the myelodysplastic syndromes, which cytogenetically typically feature deletions or additions, what is the general category of cytogenetic abnormalities seen in AML?**

AML typically features translocations.

❏❏ **Describe the French American British (FAB) classification of AML.**

M0 - minimally differentiated
M1 - AML without maturation
M2 - AML with maturation
M3 - acute promyelocytic leukemia
M4 - acute myelomonocytic leukemia
M5 - acute monocytic leukemia
M6 - acute erythroleukemia
M7 - acute megakaryocytic leukemia.

❏❏ **What is the most frequent FAB subtype of AML seen?**

M2 (AML with maturation) accounts for approximately 40% of AML followed in frequency by M1 (AML without maturation) and M4 (acute myelomonocytic leukemia), each of which account for about 20% of cases.

❏❏ **Which is the least common class of AML?**

Acute megakaryocytic leukemia (M7) at an approximate incidence of 1%.

❏❏ **Which class of AML is associated with abnormalities of chromosome 16?**

Approximately one fourth of cases of M4 feature an abnormal chromosome 16.

❏❏ **Besides CML and some cases of ALL, what type of acute leukemia can also feature the Philadelphia chromosome?**

Some 10% of AML without maturation (M1) demonstrate the Philadelphia chromosome and carry a poor prognosis.

❏❏ **A blast which is negative with peroxidase staining and strongly positive with nonspecific esterase is consistent with what type of blast?**

Monoblast.

❏❏ **Describe the characteristic eosinophil findings in a case of AML M4 with increased marrow eosinophilia.**

The bone marrow contains more than 3% eosinophils at least some of which contain abnormal granules which are often basophilic. Cytochemical stains show these abnormal granules to react with chloroacetate esterase and periodic acid-Schiff (PAS) which is unlike normal eosinophils.

❏❏ **What chromosomal abnormality is associated with M4 with increased marrow eosinophilia?**

Abnormalities of chromosome 16 are associated with M4 eosinophilia. This can be in the form of a translocation (16;16)(p13;q22) or an inversion (16)(p13;q22).

❏❏ **What is the term used to describe a leukemic infiltrate into tissue producing a mass?**

Granulocytic sarcoma or chloroma.

❏❏  **An 82-year-old male presents with a white count of 150,000 per microliter and the peripheral blood smear shows many "smudge" cells. What is the most likely diagnosis?**

Chronic lymphocytic leukemia (CLL).

❏❏  **What type of lymphocyte makes up essentially all cases of chronic lymphocytic leukemia?**

Almost all cases are B-cell.

❏❏  **What are some of the complications which can result in a case of long-standing CLL?**

Patients can develop a warm antibody autoimmune hemolytic anemia, hypogammaglobulinemia with subsequent bacterial susceptibility and infiltration of other organs, such as the prostate in males.

❏❏  **What is the typical survival time in a patient with CLL?**

The median survival time is 3 to 7 years. The course is indolent but steady and treatment is largely ineffective.

❏❏  **What genes are involved in the various translocations which are seen in virtually all cases of B-cell ALL?**

The c-myc oncogene is located on chromosome 8. The major translocation seen in B-cell ALL, t(8;14) results in the immunoglobulin heavy chain locus on chromosome 14 being juxtaposed with c-myc oncogene on chromosome 8. The kappa (chromosome 2) and lambda (chromosome 22) light chain loci are juxtaposed to c-myc oncogene in the translocations involving chromosomes 2 and 8 and 8 and 22 which are sometimes seen in B-cell ALL.

❏❏  **What is the term used to describe an aggressive transformation of an indolent B-cell lymphoma to a high grade lymphoma?**

Richter transformation.

❏❏  **In addition to pan B-cell antigens expressed in B-cell CLL, what other classic antigen is expressed by these cells?**

Most cases of B-cell CLL express CD5 which is typically a pan T-cell antigen.

❏❏  **In CLL, what happens to natural killer (NK) cells and T-helper cells?**

NK function is diminished or even absent even though absolute numbers of NK cells may, in fact, be increased. The T-helper to suppressor ratio is inverted and the T-helper function is often diminished as well.

❏❏  **Describe the morphologic appearance of a prolymphocyte.**

Prolymphocytes are larger than typical CLL lymphocytes, have more abundant basophilic cytoplasm and prominent, often centrally located nucleoli.

❏❏  **How many patients with CLL will develop a "prolymphocytoid transformation"?**

About 15%.

❏❏  **What percentage of prolymphocytes is generally necessary to designate a leukemia as chronic lymphocytic leukemia/prolymphocytic leukemia?**

CLL has fewer than 10% prolymphocytes and prolymphocytic leukemia has greater than 55% prolymphocytes, thus those cases which fall between these two ranges should be designated as CLL/PLL.

❑❑  **What percentage of cases of PLL are B-cell origin?**

Approximately 80%.

❑❑  **What is the causative agent of adult T-cell leukemia/lymphoma?**

Human T-cell leukemia virus-1 (HTLV-1).

❑❑  **What is mycosis fungoides compared to Sezary syndrome?**

Sezary syndrome is characterized by circulating tumor cells (T-cells) which have very convoluted cerebriform nuclei in association with a diffuse exfoliative erythroderma while mycosis fungoides is simply a primary lymphoma of the skin which is of T-cell phenotype.

❑❑  **What are the syndromes which fall under the title of myeloproliferative disorders?**

CML, polycythemia vera, myelofibrosis with myeloid metaplasia, and essential thrombocythemia.

❑❑  **What are the characteristic cytogenetic abnormalities seen in myelofibrosis?**

Sorry, there are none.

❑❑  **What do the bone marrow aspirations in patients with myelofibrosis have in common with those with hairy cell leukemia?**

Both often result in a "dry tap".

❑❑  **In a bone marrow core biopsy of myelofibrosis, what would one expect to find early in the course of disease?**

Hypercellularity with abnormal megakaryocytes in clusters.

❑❑  **If one sees a hypercellular bone marrow and the leukocyte alkaline phosphatase (LAP) score is low, what would you suspect as the diagnosis?**

CML; however, in myelofibrosis the LAP may be high, normal or low and early in the disease the bone marrow is hypercellular so it cannot be ruled out.

❑❑  **What is the classic red cell morphology associated with myelofibrosis?**

Tear drop forms (dacryocytes).

❑❑  **Polycythemia vera (PV) is characterized by excessive production of which cell line(s)?**

All three - red blood cells, leukocytes, and megakaryocytes.

❑❑  **Are patients with PV at increased risk for development of acute leukemia?**

Yes, or I would not have asked.  It is also higher in those patients treated with chemotherapy compared to those treated with phlebotomy alone.

❑❑  **What are the most common cytogenetic abnormalities of PV?**

+8, +9, and 20q-.

❑❑  **Is a man or a woman more likely to have hypereosinophilic syndrome?**

It is 9:1 more common in men.

❏❏  **How does CML occurring in a 16-year-old differ from that occurring in a 1-year-old?**

Juvenile CML is defined as that which occurs in very young children, typically less than 2, and it differs from the adult type CML occurring in a young person in that JCML is Philadelphia chromosome negative, pursues an aggressive course more like AML than CML and the patients feature a markedly increased hemoglobin.

❏❏  **What are some causes of secondary polycythemia vera?**

Chronic hypoxia (secondary to pulmonary disease, congenital heart disease, high elevations, smoking), increased erythropoietin production (secondary to polycystic kidney disease, renal cell carcinoma, hepatocellular carcinoma, cerebellar hemangioma), pheochromocytoma, and adrenal adenoma with Cushing's syndrome.

❏❏  **Which of the myelodysplastic syndromes often results in extramedullary hematopoiesis (EMH)?**

Myelofibrosis patients often exhibit EMH particularly in the liver and spleen.

❏❏  **What type of lymphocytes are infected by EBV in mononucleosis?**

B-lymphocytes.

❏❏  **The atypical lymphocytes seen in the peripheral blood in mononucleosis are of what type?**

They are T-lymphocytes (CD8+).

❏❏  **What is the classic cell associated with Hodgkin's disease?**

The Reed-Sternberg cell.

❏❏  **What is the morphologic appearance of Reed-Sternberg cells?**

The classic RS cell is bilobated with large eosinophilic inclusion-like nucleoli; however, variants may be mononucleated or multilobated.

❏❏  **According to the Rye classification, what are the different types of Hodgkin's disease?**

Lymphocyte predominance, mixed cellularity, lymphocyte depleted, and nodular sclerosis.

❏❏  **What is the RS cell variant seen in lymphocyte predominance Hodgkin's disease?**

The so-called L&H cell which has a "popcorn" appearance.

❏❏  **What is the RS cell variant seen in mixed cellularity type of HD?**

Mononuclear variants of RS cells as well as classic RS cells are seen.  The background contains a mixed infiltrate of eosinophils, histiocytes, and plasma cells.

❏❏  **What is the classic RS cell variant seen in nodular sclerosis Hodgkin's disease?**

RS cells, often mononuclear, are present with large spaces surrounding them, hence they have been given the term lacunar cells.

❏❏  **Of the types of HD in the Rye classification, which has the poorest prognosis?**

Lymphocyte depletion.

❑❑ **What is the most common variant of Hodgkin's disease?**

Nodular sclerosis.

❑❑ **What is the least common variant of Hodgkin's disease?**

Lymphocyte depletion.

❑❑ **Is extranodal involvement by tumor more common in Hodgkin's disease or non-Hodgkin's lymphoma (NHL)?**

Non-Hodgkin's lymphoma.

❑❑ **What general cell type is the RS cell derived from?**

It is lymphoid as opposed to monocytic or histiocytic.

❑❑ **What infectious agent is detected in some cases of Hodgkin's disease?**

EBV.

❑❑ **What is a long term risk in patients treated with radiotherapy for Hodgkin's disease?**

As is often the case, long term survivors of previous radiation therapy or chemotherapy suffer from an increased risk for a second malignancy. Most commonly they are AML, lung cancer, non-Hodgkin's lymphoma, melanoma, and breast cancer.

❑❑ **What is a typical patient profile of someone with lymphocyte predominance Hodgkin's disease?**

They are typically of low stage, asymptomatic, and young. Thus, as would be expected, they have a good prognosis and respond to therapy.

❑❑ **Give a similar patient profile of someone with lymphocyte depletion type Hodgkin's disease.**

These patients are older, higher stage and symptomatic, and thus have a poor prognosis.

❑❑ **What are some of the clinical signs that are referred to as "constitutional symptoms"?**

Fever, weight loss, and night sweats.

❑❑ **Compare the typical age of a patient with Hodgkin's disease versus non-Hodgkin's lymphoma.**

Hodgkin's disease is mainly a disease of the young (30 or less) while non-Hodgkin's lymphoma occurs in older people (greater than 40).

❑❑ **Compare the incidence of bone marrow involvement in follicular lymphoma vs. Hodgkin's disease.**

Follicular lymphoma very commonly involves the bone marrow in a paratrabecular pattern, while Hodgkin's disease involves the bone marrow in only about 10% of cases.

❑❑ **What happens to cellular immunity in patients with Hodgkin's disease?**

Patients with HD have varying degrees of deficiency or suppression of cellular immunity. Cytokine production by the Hodgkin's tumor itself may play a role in this observation.

❑❑  **Briefly describe the staging classification for Hodgkin's disease.**

Stage I - single lymph node involvement
Stage II - two or more lymph node regions from one side of the diaphragm
Stage III - lymph node involvement on both sides of the diaphragm
Stage IV - involvement of extranodal sites

❑❑  **What is the primary treatment for localized Hodgkin's disease?**

Radiotherapy.

❑❑  **What are the two main patterns seen in non-Hodgkin's lymphoma?**

Follicular (nodular) and diffuse.

❑❑  **In general, which of the two basic patterns carries a better prognosis?**

Follicular.

❑❑  **What is the working formulation of lymphoma?**

This is one of several organizational schemes of non-Hodgkin's lymphoma.  It is divided into low, intermediate, and high grade.  Low grade includes small lymphocytic, follicular small cleaved, and follicular mixed. Intermediate grade includes follicular large cell, diffuse small cleaved, diffuse mixed cell. High grade lymphoma includes immunoblastic, diffuse large cell, small non-cleaved (Burkitt's and non-Burkitt's), and lymphoblastic.

❑❑  **What type of non-Hodgkin's lymphoma is associated with an occasional monoclonal spike (IgM) and amyloidosis?**

Small lymphocytic lymphoma.

❑❑  **In general, what is the expected clinical course in a patient with a low grade or indolent lymphoma compared to a high grade lymphoma?**

Low grade lymphomas, as the name indicates, are slowly progressive and have low proliferation rates while the high grade lymphomas have high proliferation rates and can progress rapidly.  However, owing to the proliferation rates, the high grade lymphomas may respond better to treatment and therefore have higher rates of "cure".  In contrast, low grade lymphomas do not respond well to therapy and although the disease course may be many years, they are not "curable" and the patient will eventually die.

❑❑  **Describe the most frequent translocation seen in Burkitt's lymphoma.**

t(8;14)(q24;q32).  Remember, chromosome 8 is the site of proto-oncogene  c-myc and the heavy chain gene locus is on chromosome 14.

❑❑  **What non-Hodgkin's lymphoma is considered the lymphoma counterpart to CLL?**

Small lymphocytic lymphoma (SLL).

❑❑  **How frequently is there bone marrow involvement at the time of diagnosis of follicular lymphoma?**

About 75% of the time.

❑❑  **What is the characteristic translocation associated with follicular lymphomas?**

t(14;18). Remember, 14q32 is the location of the IgH heavy chain gene involved in Burkitt's lymphoma. 18q21 is the site of bcl-2 which normally prevents programmed cell death (apoptosis). Hence, the translocation results in overexpression of the bcl-2 protein and prolonged cell life.

❏❏ **Which high grade lymphoma has a classic presentation as a jaw mass in a child in Africa?**

Small non-cleaved lymphoma (Burkitt's).

❏❏ **What viral agent has a distinct causative relationship with Burkitt's lymphoma?**

EBV.

❏❏ **What cell type creates the starry sky pattern in Burkitt's lymphoma?**

Macrophages.

❏❏ **What percentage of B-immunoblastic lymphomas are seen in association with an immunologic disorder?**

50%.

❏❏ **What cytogenetic abnormality characterizes mantle zone lymphoma?**

t(11;14).

❏❏ **What type of T-cells are involved in mycosis fungoides?**

T-helper cells (CD4+).

ANAPLASTIC LARGE CELL LYMPHOMA ANTI-ALK IMMUNOPEROXIDASE

❏❏ **What is the characteristic translocation of anaplastic large cell lymphoma (ALCL) as shown above?**

t(2;5)(p23;q35).

❏❏ **What are the two major types of post transplantation lymphoproliferative disorders (PTLD)?**

Polymorphous and monomorphous.

❏❏ **What is the causative agent found in essentially 100% of PTLD?**

EBV.

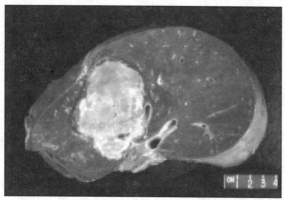

**POST-TRANSPLANT LYMPHOPROLIFERATIVE DISORDER (PTLD)**

❑❑  **Given the gross appearance of this tumor in a small bowel transplant recipient, would you expect this PTLD to be of the monomorphous or polymorphous type?**

Obviously you cannot be sure, but the point is that the monomorphous type is more likely to exhibit vast areas of necrosis as seen in this tumor.

❑❑  **What are Bence-Jones proteins?**

They are free light chains produced in plasma cell dyscrasias.

❑❑  **What is the most common immunoglobulin produced in multiple myeloma?**

IgG occurs in over half of cases followed in frequency by IgA.

❑❑  **What are the major criteria used in the diagnosis of multiple myeloma?**

Greater than or equal to 30% of the bone marrow is plasma cells; serum IgG greater than or equal to 3.5 g/dl or IgA greater than or equal to 2 g/dl; urinary kappa or lambda greater than or equal to 1 g/24 hrs; biopsy proven plasmacytoma.

❑❑  **What serum marker has been used to gauge prognosis in multiple myeloma?**

Serum beta-2 microglobulin elevation indicates a high tumor burden.

❑❑  **What is the term used to describe the presence of a monoclonal gammopathy in a patient who does not have indications of a classic monoclonal gammopathy?**

Monoclonal gammopathy of undetermined significance (MGUS).

❑❑  **How frequently does amyloidosis develop in patients with multiple myeloma?**

10-20% of cases.

❑❑  **What is the major cause of death in patients with multiple myeloma?**

Infection.

❑❑  **What is the second most common cause of death in patients with multiple myeloma?**

Renal insufficiency.

❏❏ **What is the most common monoclonal gammopathy?**

MGUS.

❏❏ **What characteristic finding does one see in the red blood cells in a peripheral blood smear of a patient with multiple myeloma?**

Rouleaux formation.

❏❏ **What is Waldenstrom's macroglobulinemia?**

This is a monoclonal gammopathy that produces immunoglobulin M in association with a plasmacytoid lymphoma.

❏❏ **What are the three variants of heavy-chain disease?**

Gamma-chain disease, alpha-chain disease, and mu-chain disease.

❏❏ **Of the heavy-chain disease variants, which is the most common and typically found in young adults?**

Alpha-chain disease, particularly in people from the Mediterranean.

❏❏ **Of the heavy-chain disease variants, which is the least common?**

Mu-chain, it is typically found in patients with CLL.

❏❏ **Historically, what are the three entities which comprise the general category of Langerhans cell histiocytosis?**

Letterer-Siwe syndrome, Hand-Schuller-Christian disease, and eosinophilic granuloma.

❏❏ **What is the characteristic ultrastructural finding in a Langerhans histiocyte?**

Bierbeck granule.

❏❏ **What is the characteristic clinical finding in the Letterer-Siwe variant?**

This occurs in infants, although it can occur in adults, and is characterized by a skin rash over the trunk and scalp as well as hepatosplenomegaly.

❏❏ **What three clinical findings are referred to as the Hand-Schuller-Christian triad?**

Diabetes insipidus, exophthalmos, and calvarial bone lesions.

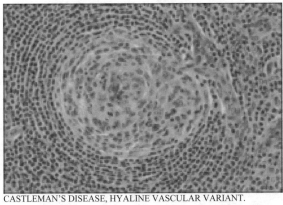

CASTLEMAN'S DISEASE, HYALINE VASCULAR VARIANT.

❏❏ **In the localized type of Castleman's disease, what is the natural course following resection of the lesion?**

The symptoms and abnormal laboratory values return to normal.

❏❏ **Which cytokine stimulates differentiation of eosinophilic precursor cells in certain infections resulting in an eosinophilic leukocytosis?**

IL-5.           Hot T-Bone stEAk

❏❏ **Based on expression of immunoglobulin, what is the difference between a pre-B cell and a B cell?**

A pre-B cell expresses cytoplasmic immunoglobulin while a B cell expresses surface immunoglobulin. In addition, the B cell expresses CD21 and 22 not seen in the pre-B cell and does not express CD10 (CALLA) which is seen in the pre-B cell.

❏❏ **What are the most common chromosomal abnormalities seen in SLL?**

Trisomy 12, 11q-, and deletions of 13q12-14 with trisomy 12 and deletions of 11q being associated with the worst prognosis.

❏❏ **In body cavity large B-cell lymphomas, what virus is seen in the tumor cells in essentially all cases?**

Human herpesvirus 8.

❏❏ **What is the name given to the PAS positive inclusions which contain immunoglobulin within plasma cells in conditions such as Waldenstrom's macroglobulinemia?**

When in the cytoplasm they are called Russell bodies and when in the nucleus they are called Dutcher bodies. When they comprise "grape-like" masses within the cytoplasm they are referred to as Mott cells.

# NEOPLASIA

☐☐ **What embryologic cell lines are carcinomas derived from?**

Ectoderm and endoderm.

☐☐ **What embryologic tissue are sarcomas derived from?**

Mesoderm.

☐☐ **What does the term anaplasia mean?**

This refers to the loss of the typical functional and microscopic appearance of a cell or tissue.

☐☐ **What does the word tumor mean?**

A swelling. Therefore, it includes benign and malignant processes; however, it has unfortunately become synonymous with "cancer".

☐☐ **What is the term used to describe the collagenous reactive change seen in the stroma of some invasive tumors?**

Desmoplasia.

☐☐ **What is the general term used to describe the tumor which is composed of numerous different cell types, originating from more than one embryologic germ cell layer?**

Teratoma.

☐☐ **What is the term which describes an overgrowth of disordered cells or tissue which are normally found in that area?**

Hamartoma.

☐☐ **What is the term which describes variation in size and shape of cells or nuclei?**

Pleomorphism.

☐☐ **Does dysplasia always progress to cancer?**

No, the majority of dysplasias seen in the uterine cervix, for example, will not subsequently develop into a squamous cell carcinoma.

☐☐ **What is tumor doubling time?**

This is the amount of time that a particular tumor takes in order for it to double the number of cells comprising it.

☐☐ **What is the growth phase of a tumor?**

These are cells that are undergoing replication and thus are most vulnerable to the effects of chemotherapy.

☐☐ **In general, what is the pattern of growth of a benign tumor?**

Benign tumors tend to grow as cohesive, expansile masses, compared to malignant tumors which tend to be poorly circumscribed and infiltrate.

❑❑  **What structure is breached thus separating an in situ lesion from an invasive one?**

The basement membrane.

❑❑  **What are the three ways by which a malignant tumor can spread?**

1. Direct extension or seeding
2. Lymphatic space invasion
3. Hematogenous spread

❑❑  **What is the most common route by which carcinomas spread?**

Lymphatics.

❑❑  **In general, compare the spread of carcinomas to sarcomas.**

Carcinomas tend to spread via lymphatics and sarcomas tend to spread hematogenously.

❑❑  **Name a sarcoma which is an exception to the previous rule and tends to spread via lymphatics.**

Synovial sarcoma.

❑❑  **What growth factor may be responsible for the desmoplastic tissue response seen in some invasive malignancies?**

Many neoplastic cells secrete TGF-beta.

❑❑  **What effect does TGF-beta have on many epithelial cells?**

It inhibits them; however, many neoplasms appear to be resistant to its effect.

❑❑  **What is a choristoma?**

This is normal tissue appearing in a site where it is not indigenous.

❑❑  **What growth factor produced by many tumors also aids in neovascularization to help support the growth of the tumor?**

TGF-b.

❑❑  **What are some of the proteases that tumor cells secrete which may help in destruction of the basement membrane and subsequent invasion?**

Transin, fibrinolysin, and collagenases.

❑❑  **What role do inflammatory cells play in tumor invasion and metastasis?**

Many inflammatory cells secrete proteases and growth factors, thus they may aid in the destruction of the basement membrane and subsequent invasion and even metastasis.

❑❑  **What are two examples of carcinomas that tend to spread via vascular invasion as opposed to lymphatic invasion?**

Renal cell carcinoma (renal vein) and hepatocellular carcinoma (hepatic vein).

❏❏ **Which is more important in prognosis, stage or grade of tumor?**

Stage.

❏❏ **What is the second leading cause of death in the United States?**

Cancer.

❏❏ **How does the incidence of cancer differ worldwide compared to the United States?**

Cancer is much less common worldwide, particularly in underdeveloped countries where malnutrition and infectious disease such as malaria are more frequent causes of death than cancer.

❏❏ **What are four general categories of risk factors for cancer?**

Age, diet, environment, and genetics.

❏❏ **In the 1-14 year old age group, what are the top two causes of death?**

Accidental death is number one followed by cancer (11% of deaths).

❏❏ **What is the most common type of cancer found in males?**

Prostate.

❏❏ **What is the most common type of cancer found in females?**

Breast.

❏❏ **What is the leading cause of cancer death in males?**

Lung.

❏❏ **What is the leading cause of cancer death in females?**

Lung.

❏❏ **What does the grade of the tumor refer to?**

Grade refers to the degree of differentiation, that is, a well-differentiated tumor is much like normal tissue where a poorly-differentiated tumor lacks distinctive features to indicate its origin.

❏❏ **What does anaplasia mean?**

This refers to a high grade tumor which is poorly-differentiated or lacks differentiation.

❏❏ **What effect does the process of "smoking" food have on cancer incidence?**

Smoking of food results in the production of chemical carcinogens and may be a part of why people in Iceland, who consume large quantities of smoked fish products, have an increased rate of carcinoma of the esophagus.

❏❏ **How does the amount of fiber and fat relate to colon cancer?**

A diet high in fat and low in fiber appears to be related to an increased incidence of colon cancer, although the details of this subject remain highly debatable.

❏❏ **What is one proposed mechanism for the increased incidence of hepatocellular carcinoma in people in Africa?**

The prevalence of hepatitis B virus infection is quite high and is known to be related to an increased incidence of hepatocellular carcinoma.

❏❏ **Name several types of malignancies that are increased in incidence in a setting of alcohol abuse.**

Oropharyngeal, laryngeal, esophageal, and hepatocellular carcinoma (following cirrhosis).

❏❏ **Name several types of cancer that are increased secondary to smoking.**

Oropharyngeal, laryngeal, esophageal, pancreatic, bladder, and of course, lung.

❏❏ **How does sexual intercourse relate to the incidence of cervical cancer?**

The incidence of cervical cancer is increased with a younger age at first intercourse and a high number of sexual partners.

❏❏ **Given the association of intercourse history and cervical cancer, what is at least one postulated mechanism behind this?**

Infection with human papillomavirus (HPV) of certain serotypes increases the incidence of cervical cancer. Early and frequent intercourse and multiple sexual partners increases the risk of HPV infection and therefore cervical carcinoma.

❏❏ **What hematologic malignancy are patients with Down's syndrome at increased risk for developing?**

Acute leukemia is up to 30 times more common in patients with Down's syndrome.

❏❏ **What type of malignancy is associated with an increased incidence in children with immunodeficiencies?**

Lymphomas.

❏❏ **What is the phrase used to describe the process of CD8+ T-cells killing tumor cells in the body?**

Immune surveillance.

❏❏ **In young children, other than acute leukemia, what is the organ system most commonly involved in primary malignancies?**

Central nervous system.

❏❏ **What is the incidence of colon carcinoma in a patient with familial adenomatous polyposis?**

This is an autosomal dominant mutation present at birth resulting in numerous adenomas of the colon which will develop into carcinoma of the colon in essentially all people afflicted by the age of 50.

❏❏ **Are all inherited cancer syndromes autosomal dominant in nature?**

No, xeroderma pigmentosum, for example, is autosomal recessive.

❏❏ **How can one explain the fact that all members of the family are not afflicted when they inherit an autosomal dominant gene associated with a cancer syndrome?**

Low penetrance.

☐☐ **List some examples of autosomal recessive cancer syndromes involving defective repair of DNA.**

Xeroderma pigmentosum, ataxia-telangiectasia, Bloom's disease, and Fanconi's syndrome.

☐☐ **List some examples of autosomal dominant inherited cancer syndromes.**

Familial retinoblastoma, familial adenomatous polyposis, the multiple endocrine neoplasia syndromes, neurofibromatosis, and Von Hippel-Lindau syndrome.

☐☐ **Of the noninherited, sporadic adenomatous polyps of the colon, which type is associated with the highest risk for development of cancer?**

Villous adenomas.

☐☐ **What is the malignant counterpart of the leiomyoma?**

Leiomyosarcoma.

☐☐ **What is the benign counterpart of osteosarcoma?**

Osteoid osteoma.

☐☐ **Would you expect a tumor with a high mitotic rate, extensive necrosis, marked pleomorphism, and existance as individual cells, in solid sheets and clusters to be high or low grade?**

High grade.

☐☐ **Can a benign tumor result in death?**

Of course, by local effects such as compression of vital structures.

☐☐ **What is the term used to describe a bone fracture secondary to a malignancy?**

Pathologic fracture.

☐☐ **Are malignant tumors monoclonal or polyclonal?**

Monoclonal, that is, derived from one parent cell.

☐☐ **What is the term used to describe the characteristic whereby neoplastic cells proliferate in an otherwise uncontrolled manner?**

Autonomy.

☐☐ **What are some conditions that are considered precancerous?**

Ulcerative colitis, chronic gastritis, Barrett's esophagus, villous adenomas with high grade dysplasia, cervicovaginal dysplasia and many others.

☐☐ **In general, do benign neoplasms "transform" into malignancies over time?**

No.

☐☐ **What are two manners by which a genetic mutation resulting in a cancer occur in cells?**

Acquired (somatic cells) or inherited (germ line).

☐☐  **What types of environmental agents can cause somatic mutation?**

Chemicals, viruses, and radiation.

☐☐  **As a tumor outgrows its blood supply, what type of necrosis does one see?**

Ischemic necrosis.

☐☐  **What are the factors that are associated with endothelial cell proliferation and subsequent neovascularization of a tumor?**

Tumor angiogenesis factor, TGF-a, TGF-b, EGF, PDGF, and VEGF.

☐☐  **In general how does the cell to cell adherence in tumors compare to normal tissue?**

Tumors tend to be less adherent thus aiding in invasion.

☐☐  **How does the calcium content of tumor cell walls compare to normal cell walls?**

Decreased.

☐☐  **In general, what is the nature of the cell surface charge found in malignant cells?**

They tend to have a high negative surface charge and increased cell to cell repulsion.

☐☐  **What is the term used to describe an abnormal DNA content?**

Aneuploid.

☐☐  **For at least some tumors, how does the presence of aneuploid DNA seem to relate to overall prognosis?**

At least for some, aneuploidy seems to confer a worse prognosis.

☐☐  **What is an oncogene?**

These are genes which, in general, encode growth factors and growth factor receptors which tend to stimulate growth.

☐☐  **What is a tumor-suppressor gene?**

This is a gene which encodes negative growth regulators, thus inhibiting growth.

☐☐  **What are two oncogenes which are associated with lung carcinoma?**

L-myc and K-ras.

☐☐  **What is the location and name of the oncogene involved in Burkitt's lymphoma, among other things?**

C-myc on chromosome 8q24.

☐☐  **What is the name and location of the tumor suppressor gene associated with renal cell carcinoma and Von Hippel-Lindau syndrome?**

VHL on chromosome 3p25.

❏❏  **Which tumor suppressor gene is associated with numerous cancers including colon, lung, and breast, is located on the nucleus, acts via a transcription factor, and is associated with Li-Fraumeni syndrome?**

p53 found on chromosome 17p13.

❏❏  **What is the name and location of the tumor suppressor gene associated with retinoblastoma?**

Rb on chromosome 13q14.

❏❏  **What is the significance of the NF1 gene?**

It is a tumor suppressor gene associated with neurofibromas (type I neurofibromatosis) which acts via a GTPase activation mechanism.

❏❏  **What is the term which refers to homologous cellular genes which are present in the DNA of most organisms and are closely related to retrovirus-derived oncogenes?**

Protooncogenes or cellular oncogenes.

❏❏  **How many somatic cellular oncogene mutations are required for neoplastic transformation?**

It varies, at least in some cells two or more control points must be mutated or overridden in order for neoplastic transformation to occur.

❏❏  **What are some of the different things that cellular oncogenes encode for?**

Growth factors, receptors for extracellular growth factors, polypeptide signal transducers, cytoplasmic hormone receptors, and polypeptides which bind certain DNA regulatory regions thus regulating transcription and ultimately replication.

❏❏  **What is the action of the oncogene product of c-abl, c-ras, and c-src?**

They encode for proteins which act as signal transducers between the cell membrane and cytoplasmic proteins.

❏❏  **What is insertional mutagenesis?**

This is disregulated expression of a protooncogene following insertion of a retroviral promoter very near to it.

❏❏  **What are the two methods by which a protooncogene may become oncogenic?**

Via retroviral transduction or disregulation in situ resulting in conversion into cellular oncogenes.

❏❏  **Which oncogene is most commonly mutated amongst the dominant oncogenes in human malignancies?**

ras is mutated in almost 1/3 of human tumors.

❏❏  **What are the two patterns of gene amplification?**

Double minutes and homogeneous staining regions (HSR).

❏❏  **Who proposed the "two hit" hypothesis of oncogenesis?**

Knudsen.

❏❏   **What is the "two hit" hypothesis?**

This refers to the idea that a germ cell mutation ("first hit") is inherited from a parent and is therefore present in all of the cells in the body and a second mutation ("second hit") must then occur in a cell with the first hit in order to develop the malignancy.  He developed this hypothesis specifically regarding retinoblastoma.

❏❏   **How does the "two hit" theory apply in a sporadic (not familial) case of retinoblastoma?**

It still holds.  Both "hits" or mutations must occur in a cell and result in loss of both retinoblastoma gene alleles.

❏❏   **What does the phrase "loss of heterozygosity" mean?**

This simply means that a cell becomes homozygous for a mutant allele where before it was heterozygous, or contained one normal gene.

❏❏   **How are the APC and NF-1 genes similar?**

They are both involved in hereditary development of tumors which are benign, but they progress to malignancies.  APC results in development of adenomatous colonic polyps and NF-1 results in benign neurofibromas.

❏❏   **What are three tumor suppressor genes which are found in the nucleus?**

Rb, WT-1, and p53.

❏❏   **What is the action of the retinoblastoma gene product (pRb) in its active, hypophosphorylated form?**

It binds transcription factors thus preventing replication.

❏❏   **What common tumor suppressor gene reacts to mutagenic agents by undergoing post translational modifications, stabilizing, accumulating, and then causing cell arrest in the G1 phase of the cell cycle?**

p53.

❏❏   **What is the reason for p53 to normally cause cell arrest in the G1 phase?**

This allows the cell to make critical repairs to DNA that may have been damaged due to a mutagenic agent.

❏❏   **If p53 fails in its bid to allow cell repair of DNA damage via cell cycle arrest, what action does p53 then have?**

It seems to trigger apoptosis.

❏❏   **What action does bcl-2 have that it plays such a key role in follicular lymphomas?**

It prevents programmed cell death.

❏❏   **Where is bcl-2 located within the cell?**

In the mitochondrial membrane.

❏❏   **What does the presence of consistent chromosomal deletions in a specific tumor indicate?**

The presence of a tumor suppressor gene.

❏❏  **In general, how do growth factors act on a cell?**

They bind specific plasma membrane receptors which then cause transduction of a signal.

❏❏  **What are the phases of a tumor cell cycle?**

The same as any cell - G0, G1, S, G2, M.

❏❏  **How does the cell cycle time for tumors compare to normal tissue?**

It is usually the same as or even longer than a normal tissue's cell cycle time, perhaps contrary to one's intuition.

❏❏  **What are some tumor-derived angiogenic factors?**

Fibroblast growth factor (FGF), TGF-a, TGF-b, endothelial growth factor (EGF), platelet-derived growth factor (PGF), and vascular endothelial growth factor (VEGF).

❏❏  **What percentage of deaths due to cancer are related to the use of tobacco products?**

Almost 1/3.

❏❏  **What are the two major mechanisms of chemical carcinogenesis?**

Genotoxic carcinogens and non-genotoxic carcinogens.  Genotoxic carcinogens produce covalent modifications of various cell components like DNA while non-genotoxic carcinogens do not.

❏❏  **Do all assaults on DNA via various toxic substances result in detectable and mutagenic damage?**

No, because the body has the ability to excise or repair these areas of DNA.

❏❏  **What is a promoter as it applies to carcinogenesis?**

These are agents that are not carcinogenic in and of themselves but do serve to facilitate and enhance the development of a tumor.

❏❏  **List some examples of chemical carcinogens which are genotoxic.**

Benzopyrine, nitrogen mustard, mitomycin C, aflatoxin B, safrole, cycasin, and many others.

❏❏  **Name some metals which are carcinogenic in humans.**

Arsenic, beryllium, chromium, and nickel.

❏❏  **What is the inherent abnormality in xeroderma pigmentosa which results in an increased incidence of cancer?**

Defective DNA repair.

❏❏  **Given that cancer is a clonal disease, are all progeny of the original tumor cells identical morphologically and biochemically?**

No, various subclones, sometimes more aggressive, are produced throughout the course of the tumor.

❏❏  **With regard to neoplasia, what does the term initiator refer to?**

An initiator is something that changes DNA structure and is mutagenic.

❑❑  **In the theory of neoplasia, which is the first step, initiation or promotion?**

Initiation is the primary insult.

❑❑  **How much more likely is someone who is positive for hepatitis B virus to develop hepatocellular carcinoma?**

200 times.

❑❑  **What malignancy is aflatoxin classically associated with?**

Hepatocellular carcinoma.

❑❑  **What percentage of people with hepatocellular carcinoma are positive for hepatitis C virus and negative for hepatitis B virus?**

Approximately 1/2.

❑❑  **What tumor has a high incidence in China and is associated with the presence of DNA from Epstein-Barr virus?**

Nasopharyngeal carcinoma.

❑❑  **What two oncogenes are important in tumor genesis caused by human papillomavirus (HPV)?**

E6 and E7 proteins.

❑❑  **What is the mechanism of action of the E6 and E7 proteins in HPV?**

They most likely bind and activate the gene products of p53 and the retinoblastoma gene.

❑❑  **What types of HPV are associated with malignant tumor development?**

Most commonly types 16 and 18.

❑❑  **Are immunoincompetent patients more susceptible to the development of malignancies?**

Yes.

❑❑  **What types of malignancies are immunoincompetent patients most likely to develop?**

Lymphoproliferative disorders/lymphomas.

❑❑  **What is the gene which is often amplified in the case of tumor resistance to therapy?**

Multidrug resistance gene (MDR1).

❑❑  **How does the death rate for gastric carcinoma in Japan compare to the United States?**

It is approximately six times higher in Japan.

❑❑  **How does the cancer death rate in Japan for breast and prostate carcinoma compare to that in the United States?**

These are quite rare in Japan.

❑❑  **Patients with ataxia telangiectasia have an increased incidence of what tumors?**

Leukemia and lymphomas.

❑❑ **What is a chromosomal inversion?**

This is when a portion of DNA becomes oriented opposite to its original, natural direction.

❑❑ **What virus is greatly associated with cancer of the uterine cervix?**

Human papilloma virus (HPV).

❑❑ **What chemical carcinogen is classically associated with angiosarcoma of the liver?**

Vinyl chloride.

❑❑ **What type of cancer is classically associated with polycyclic hydrocarbons (like soot)?**

Scrotal cancer.

❑❑ **What chemical carcinogen is classically associated with lung cancer and mesothelioma?**

Asbestos.

❑❑ **What type of cancer is classically associated with the aromatic amines?**

Bladder.

❑❑ **What is the term used to describe the "wasting" effect or significant weight loss seen in patients with cancer?**

Cachexia.

❑❑ **What factor is associated with tumor related cachexia?**

Cachectin (tumor necrosis factor).

❑❑ **What is the term used to describe the condition where a substance produced by a tumor causes certain symptoms, not related to direct or metastatic spread of the tumor?**

Paraneoplastic syndrome.

❑❑ **What types of tissues are considered mesenchymal?**

Bone, smooth muscle, fat and fibrous tissue.

❑❑ **What types of cells in the body can potentially destroy tumor cells?**

Cytotoxic T-cells (CD8+), killer cells, natural killer cells, and macrophages.

❑❑ **What are some of the options for treatment of cancer?**

Surgical excision, chemotherapy, radiotherapy, and immunotherapy.

❑❑ **What effect can cancer have on the clotting system?**

Patients can become hypercoagulable.

❑❑ **Is there an increased incidence of malignancy in patients with acquired immunodeficiency syndrome (AIDS)?**

Yes, any condition which results in immunosuppression increases the risk of malignancy.

❑❑  **What types of malignancies have a higher incidence in China or Japan as opposed to the United States?**

Nasopharyngeal carcinoma, gastric carcinoma, hepatocellular carcinoma, and choriocarcinoma.

❑❑  **What is Trousseau's phenomenon?**

This is a migratory thrombophlebitis which is classically associated with adenocarcinoma of the pancreas but can also be seen in association with other malignancies.

❑❑  **What is the term used to describe the action of two initiating agents working in conjunction to produce a malignancy?**

Cocarcinogenesis.

❑❑  **What is a point mutation?**

This is a single nucleotide change within a certain gene sequence.

❑❑  **What happens to epithelial cadhedrins in solid epithelial tumors like breast carcinoma?**

They are downregulated, which is to say they have decreased cell to cell adherence which allows them to "break away" from the primary tumor.

❑❑  **What are three classes of proteases that aid tumor cells in invasion?**

Matrix, cystine, and serine metalloproteinases.

❑❑  **What is the importance of type IV collagenase?**

It is a metalloproteinase that cleaves the type IV collagen of basement membranes and aids in tumor invasion.

❑❑  **What is cathepsin D?**

A cystine proteinase which serves to aid in degradation of the extracellular matrix.

❑❑  **What effect do some of the matrix components which are cleaved by tumor cells in the process of invasion have on tumor cells?**

They seem to be chemotactic.  Some growth factors like insulin-like growth factor also seem to be chemotactic for tumors.

❑❑  **What is a complete carcinogen compared to an incomplete carcinogen?**

Complete carcinogens are those chemicals which can serve both as an initiator and a promoter; therefore, they can cause cancer in and of themselves without outside influences.  Incomplete carcinogens are initiators and still need promoters to cause cancer.

❑❑  **What is the Ames test?**

This is a test whereby a chemical's ability to cause mutations in a bacterium (Salmonella typhimurium) is assessed to determine its mutagenic potential.

❑❑  **Promoters do not cause genetic mutations, so what is their function in tumor development?**

They induce cell proliferation.

❑❑ **What human malignancy is beta-naphthyllamine associated with in the exposed workers (aniline dye and the rubber industry)?**

Bladder cancer.

❑❑ **Where does the aflatoxin B toxin and aflatoxin B1 that causes hepatocellular carcinoma come from?**

Aspergillus flavus.

❑❑ **How does UVB light cause cancer?**

Through the formation of pyrimidine dimers.

❑❑ **Which serotypes of human papillomavirus (HPV) have been associated with invasive squamous cell carcinoma of the cervix?**

16, 18, 31, 33, 35, and 51.

❑❑ **With regard to EBV, what does latent membrane protein-1 (LMP-1) interact with?**

blc-2 gene.

❑❑ **What are tumor specific antigens?**

These are antigens which are present on tumor cells, but not normal cells and result in an immune response.

❑❑ **What are tumor associated antigens?**

These are antigens which are expressed not only by tumor cells but also by normal cells.

❑❑ **What are the three general categories of tumor associated antigens?**

1. Tumor associated carbohydrate antigens (TACA)
2. Oncofetal antigens
3. Differentiation specific antigens

❑❑ **What is the most common manifestation of a paraneoplastic syndrome?**

Hypercalcemia.

❑❑ **Of the endocrinopathies that result from a paraneoplastic syndrome, what is the most common syndrome to develop?**

Cushing's syndrome.

❑❑ **Of patients with Cushing's syndrome as a paraneoplastic syndrome, what tumor are these patients most likely to have?**

50% have lung cancer, usually small cell type.

❑❑ **What is the most common tumor associated with hypercalcemia?**

Squamous cell carcinoma of the lung.

□□  **In patients over the age of 40, what is acanthosis nigricans often associated with?**

50% of these patients have some type of cancer.

□□  **What two tumors is acute disseminated intravascular coagulation (DIC) classically associated with?**

Acute promyelocytic leukemia (AML FAB 3) and adenocarcinoma of the prostate.

□□  **What are the three components of the American Joint Committee on Cancer's staging system?**

Evaluation of the tumor (T), evaluation of the lymph nodes (N), and evaluation of metastatic disease (M).

□□  **What are some laboratory methods of diagnosing malignancy which are short of resection of the mass?**

Fine needle aspiration, biopsy, exfoliative cytology, molecular and cytogenetic analysis, measurement of serum tumor markers, and flow cytometry.

□□  **What malignancy is the tumor marker CA-125 associated with?**

Ovarian cancer.

□□  **What is the tumor marker CA-19-9 associated with?**

Colon and pancreatic cancer.

□□  **What is the tumor marker CA-15-3 associated with?**

Breast cancer.

□□  **What is the tumor marker alpha-fetoprotein associated with?**

Hepatocellular carcinoma and non-seminomatous germ cell tumors of the testis.

□□  **What is the tumor marker calcitonin associated with?**

Medullary carcinoma of the thyroid.

□□  **What is the tumor marker human chorionic gonadotropin associated with?**

Trophoblastic tumors and non-seminomatous tumors of the testis.

□□  **What phase of the cell cycle is arrested by the normal action of p53?**

The late G1 phase.

# IMMUNITY

☐☐ **What are the two general categories of immune response?**

Cellular immunity and humoral immunity.

☐☐ **What cell is the mediator of cellular immunity?**

T lymphocytes.

☐☐ **What cell is the mediator of the humoral immune response?**

B lymphocytes.

☐☐ **What is an immunogen?**

This is any substance that elicits an immune response.

☐☐ **What is an antigen?**

This is a substance which reacts with the products of the immune response.

☐☐ **What is a complete antigen?**

This is an antigen that not only reacts with the products of the immune response but also can be immunogenic itself.

☐☐ **What is a hapten?**

This is an antigen which can elicit an immune response when joined to a larger, carrier molecule which is immunogenic.

☐☐ **In the circulating blood, what percentage of lymphocytes are T-cells?**

About 2/3 are T-cells.

☐☐ **Where are T lymphocytes normally found in tissue?**

They are found in the periarteriolar sheaths of the spleen and the paracortex of lymph nodes.

☐☐ **Describe the components of the most common T-cell receptor (TCR).**

95% of T-cells have a TCR which is made up of an alpha and beta chain bound by a disulfide link.

☐☐ **What is the second most common TCR?**

A gamma and delta chain bound by disulfide bonds.

☐☐ **Where does one tend to find the TCR gamma delta cells?**

Near epithelial interfaces, like the respiratory and gastrointestinal tracts.

❏❏ **What CD molecule is expressed by T-helper/inducer cells?**

CD4.

❏❏ **What molecule is expressed by cytotoxic/suppressor T-cells?**

CD8.

❏❏ **What is the normal ratio of CD4 to CD8 positive cells?**

2:1.

❏❏ **What molecule is recognized by CD4 cells compared to CD8 cells?**

CD4+ cells bind to the class II major histocompatibility complex (MHC) while CD8+ cells bind to the class I MHC.

❏❏ **Which T-cell subset is gradually diminished in acquired immunodeficiency syndrome (AIDS)?**

CD4+ T-cells.

❏❏ **What is the difference between the two recently recognized subsets of CD4+ T-cells?**

T-helper-1 cells produce and secrete interleukin-2 (IL-2) and interferon-gamma (IFN-g), while T-helper-2 cells produce IL-4 and IL-5 but not IL-2 or IFN-g. Thus, T-helper-1 cells are not involved in macrophage-dependent immune responses, while T-helper-2 cells help in production of other antibody classes.

❏❏ **Once stimulated, what do B-lymphocytes ultimately become?**

Plasma cells.

❏❏ **Of the 5% of T-cells which have a gamma-delta TCR, is CD4 or CD8 expressed on their surface?**

Neither.

❏❏ **What are the components of T-cell receptor messenger RNA?**

Variable, joining and constant regions. In addition, the TCR beta chain contains a diversity region between the variable and joining regions.

❏❏ **What cell expresses CD19?**

This is a transducing molecule which is expressed early in B-cell differentiation.

❏❏ **What are some functions of macrophages?**

Antigen presentation to T-cells, cytokine production, and tumor lysis via toxic metabolites and proteolytic enzymes.

❏❏ **How effective are Langerhans cells and dendritic cells in phagocytosis?**

Poorly, if at all.

❏❏ **List some substances which are produced and secreted by T-cells.**

Cytokines including IL-2, IL-3, IL-4, IL-5, IL-6, and gamma interferon (IFN-g).

❑❑ **What cytokine stimulates hematopoietic stem cells, inhibits fibroblasts, and assists the maturation of T and B-cells?**

IL-6.

❑❑ **What are some of the actions of IL-4?**

It upregulates class II major histocompatibility complex (MHC) and acts as a growth factor for mast cells, B-cells and activated T-cells.

❑❑ **Where are B-cells normally found in tissue?**

Germinal centers and the superficial cortex of lymph nodes, the lymphoid follicles of the splenic white pulp, and in the bone marrow.

❑❑ **What cells in the immune system do not have surface immunoglobulin or T-cell receptors, and have an ability to lyse some cells without prior sensitization?**

Natural killer (NK) cells.

❑❑ **What are the five types of immunoglobulins produced by B-cells?**

IgG, IgA, IgM, IgD, and IgE.

❑❑ **What is the name of the immunoglobulin region which is heterogeneous and binds antigen?**

The variable region.

❑❑ **What is the name of the immunoglobulin region which controls the binding of complement?**

Constant region.

❑❑ **In the development of heavy chain messenger RNA and subsequently the heavy chain itself, what is the order of the variable (V), diversity (D), and joining (J) gene rearrangements?**

D-J joining, then V-D/J joining, then transcription, then RNA splicing with V/D/J-C joining followed by translation and production of the immunoglobulin heavy chain.

❑❑ **What is the order of the gene rearrangements of the variable (V), joining (J), and constant (C) regions of light chain production?**

V-J joining, transcription, V/J-C joining, translation, and light chain production.

❑❑ **What is the main function of the histocompatibility antigens?**

They bind portions of foreign proteins such that they may be presented to specific T-cells.

❑❑ **On what chromosome is the major histocompatibility complex (MHC), which is also known as the human leukocyte antigen complex (HLA), locus located?**

Short arm of chromosome 6.

❑❑ **In the classic pathway of complement, what is the initial step?**

Direct binding of C1 to an antigen-antibody complex.

❑❑ **What makes up the membrane attack complex?**

C5b bound with C6 through C9.

❑❑  **Which cells express class I MHC antigens?**

All nucleated cells and platelets.

❑❑  **What are the three major loci of class II MHC antigens?**

HLA-DP, HLA-DQ, and HLA-DR.

❑❑  **Which T-cell subtype is restricted to antigens in association with MHC class II molecules?**

CD4+.

❑❑  **Name some major diseases and HLA allele associations.**

Ankylosing spondylitis, post gonococcal arthritis and acute anterior uveitis with B27; "chronic-active" hepatitis and Sjogren's syndrome with DR3; rheumatoid arthritis and DR4; hemochromatosis and A3; 21-hydroxylase deficiency and BW47; insulin-dependent diabetes mellitus and DR3, DR4 and DR3/DR4.

❑❑  **What are the four major hypersensitivity reactions?**

Type I - immediate hypersensitivity
Type II - antibody-mediated cytotoxicity
Type III - immune complex disease
Type IV - cell-mediated hypersensitivity.  (delayed)

❑❑  **What type of main hypersensitivity reaction is Goodpasture's syndrome?**

Type II antibody-mediated cytotoxicity.

❑❑  **What type of hypersensitivity is systemic lupus erythematosus and the Arthus reaction?**

Type III immune complex disease.

❑❑  **What type of hypersensitivity reaction is acute rejection of a solid organ transplant?**

Type IV cell-mediated (delayed).

❑❑  **What antibody and which cells are the mediators of a type I (anaphylactic) hypersensitivity reaction?**

IgE and mast cells and basophils.

❑❑  **What causes degranulation of mast cells and basophils in immediate hypersensitivity?**

Bridging of the bound antigen by two adjacent IgE molecules on a mast cell or basophil.

❑❑  **What are some primary mediators (granules) of mast cells?**

Histamine, eosinophil chemotactic factor, neutrophil chemotactic factor, proteases, and proteoglycans.

❑❑  **What is the general mechanism of action of a type II hypersensitivity reaction?**

An antibody (typically IgM or IgG) binds to a cell surface antigen resulting in either complement-mediated cytotoxicity or an antibody-mediated cytotoxicity.

❑❑  **What are the two general categories of type III hypersensitivity reaction sites?**

1. Systemic immune complex disease
2. Local immune complex disease (Arthus reaction)

❑❑  **What is the Arthus reaction?**

This is a reaction described many years ago whereby a foreign antigen is injected into the body and an antibody response is mounted. Later, injection at a subcutaneous site of the same antigen results in edema, erythema, and hemorrhage at that site secondary to the action of preformed antibodies against the injected antigen.

❑❑  **What subset of lymphocytes mediates the type IV hypersensitivity reaction (cell-mediated)?**

T-lymphocytes.

❑❑  **Which MHC class has beta-2-microglobulin within its glycoprotein structure?**

Class I.

❑❑  **Which hypersensitivity reaction is in effect during atopic dermatitis?**

Type I (immediate hypersensitivity).

❑❑  **Where are the three main sites of damage in graft versus host disease?**

Gastrointestinal tract, liver, and skin.

❑❑  **What are the three basic phases of systemic immune complex disease?**

1. Antigen-antibody complex formation in the circulation
2. Deposition of immune complexes
3. Inflammatory response secondary to immune complex deposition

❑❑  **What is the mechanism of tissue damage in immune complex disease?**

The damage is secondary to activation of the complement cascade.

❑❑  **What is the main immunologic response (type I-IV) to Mycobacterium tuberculosis and contact dermatitis secondary to chemical agents?**

Type IV hypersensitivity (cell-mediated).

❑❑  **What hypersensitivity reaction is involved in polyarteritis nodosa?**

Type III (immune complex).

❑❑  **Chronologically, when does hyperacute rejection occur in solid organ transplantation?**

Usually within minutes of transplantation secondary to pre-existing antibodies to donor antigens.

❑❑  **The inflammatory reaction shown below is an example of what type of hypersensitivity reaction?**

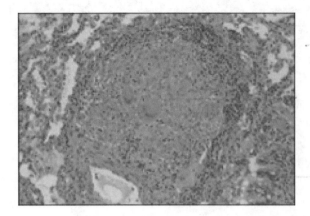

This is a granuloma and the granulomatous response is a type IV hypersensitivity reaction.

❑❑ **Describe the role that IFN-g plays in development of fibrosis following a delayed-type hypersensitivity reaction?**

IFN-g activates macrophages, thus enhancing their ability to kill microorganisms, and causing them to secrete several growth factors such as platelet-derived growth factor and TGF-b. TGF-b stimulates fibroblasts and ultimately collagen synthesis, thus if the offending agent is not removed the sustained hypersensitivity reaction ultimately results in fibrosis.

❑❑ **Is HLA matching used in liver transplantation?**

No.

❑❑ **What is the term for the site on the antibody where the antigen binds?**

Paratope.

❑❑ **What is the nature of the bond that holds the heavy and light chains together in the antibody molecule?**

Disulfide bonds.

❑❑ **How are the HLA antigens expressed?**

Codominantly.

❑❑ **What is the structure of the HLA class I molecule?**

It is composed of an alpha1 and alpha2 domain (variable) and an alpha3 domain and a beta-2-microglobulin (conserved).

❑❑ **What is the structure of the HLA class II molecule?**

It is composed of an alpha1 and beta1 domain (variable) with a peptide binding site between the alpha2 and beta2 domain (constant).

❑❑ **What are the clinical features of atopic allergy?**

Pruritus, cutaneous wheal and flare, sneezing, and dyspnea.

❑❑ **What is clonal anergy?**

This is when, under certain conditions, lymphocytes face an extended and even permanent inactivation following exposure to antigens.

❑❑ **What is the term used to describe the body's normal ability to recognize self-antigens, and thus not elicit an immune response?**

Immunologic tolerance.

❑❑ **What is the mechanism by which autoimmunity develops?**

It is unknown, several mechanisms have been postulated, including an imbalance of suppressor and helper T-cell function, other effects of microbial agents, and genetic factors.

❑❑ **In general, are autoimmune disorders more common in men or women?**

Women.

❑❑ **What are some of the criteria used to diagnose systemic lupus erythematosus (SLE)?**

Malar or discoid rash, photosensitivity, oral ulcers, arthritis, serositis, renal problems, neurologic disorders, hematologic disorders, immunologic disorders, and an abnormal antinuclear antibody titer.

❑❑ **Of the antinuclear antibodies, which is most specific and frequent in SLE?**

Anti double-stranded DNA.

❑❑ **Which autoantibody is present in over 95% of patients with mixed connective tissue disorder (MCTD)?**

Anti-mRNP.

❑❑ **Which autoantibody is present in over 70% of patients with CREST?**

Anti-centromere antibody.

❑❑ **What two antibodies are positive in more than 95% of cases of drug-induced lupus erythematosus?**

Generic antinuclear antibody and antihistone.

❑❑ **What disease is associated with anti-Smith antibody in about 25% of cases?**

SLE.

❑❑ **What false positive test result can result from binding antiphospholipid antibodies and cardiolipin antigen in patients with SLE?**

Syphilis.

❑❑ **What are some drugs which can induce an SLE-like response?**

Hydralazine, procainamide, and D-penicillamine.

❑❑ **Are cationic or anionic anti-DNA antibodies more likely to deposit in the kidneys and cause damage?**

Cationic anti-DNA antibodies.

❏❏  **What is the term given to the vegetation sometimes seen on cardiac valves in SLE?**

Libman-Sacks endocarditis.

❏❏  **In patients with HLA-DR4, what drug is associated with an increased risk of developing lupus erythematosus?**

Hydralazine.

❏❏  **What particular HLA types are associated with an increased risk of systemic lupus erythematosus?**

HLA-DR2, DR3, A1, and B8.

❏❏  **Which disease is anti-SS-B highly specific for?**

Sjogren's syndrome.

❏❏  **Which complement components are often deficient in patients with SLE?**

C2 and C4.

❏❏  **What is the immunofluorescence pattern seen in SLE?**

A "full house" of IgG, IgA, IgM, and C1q and C3.

❏❏  **What is Sjogren's syndrome?**

This autoimmune disease is associated with dry eyes and a dry mouth secondary to a lymphocytic infiltrate involving the salivary and lacrimal glands.

❏❏  **What is the term used to describe the dry eyes and dry mouth of Sjogren's syndrome?**

SICCA complex.

❏❏  **What type of malignancy are patients with Sjogren's syndrome at increased risk for?**

Lymphoma.

❏❏  **Can patients with Sjogren's syndrome have elevated titers of rheumatoid factor?**

Yes, and ANA.

❏❏  **What HLA antigen types are associated with Sjogren's syndrome?**

HLA-DR3, HLA-DQA1, and HLA-DQB1.

❏❏  **What percentage of patients with Sjogren's syndrome have another autoimmune disorder?**

60%.

❏❏  **Where would one biopsy to attempt to make the diagnosis of Sjogren's syndrome?**

The lip, to evaluate the minor salivary glands.

❏❏  **What does CREST syndrome include?**

Calcinosis, Raynaud's phenomenon, esophageal dysmotility, sclerodactyly, and telangiectasia.

❏❏  **What does the antibody SS-B found in Sjogren's syndrome bind with?**

Epstein-Barr virus RNA.

❏❏  **What is the most common autoantibody found in patients with systemic sclerosis (scleroderma)?**

Anti-Scl-70.

❏❏  **What is the Scl-70 antigen?**

It is a nonhistone nuclear protein.

❏❏  **What is POEMS?**

This is a disorder related to scleroderma which includes plasma cell dyscrasia with polyneuropathy, organomegaly, endocrinopathy, monoclonal protein and skin disease (POEMS).

❏❏  **How often are the lungs involved in progressive systemic sclerosis?**

More than half the time, often giving a picture similar to idiopathic pulmonary fibrosis.

❏❏  **Which disease has a classic rash composed of a lilac discoloration of the upper eyelids with associated periorbital edema?**

Dermatomyositis.

❏❏  **What are the scaly, erythematous patches over the knuckles, elbows and knees in dermatomyositis?**

Grotton's lesions.

❏❏  **What muscle groups are affected in dermatomyositis?**

The proximal muscles initially.

❏❏  **How does polymyositis differ from dermatomyositis?**

It has no cutaneous manifestation, occurs predominantly in adults, and has a slight increased risk of development of solid tumors.

❏❏  **Of the autoantibodies, which appears to be most specific for inflammatory myopathies?**

Anti tRNA synthetases.

❏❏  **What types of infections are common in patients with Bruton's X-linked agammaglobulinemia?**

*B - cell def.*

Pyogenic infections, such as streptococci and staphylococci..

❏❏  **What is the status of the total number of circulating B-cells in patients with common variable immunodeficiency?**

They have normal numbers of B-cells in spite of being hypogammaglobulinemic.

❏❏  **What happens to the incidence of associated autoimmune disease in patients with common variable immunodeficiency and X-linked agammaglobulinemia?**

Both have increased incidence of autoimmune disease.

❏❏  **What is the most frequent common variable immunodeficiency (CVI)?**

Isolated IgA deficiency.

❏❏  **What happens to T-cell function in patients with CVI?**

Some patients have abnormal T-cell regulatory function.

❏❏  **What are some of the clinical manifestations of selective IgA deficiency?** *secretion*

Other autoimmune disease, sinopulmonary infections, diarrhea, and IgE-mediated allergies.

❏❏  **How common are antibodies to IgA in patients with isolated IgA deficiency?**

40% of patients.

❏❏  **What oropharyngeal pouches form the thymus gland?**

Third and fourth.

❏❏  **What are the clinical manifestations of patients with DiGeorge's syndrome?**    *T + B*

Absence of cell-mediated immunity, tetany, cardiac defects, and abnormal facies.

❏❏  **What is the most common ultimate cause of death in patients with DiGeorge's syndrome?**

Death is usually related to the cardiac problems or tetany rather than recurrent infections.   *← PT*

❏❏  **How common is complete absence of the thymus?**

This is rare, usually there is at least a very small thymus present even if it is in an abnormal location.

❏❏  **How is the form of severe combined immunodeficiency (SCID) where there is near total absence of both B and T-cells inherited?**

Autosomal recessive.

❏❏  **In the X-linked form of SCID, how does the number of B-cells compare to the number of T-cells?**

There is a severe and progressive deficiency of T-cells, while the number of B-cells might actually be elevated.

❏❏  **What percentage of patients with SCID have the X-linked form?**

50%.

❏❏  **In the autosomal recessive form of SCID, what enzyme are many patients lacking?**

Adenosine deaminase (ADA) is absent in 40% of patients.

❏❏  **What is Omen's syndrome?**

Splenomegaly and lymphadenopathy, erythroderma, and activated T-lymphocytes in the peripheral blood, spleen and skin.

❏❏ **What are the clinical manifestations of Wiskott-Aldrich syndrome?**

Recurrent infections, eczema, and thrombocytopenia with an early death.

❏❏ **In patients with Wiskott-Aldrich syndrome, what does one typically see in the levels of various isotypes of immunoglobulins?**

IgM is low, IgG is usually normal, and IgA and IgE are often elevated.

❏❏ **What is the causative agent of X-linked lymphoproliferative disorder (XLP)?**

EBV.

❏❏ **What is the deficiency in patients with hereditary angioedema?**

C1 esterase inhibitor.

❏❏ **What is the result of absence of C1 esterase inhibitor in patients with hereditary angioedema?**

This results in excessive C1 esterase activation, resulting in production of vasoactive C2 kinin, and recurrent episodes of localized edema of skin and mucous membranes.

❏❏ **What are some of the patient groups who are at risk for contraction of HIV and subsequently AIDS?**

Homosexual or bisexual males, intravenous drug users, hemophiliacs, recipients of blood, blood components and organs, heterosexuals who have contacted other high risk group members.

❏❏ **What general type of virus is HIV?**

It is a retrovirus.

❏❏ **What type of T-lymphocyte is the target of HIV?**

CD4+.

❏❏ **What glycoprotein is used by HIV to enter T-cells?**

GP120.

❏❏ **What are the two classic tests used to screen and then confirm HIV?**

ELISA (screen) and Western blot (confirmatory).

❏❏ **What are some of the cellular components of HIV-1?**

Envelope proteins GP120 and GP41, core proteins p17, p18, and p24.

❏❏ **Which envelope glycoprotein in HIV is transmembrane?**

GP41.

❏❏ **Once the HIV-1 has entered the cell, how does it transcribe its RNA into DNA?**

Via reverse transcriptase.

❏❏ **AIDS patients are at risk for numerous malignancies, what are some of them?**

Kaposi's sarcoma, non-Hodgkin's lymphoma, Hodgkin's disease, and even carcinoma.

❏❏ **What are some of the infectious agents which are fairly commonly found in AIDS patients?**

Pneumocystis carinii, Toxoplasma gondii, Mycobacterium avium-intracellulare, Cryptosporidium, a variety of fungi including Aspergillus, a variety of viruses including cytomegalovirus, EBV, herpes simplex, and herpes zoster.

❏❏ **What is the causative agent of bacillary angiomatosis?**

Bartonella henselae.

❏❏ **What genes of the HIV-1 code for the core proteins, reverse transcriptase, and envelope proteins?**

Gag, pol, and env, respectively.

❏❏ **What are some of the genes in HIV-1 which control the synthesis of the viral particles?**

Tat, rev, vif, nef, vpr, and vpu.

❏❏ **Besides CD4+ T-cells, what other cell is commonly infected by HIV?**

Macrophages, because they also have a CD4 molecule which has a high affinity receptor for HIV.

❏❏ **Which immunodeficient state is classically associated with infection by Giardia lamblia?**

Common variable immunodeficiency.

❏❏ **In a patient with AIDS and cytopenias, what would you expect the bone marrow cellularity to be?**

Normal or hypercellular in 90% of cases.

❏❏ **What is the nature of the anemia seen in patients with AIDS?**

Typically, it is an anemia of chronic disease (normocytic, normochromic).

❏❏ **What type of hypersensitive reaction occurs in hyperacute rejection of a solid organ transplant?**

Type II.

❏❏ **Why do the symptoms of X-linked agammaglobulinemia not appear until after age six months typically?**

Because of residual circulating maternal antibodies.

❏❏ **What is the typical level of gammaglobulins in a patient with AIDS?**

Interestingly, they are typically hypergammaglobulinemic due to a polyclonal activation of B-cells.

❏❏ **What is the ultrastructural appearance of amyloid?**

It is composed of nonbranching fibrils with a diameter of 7.5 - 10 nanometers which show a beta-pleated sheet configuration by X-ray crystallography.

❑❑  **What is the minor second component of amyloid, comprising approximately 5% of the structure?**

P component.

❑❑  **What are the two most common forms of amyloid proteins?**

Amyloid light chain (AL) and amyloid associated (AA).

❑❑  **What is the major amyloid fibril protein found in Alzheimer's disease?**

beta-2-amyloid protein.

❑❑  **What is the major amyloid fibril protein found in hemodialysis-associated amyloidosis?**

Amyloid beta-2-microglobulin.

❑❑  **What cell produces the AA protein of amyloid?**

Hepatocytes.

❑❑  **What cell produces the AL protein of amyloid?**

Plasma cells.

❑❑  **What is the most sensitive screening stain for amyloid?**

Thioflavin T or S.

❑❑  **What is the most specific cytochemical stain for amyloid?**

Congo red.

❑❑  **How common is AL amyloidosis in patients with multiple myeloma?**

Approximately 1 in 5 patients will develop it.

# INHERITED AND METABOLIC DISEASE

❑❑ **What is the term used to describe a normal number of chromosomes present in humans?**

Diploid (46 chromosomes).

❑❑ **What is mosaicism?**

This is the case where an individual has two cell lines, one containing the normal complement of chromosomes and the other with an abnormal complement.

❑❑ **What is the most common cause of aneuploidy?**

Meiotic nondisjunction.

❑❑ **What is the term used to describe loss of part or (rarely) an entire chromosome?**

Deletion.

❑❑ **What is a reciprocal or balanced translocation?**

It is an exchange of chromosomal material between two chromosomes which results in no lost genetic material.

❑❑ **What is a Robertsonian translocation?**

This is when two acrocentric chromosomes (very short p arms) join with a common centromere, thus losing the p (short) arms.

❑❑ **What is lyonization?**

This is the idea that all but one X chromosome are inactivated randomly early in development.

❑❑ **What is a Barr body?**

This is the inactivated X chromosome which appears as a clump of chromatin in somatic cells of females.

❑❑ **What percentage of spontaneous abortions have a demonstrable chromosomal abnormality?**

50%.

❑❑ **What is the phrase used to describe a single nucleotide base substitution?**

Point mutation.

❑❑ **What is the most common chromosomal abnormality?**

Trisomy 21 (Down's syndrome).

❑❑ **What is the most significant risk factor for having a child with trisomy 21?**

Increased maternal age.

**❑❑  Is there a "familial" form of Down's syndrome?**

Yes, or I would not have asked.  This accounts for less than 5% of the cases and is a result of a translocation creating three chromosomes with material from chromosome 21.  In contrast to the more common non-familial form, this has no association with maternal age as a risk factor.

**❑❑  What are some of the clinical findings and appearances in Down's syndrome?**

Severe mental retardation, Brushfield's spots (small white spots on the edge of the iris), broad nasal bridge, epicanthal folds, macroglossia, low set ears, and a single palmar crease (simian crease).

**❑❑  What are some of the cardiac abnormalities associated with Down's syndrome?**

Almost half have congenital heart disease, including endocardial cushion defects, ventricular septal defects, atrial septal defects, valve malformations, and ostium primum.

**❑❑  What are some of the other diseases or conditions that patients with Down's syndrome are at increased risk for developing?**

Acute leukemia (usually lymphoblastic), Alzheimer's disease, and increased rate of infection.

**❑❑  What is the chromosomal abnormality in cri du chat?**

Deletion of the short arm of chromosome 5 (5p-).

**❑❑  What are some of the phenotypic abnormalities in 5p- syndrome?**

Profound mental retardation, microcephaly, hypertelorism from epicanthal folds, low set ears, and a "catlike" cry.

**❑❑  What is the chromosomal abnormality in Edwards' syndrome?**

Trisomy 18.

**❑❑  What are some of the characteristic phenotypic abnormalities in trisomy 18?**

Micrognathia, "rocker bottom" feet, mental retardation, and congenital heart disease.

**❑❑  What is the chromosomal abnormality in Patau's syndrome?**

Trisomy 13.

**❑❑  What are some of the clinical manifestations of Patau's syndrome?**

Cleft lip and palate, microphthalmia, microcephaly, mental retardation, polydactyly, cardiac and renal abnormalities, and "rocker bottom" feet.

**❑❑  Where is the gene located that determines testicular development?**

It is found on the distal short arm of the Y chromosome, thus when a Y chromosome is present that determines a male sex.

**❑❑  What is the name of the gene on the distal short arm of chromosome Y which determines testicular development?**

Sry.

□□ **What is the classic karyotype in Klinefelter's syndrome?**

47, XXY (approximately 80% of cases).

□□ **List some of the clinical manifestations of Klinefelter's syndrome.**

Atrophic testes, tall stature, lack of secondary male characteristics, slightly lower intelligence quotient (IQ), and gynecomastia in a "eunichoid" body habitus.

□□ **What is the most common karyotype seen in Turner's syndrome?**

45X.

□□ **What is the most common cause of primary amenorrhea?**

Turner's syndrome.

□□ **What is the cause of the "webbed neck" seen in Turner's syndrome?**

A cystic hygroma or markedly dilated lymphatics as an infant with persistent neck "webbing" and loose skin on the neck later in life.

□□ **What are the cardiac abnormalities seen in Turner's syndrome?**

Coarctation of the aorta and sometimes aortic stenosis.

□□ **What is the appearance of the ovaries in Turner's syndrome?**

They have "streak ovaries".

□□ **In females with more than one X chromosome, what is the relationship to mental retardation?**

In general terms, the number of extra X chromosomes correlates with the degree of mental retardation. The greater the number of additional X chromosomes, the more severe the retardation.

□□ **What is the second most common cause of mental retardation?**

Fragile X syndrome.

□□ **What does the term true hermaphrodite mean?**

This is the presence of both ovarian and testicular tissue.

□□ **What is a pseudohermaphrodite?**

This is when the phenotypic and gonadal sex differs within the same patient.

□□ **What is testicular feminization?**

This is a cause of male pseudohermaphrodism in which there is complete androgen insensitivity.

□□ **What is the distinctive phenotypic abnormality seen in most males with fragile X syndrome?**

Macro-orchidism.

□□ **What is the chromosomal abnormality in Prader-Willi syndrome?**

del(15)(q11q13).

❏❏  **What is unique about the affected chromosome 15 in patients with Prader-Willi syndrome?**

The deletion affects the paternally derived chromosome 15 only.

❏❏  **What are some of the phenotypic characteristics of Prader-Willi syndrome?**

Mental retardation, short stature, obesity, hypogonadism, and small hands and feet.

❏❏  **What is the syndrome whose affected patients are called "happy puppets"?**

Angelman syndrome.

❏❏  **What chromosome is affected in Angelman syndrome?**

The same region of chromosome 15 as in Prader-Willi; however, the deletion involves the maternally derived chromosome 15.

❏❏  **What are some of the clinical findings in patients with Angelman syndrome?**

Mental retardation, ataxia, seizures, and excessive, inappropriate laughter.

❏❏  **What does variable number of tandem repeats (VNTR) refer to?**

These are short sequences of DNA that are arranged one after another (head to tail) and repeated numerous times.

❏❏  **What does the phrase "reduced penetrance" refer to?**

This is when someone has an abnormal gene but appears phenotypically normal.

❏❏  **What is variable expressivity?**

This is when a person has an abnormal gene and expresses a certain trait; however, the trait is expressed differently among different people carrying the same abnormal gene.

❏❏  **What enzyme deficiency is associated with phenylketonuria?**

Phenylalanine hydroxylase.

❏❏  **What enzyme deficiency is associated with Tay-Sachs disease?**

Hexosaminidase.

❏❏  **What enzyme deficiency is associated with severe combined immunodeficiency?**

Adenosine deaminase.

❏❏  **What red blood cell structural components are absent in hereditary spherocytosis?**

Spectrin (most commonly), ankyrin, or protein 4.1.

❏❏  **How is Marfan syndrome inherited?**

Autosomal dominant in the familial cases.

❏❏  **What is the glycoprotein that is the primary abnormality in Marfan syndrome?**

Fibrillin.

❒❒  **What are some of the clinical manifestations of Marfan syndrome?**

Tall stature, particularly the lower half of the body; bilateral subluxation or dislocation of the lens (ectopia lentis); "cystic medial necrosis" of the ascending aorta; and mitral valve prolapse.

❒❒  **In the many disorders that comprise the Ehlers-Danlos syndrome, what is the general abnormality?**

A defect in collagen synthesis or structure.

❒❒  **What is the status of the skin and joints in patients with Ehlers-Danlos syndrome?**

The skin is hyperextensible and the joints are quite hypermobile.

❒❒  **Which type of Ehlers-Danlos syndrome (EDS) is associated with colonic and large artery rupture?**

EDS type IV.

❒❒  **How are the various EDS inherited?**

They are inherited in autosomal dominant, recessive, and X-linked fashions.

❒❒  **What is the most common autosomal recessive form of EDS?**

Type VI.

❒❒  **What is the enzyme abnormality in type VI EDS?**

Reduced activity of lysyl hydroxylase.

❒❒  **What specific types of collagen are affected in type VI EDS?**

Types I and III.

❒❒  **What type of EDS is associated with retinal detachment and corneal rupture?**

Type VI.

❒❒  **What type of EDS is associated with diaphragmatic hernia?**

Type I.

❒❒  **What is the abnormal form of collagen present in type IV EDS?**

Type III.

❒❒  **How is EDS type IX inherited?**

X-linked recessive.

❒❒  **What would you expect the copper and cerruloplasmin serum levels to be in a patient with EDS type IX?**

Low, although these patients have high levels of intracellular copper.

❒❒  **What is the abnormality found in familial hypercholesterolemia?**

There is a mutation in the gene which encodes for the receptor for low density lipoprotein (LDL), thus the levels of cholesterol increase inducing severe atherosclerosis.

❑❑ **How is hereditary hemorrhagic telangiectasia (Osler-Weber-Rendu syndrome) inherited?**

Autosomal dominant.

❑❑ **What is the enzyme deficiency in galactosemia?**

Galactose-1 phosphate uridyltransferase.

❑❑ **What is the deficient enzyme in Gaucher's syndrome?**

Glucocerebrosidase resulting in accumulation of glucocerebroside.

❑❑ **What is the deficient enzyme in Niemann-Pick syndrome?**

Sphingomyelinase which results in the accumulation of sphingomyelin.

❑❑ **What is the deficient enzyme in Hurler's syndrome?**

Alpha-L iduronidase is deficient thus resulting in accumulation of heparan sulfate and dermatan sulfate.

❑❑ **What is the enzyme deficiency in Von Gierke's disease (type I glycogenosis)?**

Glucose-6-phosphatase resulting in the accumulation of glycogen.

❑❑ **What are the common names of the types II and III glycogenoses?**

Pompe's disease (deficient in a-1,4-glucosidase) and Cori's disease (deficient in amylo-1,6-glucosidase), respectively.

❑❑ **What is McArdle's syndrome?**

This is the deficiency of muscle phosphorylase which is also called type V glycogenosis.

❑❑ **What is the enzyme deficiency in alkaptonuria?**

Homogentisic acid.

❑❑ **How is alkaptonuria inherited?**

Autosomal recessive.

❑❑ **What is the term used to describe the discolored fibrous and soft tissue in alkaptonuria?**

Ochronosis.

❑❑ **What is the most common form of gangliosidoses?**

Tay-Sachs disease.

❑❑ **What is Krabbe disease?**

This is deficiency of galactosylceramidase resulting in accumulation of galactocerebroside.

❑❑ **What is the enzyme deficiency in Fabray disease?**

alpha-galactosidase A.

❏❏ **What is the enzyme deficiency in mucopolysaccharidosis II (Hunter's syndrome)?**

L-iduronosulfate sulfatase.

❏❏ **Which disease classically has a patient with a "cherry-red spot"?**

Tay-Sachs disease.

❏❏ **What is the classic ultrastructural finding in a patient with Niemann-Pick disease?**

"Zebra bodies".

❏❏ **What is the most common variant of Niemann-Pick disease?**

Type A accounts for about three fourths of the cases.

❏❏ **Other than Tay-Sachs disease, what other metabolic disorder is associated with a "cherry-red spot" in the macula in approximately 1/2 of the patients?**

Niemann-Pick disease.

❏❏ **How is Gaucher's disease inherited?**

Autosomal recessive with the mutation located on chromosome 1q21.

❏❏ **What is the most common type of Gaucher's disease?**

Type I, which occurs in adults and accounts for over 90% of the cases. This can be associated with a normal life span and does not involve the nervous system.

❏❏ **What is the characteristic radiologic feature in the distal femur in patients with Gaucher's disease?**

Erlenmeyer-flask deformity.

❏❏ **What is another name for glycogenosis type IV?**

Andersen's disease or brancher deficiency.

❏❏ **In the mucopolysaccharidoses (MPS), what is the general abnormality in each of the types?**

Each has a deficiency of various lysosomal enzymes which, in a normal person, are present and degrade mucopolysaccharides or glycosaminoglycans.

❏❏ **What are the glycosaminoglycans that accumulate in the various MPS?**

Dermatan sulfate, heparan sulfate, keratan sulfate, and chondroitin sulfate.

❏❏ **Each of the MPS are autosomal recessive except for one, which one?**

MPS type II (Hunter's) which is X-linked.

❏❏ **What are some clinical finding in Hurler's syndrome (MPS-I)?**

The initial findings are seen at about 12 months of age and initially include coarse facial features. Later, corneal clouding, gingival hyperplasia, hepatosplenomegaly, mental retardation, CNS involvement, and cor pulmonale develop.

☐☐ **What is the usual cause of death in Hurler's syndrome?**

Death is by age 10 and typically secondary to cardiovascular problems,

☐☐ **What is the usual survival in Hunter's syndrome (MPS-II) and how does it compare to MPS-I (Hurler's)?**

It is milder than Hurler's syndrome (MPS-I) and lacks the corneal clouding seen in the former. Death is typically by age 20, in contrast to MPS-I.

☐☐ **What is another name for MPS-III?**

Sanfilippo's syndrome. Survival is similar to Hunter's syndrome.

☐☐ **What is the major organ system involved in MPS-IV (Morquio syndrome)?**

Keratan sulfate and chondroitin-6-sulfate accumulate in the skeletal system. These patients have a very hypoplastic ondontoid process and suffer atlantoaxial subluxation and die in their 20s with cardiorespiratory difficulties.

☐☐ **What is the most common glycoprotein storage disease?**

alpha-1-antitrypsin (A1A) deficiency.

☐☐ **What is the enzyme which is deficient in Farber's disease?**

Ceramidase which leads to accumulation of ceramide and other gangliosides in skin, lymph nodes, brain, and other organs.

☐☐ **Which type of glycogen storage disease affects the liver and kidney predominantly?**

von Gierke disease (type IA).

☐☐ **Which of the glycogenoses features lysosomal accumulation of glycogen, in contrast to the diffuse cytoplasmic accumulation in the other glycogenoses?**

Type II (Pompe's disease).

☐☐ **What types of glycogenoses primarily affect the muscles?**

Type V (McArdle's disease) and type VII (Tarui disease).

☐☐ **Which glycogenosis features deposition in the liver only?**

Type VI (Hers' disease) which has an excellent prognosis.

☐☐ **In patients with alkaptonuria, what happens to urine if allowed to stand for a period of time?**

The excreted homogentisic acid will oxidize causing the urine to turn black.

☐☐ **When does alkaptonuria become clinically evident?**

Alkaptonuria is typically manifest in the fourth decade of life when the pigment (ochronosis) deposition in the joints and articular cartilage takes its toll. The result is osteoarthritis which can cause a handicap although it is not life-threatening.

❏❏ **What is the enzyme deficiency in metachromatic leukodystrophy?**

Arylsulfatase A (cerebroside sulfatase) resulting in accumulation and deposition of cerebroside sulfatide predominantly in the white matter of the central and peripheral nervous systems.

❏❏ **What is the enzyme deficiency and result of that deficiency in Lesch-Nyhan syndrome?**

The enzyme deficiency is hypoxanthine-guanine-phosphoribosyltransferase (HGPRT) which results in deficient purine metabolism and overproduction of uric acid.

❏❏ **What are some of the clinical features of Lesch-Nyhan syndrome?**

Gout, mental retardation, self mutilation, and spasticity.

❏❏ **What is the inheritance of phenylketonuria?**

Autosomal recessive.

❏❏ **What are some of the clinical findings in phenylketonuria?**

In the untreated patient, mental retardation, seizures, and a "mousy odor" of the urine.

❏❏ **What conversion fails to take place in the absence of phenylalanine hydroxylase in patients with phenylketonuria?**

Phenylalanine cannot be converted to tyrosine in the liver.

❏❏ **What is the effect of the elevated levels of phenylalanine in these patients?**

It causes cerebral demyelination.

❏❏ **What is the treatment for patients with phenylketonuria?**

A phenylalanine free diet.

❏❏ **Of the glycogen storage diseases, which are lethal?**

Types II and IV (Pompe's and Andersen's).

❏❏ **What is the natural course of disease in acute tyrosinemia?**

Liver failure resulting in death within a few months.

❏❏ **How is maple syrup urine disease inherited?**

Autosomal recessive.

❏❏ **What type of amino acid is unable to be adequately metabolized in patients with maple syrup urine disease?**

The branched chain amino acids (leucine, isoleucine, and valine).

❏❏ **What is the abnormality seen in patients with cystinuria?**

They have an inability to transport cystine, ornithine, lysine, and arginine and may develop cystine calculi.

❑❑  **Which inborn error of amino acid metabolism is associated with many of the same clinical features of Marfan syndrome?**

Homocystinuria. Patients are tall, develop ectopia lentis, osteoporosis, and can also be mentally retarded.

❑❑  **What are the major organs involved in tyrosinemia?**

Liver and kidneys.

❑❑  **In patients with deficiency of argininosuccinate synthetase resulting in citrullinemia, what would you expect the levels of ammonia, arginine, and citrulline to be?**

Hyperammonemia, low plasma arginine, and high plasma citrulline.

❑❑  **What are the typical clinical manifestations of Zellweger syndrome?**

They have typical facies, neonatal seizures, ocular abnormalities, and usually die within a few months. The brain shows characteristic neuronal migration involving the cerebral hemispheres, cerebellum, and inferior olivary nucleus. There is also heterotopic cerebral cortex, defects of the corpus collosum, and demyelination. The liver may show micronodular cirrhosis and there are often renal cortical cysts.

HYPEROXALURIA (POLARIZED LIGHT)

❑❑  **What is the natural course of hyperoxaluria type I?**

These patients have a deficiency of alanine glyoxylate aminotransferase which results in oxalate crystal deposition in the kidneys, bones, heart, vessels (as shown above) and subcutis. Death occurs by age 20. Liver transplantation may be of benefit to these patients.

❑❑  **What is the gene that is involved in the development of cystic fibrosis?**

Cystic fibrosis transmembrane regulator gene (CFTR) which is located on chromosome 7.

❑❑  **How is Wilson's disease inherited?**

Autosomal recessive.

❑❑  **What is the substance which is abnormally metabolized in Wilson's disease?**

Copper.

❑❑  **What is another syndrome which results in abnormal copper metabolism?**

Menke's syndrome.

□□  **What is the typical phenotype associated with Menke's syndrome?**

Male infants have brittle hair, puffy cheeks, and typical skeletal changes including metaphyseal widening.

# ENVIRONMENTAL
# AND NUTRITIONAL

☐☐ **What is a laceration?**

This is a jagged tear of the skin, often with tissue bridging underneath, as a result of blunt trauma.

☐☐ **What is an abrasion?**

This is a superficial scrape or tearing away of epithelial cells.

☐☐ **What is a contusion?**

This is a disruption and breakage of small blood vessels in the skin or viscera secondary to blunt force.

☐☐ **What is an incision?**

This is a cut by a sharp object resulting in clean separation of tissues.

☐☐ **What is the term used to describe a contusion on the brain at the point of impact?**

Coup injury. Contrecoup is the contusion on the opposite side of the brain when the brain "recoils" after the initial impact.

☐☐ **At what distance would one expect to find soot present on an entrance wound from a handgun?**

6 to 8 inches.

☐☐ **How far out would a handgun still create stippling of the skin at the entrance wound?**

One and a half to three feet.

☐☐ **In general, what is the shape of an entrance wound compared to an exit wound?**

An entrance wound is round while the exit wound is stellate.

☐☐ **What is the shape of a contact or near contact entrance gunshot wound in an anatomic site where the skin is pulled tight over bone such as the temple?**

That may produce a stellate shaped entrance wound as gas goes between the skin and bone, lifting the skin off and causing a stellate laceration.

☐☐ **What does "manner of death" mean?**

This refers to an explanation of how the cause of death occurred, that is, either naturally (by disease only) or violently.

☐☐ **What is the mechanism of death?**

This is an etiologically nonspecific physiologic and biochemical alteration by which the cause of death results in death.

❑❑  **What is an avulsion?**

This is when tissue is torn away from a site.

❑❑  **What is frost bite?**

This refers to an extensive exposure to very cold temperatures of a body part or parts. The tissue is white from lack of circulation and may become necrotic.

❑❑  **What is hypothermia?**

This is when the core body temperature is markedly lower than normal. This induces vasoconstriction and can certainly result in death.

❑❑  **Which type of gunshot wound, entrance or exit, typically has an abrasion collar?**

Entrance.

❑❑  **What is the classification of burns?**

First degree - results in hyperemia but no permanent damage to the epithelium
Second degree - partial destruction of the epidermis with blistering of the skin
Third degree - full thickness epidermal destruction with damage of the underlying dermis and even dermal appendages resulting in scarring

❑❑  **What bacterial infection classically occurs in severe burn injuries?**

Pseudomonas aeruginosa.

❑❑  **What is the term used to describe an acute gastric ulcer which is sometimes seen in association with severe burn injuries?**

Curling's ulcer.

❑❑  **In large burns, what kind of shock may ensue?**

"Neurogenic" shock may occur almost immediately followed by hypovolemic shock secondary to marked loss of fluids and electrolytes from the burn.

❑❑  **What is the mechanism by which both generalized and even pulmonary edema may develop following a severe burn injury?**

There is marked loss of plasma protein in the pronounced exudative phase following a burn which then causes fluid to escape into the extravascular spaces.

❑❑  **What metabolic abnormality is almost always present in exertional heat stroke?**

Lactic acidosis.

❑❑  **What metabolic abnormality is seen in classic heat stroke, such as that seen in chronically ill, elderly or morbidly obese people?**

Respiratory alkalosis.

❑❑  **Which type of heat stroke is most likely to have rhabdomyolysis?**

Exertional heat stroke has rhabdomyolysis, myoglobinemia, myoglobinuria, and acute tubular necrosis in about 30% of cases.

❑❑ **In the local tissue reaction to abnormally low temperatures, what are two possible ways in which the injuries occur?**

1. Crystallization of intracellular and extracellular water
2. Circulatory changes such as vasoconstriction with subsequent increased permeability and edema

❑❑ **How can electrical injury cause death?**

It may cause cardiac arrhythmias or fatal injury to critical sites such as the respiratory center in the brain stem.

❑❑ **What are "lightning marks"?**

These are linear, branching burn marks on the skin secondary to a high current burn, such as lightning.

❑❑ **Which is more likely to cause fatal injury, alternating current or direct current electrical injury?**

Alternating current can cause severe muscular contractions which then do not allow a person to break the circuit, such as the inability to let go of a wire.

❑❑ **What is the term used to describe the commonly seen benign damage done to the superficial dermis by chronic, excessive exposure to the radiant energy of the sun?**

Solar elastosis.

❑❑ **What types of skin cancer are associated with excessive exposure to the sun?**

Squamous cell carcinoma, basal cell carcinoma, melanoma, and solar or actinic keratosis which is the dysplastic condition associated with an increased incidence of squamous cell carcinoma.

❑❑ **What are two major chemicals used in society which help destroy the ozone layer by providing active free radicals?**

Chlorofluorocarbons (CFC) and nitrogen dioxide ($NO_2$).

❑❑ **Where is radon derived from?**

It is a radioactive gas and a degradation product of uranium which is found in the soil.

❑❑ **How are radon and cigarette smoking related with regard to carcinogenesis?**

They are thought to be synergistic.

❑❑ **What is the number one cause of death related to cigarette smoking?**

Myocardial infarction.

❑❑ **What percentage of cancer deaths are attributed to smoking?**

33%.

❑❑ **What are some of the associations of cigarette smoking and pregnancy?**

Low birth weight, prematurity, spontaneous abortions, still births, and increased infant mortality.

❑❑ **Does smoking cessation reduce smoking-related mortality?**

Yes, however it does not appear to reach normal or baseline levels until at least 20 years without smoking has occurred.

❑❑ **What is the increased risk of lung cancer associated with smoking?**

10-20 times.

❑❑ **What is the classic adverse drug reaction associated with administration of an antimalarial drug (e.g., primaquine) in patients with glucose-6-phosphate dehydrogenase deficiency?**

Hemolytic anemia.

❑❑ **What anesthetic agent is classically associated with potential massive hepatic necrosis and can be fatal?**

Halothane.

❑❑ **What organ is classically severely effected by an overdose of acetaminophen?**

Liver, this is very serious and often fatal.

❑❑ **What is the mechanism of action resulting in hepatic necrosis in acetaminophen overdose?**

The acetaminophen is converted to a metabolite which is toxic to the liver and binds with glutathione. Eventually, the glutathione stores are depleted and the toxic metabolite is free to do damage resulting in massive central lobular necrosis.

❑❑ **What was the ill effect of the use of diethylstilbestrol in pregnant females who had threatened abortions which led to its discontinuance?**

Some of the female children of these patients developed vaginal adenosis and, rarely, clear cell adenocarcinoma of the vagina.

❑❑ **What is the risk of venous thromboses in patients on modern oral contraceptives ("mini pills" with estrogen and progesterone)?**

There does not appear to be any increased risk, certainly those that are less than 30 years old and do not smoke have no risk associated with the oral contraceptive.

❑❑ **What is the association with ovarian cancer and patients on oral contraceptives?**

The oral contraceptives appear to be protective and perhaps actually slightly decrease the risk of ovarian cancer.

❑❑ **What is the association of oral contraceptives and hepatic adenoma?**

There is an increased risk of hepatic adenoma with spontaneous hemorrhage.

❑❑ **What organ is the major target of cyclosporine toxicity?**

Kidney.

❑❑ **Which immunosuppressive agent is associated with potential development of interstitial pneumonitis?**

Azathioprine.

❑❑ **What are two of the major syndromes or abnormalities found in chronic alcoholic patients with thiamine deficiency?**

Wernicke's syndrome, Korsakoff's syndrome, and peripheral neuropathy.

❑❑ **What is the order in which the various parts of the central nervous system are affected in a setting of acute alcoholism?**

Cortex, limbic system, cerebellum, and lastly, the lower brain stem.

❑❑ **What are some of the clinical manifestations of chronic alcoholism?**

Alcoholic hepatitis and eventually cirrhosis, chronic pancreatitis, gastritis, rhabdomyolysis, cardiomyopathy, testicular atrophy, oral and esophageal carcinoma, and fetal alcohol syndrome.

❑❑ **What early, reversible histologic change is seen in the liver within days of consumption of even modest amounts of alcohol?**

Steatosis.

❑❑ **In general, what are the body's reserves of thiamine?**

They are very limited and found predominantly in skeletal muscle with lesser amounts in the heart, liver, kidney, and brain.

❑❑ **What are the three major functions of thiamine pyrophosphate (the phosphorylated form of thiamine) upon absorption?**

1. Oxidative decarboxylation of alpha ketoacids resulting in ATP production
2. Cofactor for transketolase in the pentose phosphate pathway
3. Maintains adequate nerve conduction and neural membranes within the peripheral nerves

❑❑ **What is the major cardiac effect of thiamine deficiency?**

Four chamber dilatation (wet beriberi).

❑❑ **What are the pathologic changes seen in the peripheral nervous system in a patient with thiamine deficiency?**

Myelin degeneration sometimes leading to axonal disruption.

❑❑ **What are the targets of the pathology in thiamine deficiency resulting in Wernicke-Korsakoff syndrome?**

Hemorrhagic necrosis in the mammillary bodies, periventricular regions of the thalamus and hypothalamus, cerebral aqueduct, floor of the fourth ventricle and anterior cerebellum.

❑❑ **What are the components of Wernicke's encephalopathy?**

Ataxia, global confusion, ophthalmoplegia, and nystagmus.

❑❑ **What effect does moderate alcohol consumption have on serum lipids?**

It tends to actually increase the level of high density lipoproteins (HDL).

❑❑ **What types of cancer are associated with arsenic exposure?**

Skin, lung, and liver.

❑❑  **What type of hematopoietic malignancy is associated with occupational exposure to benzine?**

Myelogenous leukemia.

❑❑  **What types of malignancies are associated with occupational exposure to cadmium?**

Prostate and renal carcinoma.

❑❑  **What specific malignancy is associated with the exposure to beta-naphthylamine which is seen in the rubber and dye industries?**

Bladder carcinoma.

❑❑  **What specific type of malignancy is known to occur more frequently in patients exposed to vinyl chloride?**

Angiosarcoma of the liver.

❑❑  **What are some of the malignancies that are associated with an increased exposure to chromium?**

Cancer of the nasal cavity, sinus, lung, and larynx.

❑❑  **What is the active substance in marijuana?**

D-9-tetrahydrocannabinol (THC).

❑❑  **What is the physiologic action of cocaine?**

It is a CNS stimulant which acts by blocking the reuptake of norepinephrine, dopamine, and serotonin.  In addition, it also serves to increase the synthesis of norepinephrine and dopamine and induces vasoconstriction.

❑❑  **What are some of the effects of cocaine on the heart?**

Tachycardia, hypertension, arrhythmias, myocardial infarction even in the absence of coronary atherosclerosis, myocarditis, dilated cardiomyopathy, and ruptured ascending aorta which is likely related to the hypertension induced by cocaine.

❑❑  **What are some of the effects of cocaine on a developing fetus and the pregnancy state in general?**

Increased incidence of abruptio placentae, stillbirth, preterm labor, impaired fetal development, and newborn hyperirritability.

❑❑  **What is the typical route of ingestion of heroin?**

Intravenous.

❑❑  **What are three general responses to heroin overdose?**

1. Marked, life-threatening pulmonary edema
2. Cardiac arrythmias and arrest
3. Marked respiratory depression

❑❑  **In a case of chronic carbon monoxide poisoning, what does one see microscopically in the central nervous system?**

There is diffuse neuronal loss which is most prominent in the basal ganglia, and focal cerebral demyelination.

❑❑ **What is the classic effect of methanol ingestion and poisoning?**

Blindness as a result of cell damage in the retina, optic nerve, and central nervous system.

❑❑ **What are the two main metabolites of methanol?**

Formic acid and formaldehyde.

❑❑ **What is the effect of kerosine on the CNS?**

It is a CNS depressant.

❑❑ **What is the effect of chloroform and carbon tetrachloride on the liver?**

They produce centrilobular steatosis and centrilobular necrosis.

❑❑ **What is the mechanism of action of carbon monoxide poisoning?**

Hemoglobin has 200 times the affinity for CO as it does for oxygen. Thus, oxygen delivery is severely impaired as the hemoglobin molecules hold tightly onto the CO molecules.

❑❑ **What is the characteristic gross appearance of the skin and soft tissue in someone who has died from carbon monoxide poisoning?**

They feature a bright cherry red color.

❑❑ **What is the mechanism of action in cyanide poisoning?**

Cyanide binds to cytochrome oxidase thereby inhibiting cellular respiration.

❑❑ **What is the classic scent associated with an autopsy of a patient that died from cyanide poisoning?**

Bitter almonds.

❑❑ **What is the treatment or antidote for a patient with cyanide poisoning?**

Nitrite which produces methemoglobin which then complexes with and causes dissociation of the enzyme-bound cyanide. Obviously, this must be given almost immediately.

❑❑ **If one suspected chronic arsenic toxicity, where would one look for detectable arsenic?**

Hair, nails, and skin.

❑❑ **What are the clinical signs and symptoms of mercury poisoning?**

Gastrointestinal ulceration, acute tubular necrosis, and cerebral edema in acute poisoning. Chronic gastritis and nephrotic syndrome as well as headache and memory loss are seen in chronic mercury poisoning.

❑❑ **What would you expect to find in a peripheral blood smear in a patient with lead poisoning?**

Basophilic stippling of the red cells with a hypochromic, microcytic anemia.

❑❑ **What is Fanconi's syndrome?**

This is apparent resorption of phosphate, glucose, and amino acids in the proximal renal tubule in lead poisoning.

🔲🔲  **What would you expect to see radiographically in the long bones of a pediatric patient with lead poisoning?**

Increased density of the epiphyses.

🔲🔲  **What is considered a "safe" blood lead level?**

Less than or equal to 10 mcg/dl.

🔲🔲  **What is the effect of lead on iron incorporation into the heme molecule?**

Lead blocks aminolevulinic acid dehydratase (ALA-D) and ferroketolase, thus iron is displaced and formation of zinc protoporphyrin occurs.

🔲🔲  **What would you expect the free erythrocyte protoporphyrin levels to be in a patient with lead poisoning?**

This would be elevated (greater than 50 mcg/dl) as it is a product of zinc protoporphyrin which is formed as lead interferes with iron incorporation.

🔲🔲  **What is the mechanism of action of organophosphates which results in paralysis and cardiac arrhythmias?**

They inhibit acetylcholinesterase.

🔲🔲  **What are the clinical manifestations of human exposure to polychlorinated biphenyls?**

Chloracne, impotence, visual disturbances and possibly infertility.

🔲🔲  **What are the effects of the toxin produced by the mushroom Amanita muscaria?**

It produces parasympathomimetic effects including salivation, diaphoresis, hypotension, bradycardia, and pupil constriction.

🔲🔲  **Which mushroom is more likely to cause death upon ingestion - Amanita muscaria or Amanita phalloides?**

Amanita phalloides is deadly in up to half of the cases while Amanita muscaria is associated with a full recovery.

🔲🔲  **What is the mechanism of action of the Amanita phalloides toxin?**

The toxin, amanitine, inhibits RNA polymerase.  The effects occur in 6 to 24 hours and include gastrointestinal symptoms, central lobular hepatic necrosis, acute tubular necrosis, cardiac symptoms and eventually collapse, convulsions, and coma.

🔲🔲  **What are the two major theories regarding the mechanism of action in radiation injury?**

Direct or target injury and indirect injury.  The direct theory states that the radiation acts directly on its target molecules, like DNA, resulting in damage which, if not repaired may lead to mutations or destruction of the DNA.  The indirect action theory states that the radiant energy causes damage via the formation of free radicals which then cause damage to the various components of the cell.

🔲🔲  **What are the two forms of ionizing radiation?**

Electromagnetic waves (includes x-rays and gamma rays) and particulate radiation (includes alpha and beta particles).

❏❏  **What is the phrase used to describe the period of time between radiation exposure and the appearance of its effects?**

Latency.

❏❏  **What does relative biologic effectiveness refer to?**

This compares different forms of radiation and their ability to effect the same cellular damage.

❏❏  **Which has a higher linear energy transfer value, beta particles or alpha particles?**

Alpha particles.

❏❏  **Which cell types are most sensitive to radiation injury?**

Those which have a high mitotic rate and rapid turnover such as skin, gastrointestinal tract, bone marrow, and the lymphoid system.

❏❏  **With regard to the cell cycle, when is a cell most susceptible to radiation?**

During the G2 phase of the cell cycle, while it is least sensitive in the late S phase.

❏❏  **What is one effect seen in the lungs following radiation injury?**

Pulmonary interstitial fibrosis.

❏❏  **What is the lethal range for total body radiation?**

It begins around 300 rads and is nearly 100% fatal above 500 rads.

❏❏  **What are some examples of highly radiosensitive tumors?**

Seminoma, dysgerminoma and, in general, leukemia/lymphoma.

❏❏  **What are some tumors that are relatively insensitive to radiation therapy?**

Gliomas, melanoma, renal cell carcinoma, osteosarcoma, and most large sarcomas.

❏❏  **What is Reye's syndrome?**

This occurs in children who ingest aspirin during an acute viral illness and is characterized by microvesicular steatosis in the liver and encephalopathy.

❏❏  **What size of particle can pass into and remain in the pulmonary alveoli?**

3 to 5 microns.  Smaller than that will be expired in the air and larger than that will be trapped in larger sized bronchi.

❏❏  **What is Caplan's syndrome?**

These are pulmonary nodules and rheumatoid arthritis which can occur in association with silicosis, coalworkers pneumoconiosis, or progressive massive fibrosis.

❏❏  **Which part of the lung is most commonly effected in both silicosis and coalworkers pneumoconiosis (CWP)?**

Upper lobes.

❑❑  **What is the risk of lung cancer in patients with CWP and progressive massive fibrosis (PMF)?**

There is no increase of lung cancer in either case.

❑❑  **What are the two forms of protein-calorie malnutrition?**

Marasmus (general starvation) and kwashiorkor (protein deficiency).

❑❑  **What is the typical age of a patient with marasmus?**

This typically occurs in children who are less than one year old and are not breastfeeding or supplemented adequately.  In contrast, kwashiorkor occurs in patients older than one, who are not breastfeeding and have a carbohydrate-rich but protein-poor diet.

❑❑  **What are some of the other abnormalities typically seen in kwashiorkor?**

Hepatic steatosis, severe edema, anemia, intestinal malabsorption secondary to small intestinal villus atrophy, and low serum albumin.

❑❑  **What is the clinical manifestation of deficiency of vitamin B2 (riboflavin)?**

Glossitis, dermatitis, corneal vascularization, and cheilosis.

❑❑  **What is cheilosis?**

These are skin fissures found at the corners of the mouth.

❑❑  **What is the clinical term given to deficiency of vitamin B3?**

Pellagra.

❑❑  **What is the clinical term used to describe the deficiency of vitamin C?**

Scurvy.

❑❑  **Of the water soluble vitamins, which is the only one which is stored in any appreciable quantity such that regular intake could be interrupted for a significant period of time without untoward events?**

Vitamin B12 is stored in large quantities in the liver.

❑❑  **What would you expect the bone marrow to look like morphologically in both kwashiorkor and marasmus?**

In either case, it is hypoplastic.

❑❑  **What is the "flag sign" which is sometimes seen in kwashiorkor?**

This is a band of depigmentation found in the hair which signifies a specific period of marked malnutrition.

❑❑  **What are the fat soluble vitamins?**

A, D, E, and K.

❑❑  **Which vitamin is pyridoxine?**

Vitamin B6.

❏❏ **Which vitamin is cobalamin?**

Vitamin B12.

❏❏ **Which vitamin is niacin?**

Vitamin B3.

❏❏ **What are the components of pellagra?**

Dementia, dermatitis of exposed areas, and diarrhea (the "three D's").

❏❏ **Which vitamin deficiency is associated with high output cardiac failure?**

Vitamin B1 (thiamine). This deficiency is termed beriberi or "wet beriberi" in the case of the high output cardiac failure. *dilated cardiomyopathy .*

❏❏ **What is Wernicke's triad?**

Confusion, ataxia, and ophthalmoplegia.

❏❏ **In addition to Wernicke's triad, what other characteristics are typical of Wernicke-Korsakoff syndrome?**

Marked memory loss and confabulation.

❏❏ **In addition to a deficiency of niacin, what other component must be missing in order to develop vitamin B3 deficiency?**

Tryptophan, as niacin can be synthesized from tryptophan.

❏❏ **What are the clinical characteristics of vitamin A deficiency?**

Xerophthalmia, keratomalacia, corneal scarring, and blindness. In addition, patients undergo squamous metaplasia of various sites and have impaired immune response.

❏❏ **What effect does vitamin B6 deficiency have on gamma-aminobutyric acid (GABA)?**

It is decreased as glutamate decarboxylase is dependent on pyridoxine.

❏❏ **Which inborn error of metabolism is associated with an increased need for pyridoxine (vitamin B6)?**

Homocystinuria.

❏❏ **What general type of anemia is associated with deficiency of cobalamin (vitamin B12)?**

Megaloblastic anemia.

❏❏ **What is the term used to describe the malabsorption of vitamin B12 secondary to a lack of gastric intrinsic factor?**

Pernicious anemia.

❏❏ **What parasite can also cause malabsorption of vitamin B12 and megaloblastic anemia?**

The fish tapeworm Diphyllobothrium latum.

❑❑ **Which vitamin deficiency is associated with night blindness?**

Vitamin A.

❑❑ **Describe the formation of the active form of vitamin D from 7-dehydrocholesterol.**

In the skin, 7-dehydrocholesterol is converted to cholecalciferol (vitamin D3) which is then hydroxylated in the liver to 25-hydroxyvitamin D3, followed by a second hydroxylation in the kidney to 1,25-dihydroxyvitamin D3 which is the active form of vitamin D.

❑❑ **What is the name of the disease of the bones that occurs in children and adults in vitamin D deficiency?**

In children it is called rickets and in adults it is called osteomalacia.

❑❑ **In patients with vitamin C deficiency, what is the mechanism of the pathologic effects of impaired wound healing?**

Vitamin C is a cofactor in the synthesis of hydroxyproline and hydroxylysine resulting in abnormal mesenchymal and osteoid matrix.

❑❑ **What are the clinical signs and symptoms of excess vitamin A intake?**

Alopecia, liver damage, and periosteal new bone formation.

❑❑ **What are some of the clinical manifestations seen in vitamin E deficiency?**

Spinocerebellar degeneration, particularly of the posterior columns, skeletomuscular disease, and pigmented retinopathy.

❑❑ **What happens to the clotting parameters in a patient with vitamin K deficiency?**

They are prolonged secondary to the fact that proteins C and S and factors II, VII, IX, and X are all vitamin K dependent.

❑❑ **What are some of the clinical findings in a child with scurvy?**

Subperiosteal hematomas; hemarthroses; retrobulbar, subarachnoid and intracerebral hemorrhages; abnormal bony matrix deposition; impaired wound healing, and a rash.

❑❑ **What are some of the medical problems associated with obesity?**

Insulin resistant diabetes mellitus, hypertension, hyperlipidemia, heart disease, coronary artery disease, respiratory problems, apnea, osteoarthritis, and risk of cerebrovascular accidents among other things.

# TRANSFUSION MEDICINE

❑❑  **What are the two basic categories of platelet products?**

Single donor platelets (apheresis) and random donor platelets.

❑❑  **What is the main advantage of single donor platelets over pooled platelets?**

Single donor platelets limit the antigen exposure faced in a pooled, random donor platelet product.  Thus, the patient may be less likely to become refractory.

❑❑  **One of the main reasons for use of fresh frozen plasma (FFP) is its content of the labile coagulation factors.  What are the labile coagulation factors?**

Factors V and VIII.

❑❑  **What are some of the coagulation factors present in cryoprecipitate?**

Factor VIII, von Willebrand factor (vWF), fibrinogen, factor XIII, and fibronectin activity.

❑❑  **If a person has type A blood, what antibody would you expect to find?**

Anti-B.

❑❑  **What antibody would you expect to find in type O blood?**

Anti-A and Anti-B antibodies.

❑❑  **What is the so-called "universal donor" blood type?**

Type O, because the typical antibodies of the ABO system (anti-A, anti-B, and anti-A,B) will not react with type O blood cells.

❑❑  **What is the so-called "universal red cell recipient"?**

Patients with type AB blood as they will not have serum antibodies to type A or type B red cells.

❑❑  **What is the most common blood type amongst African-Americans?**

Type O.

❑❑  **What is the most common blood type among Caucasians?**

Type O.

❑❑  **Which is more common, type A or type B blood?**

Type A is much more common in whites (40% vs. 11% for type B) and  Native Americans and slightly more common in African-Americans and Asians.

❑❑  **Amongst Caucasians, African-Americans, Native-Americans and Asians, which group has the highest percentage of type O blood?**

Native Americans have a 79% frequency of O blood type.

❏❏ **What is the precursor substance which is found on red cells upon which other antigens (A, B, or both) are added to complete the ABO blood group system?**

The H system.

❏❏ **What does a patient with type O blood have on his/her red cell surface?**

They have the H substance without the addition of either A or B antigens.

❏❏ **What is a Bombay type?**

This is a person who does not have the H gene and therefore produces no H substance, thus differing from type O blood in that regard.

❏❏ **What are the names of the two theories proposed to explain the Rh system?**

Fisher-Race and Wiener theories.

❏❏ **What is the antigen which confers Rh positivity?**

D antigen. In the absence of D antigen, the patient is termed Rh negative.

❏❏ **What is the most common cause of hemolytic disease of the newborn?**

Anti-D derived from the mother (who would obviously be Rh negative).

❏❏ **What blood group would you expect a South American Indian to have?**

Type O, essentially 100% of the time.

❏❏ **What is the predominant type of immunoglobulin molecule produced in patients with type O blood against the A and B blood groups?**

IgG, in contrast to patients with type A or B blood whose antibodies to the opposite blood group are typically IgM.

❏❏ **What type of immunoglobulin molecule comprises the so-called "cold acting" antibodies?**

IgM.

❏❏ **What type of immunoglobulin molecule comprises the so-called "warm acting" antibodies?**

IgG.

❏❏ **What is "forward typing"?**

This is the test used to determine ABO blood group type by adding known anti-A and anti-B reagents to the patient's red cells to determine the antigen present on the patient's red cells.

❏❏ **What is meant by the term "reverse typing"?**

The patient's serum is evaluated against known A and B reagent red cells to determine which antibodies are circulating in the patient's serum.

❏❏ **What is meant by an order for a "type and cross"?**

This refers to determining the ABO and Rh type of the patient's blood and then confirming its compatibility with the proposed recipient by mixing the recipient's serum with the donor's red blood cells and evaluating for agglutination.

❑❑ **What is meant by the order "type and screen"?**

Prior to surgery, a patient who may potentially receive a transfusion has his ABO and Rh type determined and an irregular antibody screen performed. However, cross match (compatibility of donor RBCs with recipient serum as above) is not performed until that time at which it is determined that a transfusion may take place.

❑❑ **What is the common name for the antiglobulin test?**

Coombs' test.

❑❑ **What are two forms of the antiglobulin or Coombs' test?**

Direct and indirect.

❑❑ **What is the utility of the direct antiglobulin test (DAT)?**

This is used to demonstrate in-vivo antibodies or complement on red blood cells.

❑❑ **What is the utility of the indirect antiglobulin test (IAT)?**

This demonstrates in-vitro reactions between red blood cells and coating antibodies.

❑❑ **What are some instances where the DAT is useful?**

It is used in many cases including evaluation of hemolytic disease of a newborn, alloimmune reactions to recently transfused RBCs, autoimmune hemolytic anemia, and drug-induced hemolysis. It is a necessary step in evaluation of transfusion reactions.

❑❑ **What are some instances in which the IAT is useful?**

The IAT is used in both identifying and detecting antibodies, blood grouping and compatibility testing.

❑❑ **How are irregular antibodies detected in a patient?**

The patient's serum is reacted with multiple panels of antigenically known RBCs. Each reaction is then evaluated for agglutination to determine if the patient's serum contains the antibody to that particular antigen.

❑❑ **What drug can classically give you a positive DAT?**

Penicillin and penicillin derivatives.

❑❑ **What is massive blood transfusion?**

This is infusion of blood products equaling the patient's blood volume within a 24 hour period.

❑❑ **What are the two main antigens found in the Kell system?**

K (Kell) and k (Cellano).

❑❑ **What are the two antigens of the Kidd system?**

Jka and Jkb.

❏❏  **What are the main antigens of the Duffy system?**

Duffy a (Fya) and Duffy b (Fyb).

❏❏  **Which blood group antigens are not truly part of the red blood cell membrane, rather are adsorbed onto the surface of RBCs from plasma?**

The Lewis antigens (Lewis a and Lewis b).

❏❏  **What type of immunoglobulin are the antibodies against the Lewis system?**

IgM, thus they are "cold reacting".

❏❏  **Which is most likely to cause death during a transfusion reaction, Kell or Lewis antibodies?**

Kell - "Kell kills, Lewis lives".

❏❏  **In the Lutheran antigen system, what happens if the cells are treated with trypsin?**

Trypsin destroys the antigens, as do several other agents such as chymotrypsin, pronase, AET, and DTT.

❏❏  **What is the acronym used to list several common cold reacting antibodies?**

"LIMPS" Lewis, I, MNS system, and P.

❏❏  **What infectious state can raise an adult's anti-I titer?**

Infection with mycoplasma organisms.

❏❏  **What particular infectious disease can cause development of cold agglutinins with anti-i specificity in adults?**

Infectious mononucleosis.

❏❏  **What are some of the infectious diseases or agents which are tested for routinely in collection of blood products?**

Syphilis, hepatitis B surface antigen, HTLV-1 antibody, HIV (including p24 antigen), hepatitis B core antibody, and hepatitis C antibody.

❏❏  **What are some of the acute complications of blood transfusion?**

Acute hemolysis, febrile nonhemolytic transfusion reaction, transfusion-related acute lung injury, allergic reaction, anaphylaxis, volume overload, nonimmune hemolysis, air embolism, massive transfusion-related complications, and sepsis.

❏❏  **What is the most common acute transfusion reaction?**

Febrile nonhemolytic and allergic reactions are the most common, each occurring at a rate of 1 per 200 transfusions.

❏❏  **How common is an acute hemolytic transfusion reaction?**

It varies from 1 in 6,000 to 25,000 transfusion reactions.

❏❏  **What is the first step in the evaluation of any transfusion reaction?**

Checking for clerical error by confirming the appropriate patient received the appropriate unit.

❏❏ **What are some of the questions which are posed to potential blood donors which may result in automatic deferral of use of the donor's blood?**

History of drug abuse, malaria, high risk sexual behavior, history of hepatitis, and a history of having received human pituitary growth hormone among other things.

❏❏ **What is the most common cause of a hemolytic transfusion reaction?**

Clerical error.

❏❏ **What are the symptoms seen in a hemolytic transfusion reaction?**

Fever, nausea, vomiting, chest pain, dyspnea and, ominously, hypotension.

❏❏ **What is the first step that one should take when a transfusion reaction is suspected?**

Stop the transfusion.

❏❏ **Beyond checking for a clerical error, what are some of the laboratory tests that should be performed in evaluation of a febrile transfusion reaction?**

Visual check for hemolysis in a pre and post transfusion specimen, a direct antiglobulin test (Coombs' test), urine for free hemoglobin and, depending on the results of the above tests, further evaluation may or may not occur.

❏❏ **What is the cause of a delayed transfusion reaction?**

A previously undetected irregular antibody.

❏❏ **When does a delayed transfusion reaction occur?**

Days following a transfusion.

❏❏ **What is the most common cause of hemolytic disease of the newborn (HDN)?**

Rh incompatibility (anti-D).

❏❏ **In HDN due to anti-D, what is the Rh status of the mother and the fetus?**

The mother is Rh-negative and the fetus is Rh-positive.

❏❏ **How common is HDN due to ABO incompatibility?**

It is uncommon and less severe than HDN secondary to Rh discrepancy.

❏❏ **In HDN secondary to ABO incompatibility, what is the blood type of the mother and fetus?**

The mother is type O, thus having anti-A and anti-B, and the fetus is either type A or B.

❏❏ **What is the significance of fetal-maternal hemorrhage (FMH)?**

This is when fetal RBCs make their way to the maternal circulation. If a mother is Rh-negative and the fetus is Rh-positive, the mother will develop anti-D antibodies. In a subsequent pregnancy, these may cross the placental membrane and cause hemolysis in utero.

❏❏ **How significant is the hemolysis that can occur due to Rh incompatibility in a mother who has been previously sensitized?**

It can range from fetal death, to hydrops fetalis, to ongoing hemolysis.

❑❑  **In ongoing hemolysis, what happens to the increased bilirubin?**

The infant can develop kernicterus by depositing unconjugated bilirubin in the basal ganglia because unconjugated bilirubin can cross the blood brain barrier.

❑❑  **If one wanted to determine how much fetal-maternal hemorrhage had occurred, what laboratory tests could be ordered?**

The rosette test, enzyme-linked antiglobulin test (ELAT), or the Kleihauer-Betke test.

❑❑  **What is the method of prevention of Rh hemolytic disease in a Rh-negative mother?**

Injection of Rh immune globulin at approximately 28 weeks gestation and following delivery of a Rh-positive infant during the immediate postpartum.

❑❑  **What is the major anticoagulant used in storage of red cells and what is its effect on calcium?**

Citrate and it chelates calcium.

❑❑  **What happens to the level of 2,3-DPG in the red blood cells when stored?**

It decreases.

❑❑  **What happens to the level of ATP in stored red blood cells?**

It decreases.

❑❑  **What happens to pH and plasma potassium in stored RBCs?**

pH is decreased and potassium is increased.

❑❑  **In a patient who has had repeated nonfebrile transfusion reactions, what would you recommend for the administration of the next blood product?**

Leukocyte depletion via a filter.

❑❑  **What is the deferral period for someone who wishes to donate blood and has just received the Rh immune globulin?**

Six weeks.

❑❑  **What are the minimum requirements regarding basic physical condition and vital signs that one must have prior to being allowed to donate blood?**

110 lbs, temperature < 99.6 degrees Fahrenheit (37.5 Celsius), pulse 50-100 beats per minute, blood pressure 180/100 mm Hg or less, hemoglobin > 12.5 g/dL.

❑❑  **How is cryoprecipitate derived?**

This is the cold-insoluble portion of plasma that remains after thawing fresh frozen plasma at temperatures of 1 to 6 degrees Celsius. It contains about half of the factor VIII, up to 40% of the fibrinogen, and some factor XIII which is present in the fresh plasma.

❑❑  **How is fresh frozen plasma collected and stored?**

FFP must be collected from the red cells and placed at -18 degrees Celsius within eight hours of collection of the original product. It must be stored at least -18 degrees Celsius and ideally -30 degrees Celsius. It can be stored for 12 months at these temperatures.

◻◻ **How are platelets stored?**

They are stored at 20-24 degrees Celsius with constant, gentle agitation for up to five days.

◻◻ **What is the primary use of irradiation of blood products?**

To prevent graft versus host disease.

◻◻ **How are FFP and cryoprecipitate thawed for use?**

Each must be thawed between 30 and 37 degrees Celsius. In each case, the sooner the product is used the better with regard to viability of the labile coagulation factors. FFP must be stored at 1 to 6 degrees Celsius and used within 24 hours of thawing. Cryoprecipitate must be transfused within six hours if its primary use is as replacement of factor VIII.

◻◻ **What percentage of the population secretes the ABO antigens in saliva and plasma?**

80%. The Se gene is dominant.

◻◻ **When it is determined that a patient is refractory to platelet concentrates, what type of platelets should be given?**

HLA-matched.

◻◻ **Does the amount of H antigen on the red cells of patients with the various blood types differ?**

Yes, or I would not have asked. O has the most H antigen, then A2 > B > A1 > A1B.

◻◻ **What is the difference between the red blood cells in patients with type A1 blood versus the variants of A including type A2, A3, and so forth?**

Antigen density. A1 cells may have close to 1,000,000 A antigen sites per red cell compared to 250,000 sites for A2 cells.

◻◻ **In a patient who has repeated allergic reactions, what might you try in order to prevent future reactions?**

Providing washed red blood cells and washed or plasma-reduced platelets if needed.

◻◻ **With regard to the H gene and the secretor gene, what is the genotype of a patient with the Bombay phenotype?**

hh sese.

◻◻ **What is the basic mechanism of action of the Kleihauer-Betke test?**

It looks for fetal hemoglobin by performing an elution of adult-type hemoglobin with an acid buffer, which then leaves the acid-resistant fetal hemoglobin intact.

◻◻ **How much Rh immune globulin should be given to a patient with suspected fetal-maternal hemorrhage?**

One ampule of Rh Ig (300 mcg) will compensate for 15 ml of fetal RBCs or 30 ml of whole blood. Thus, based on the presumed fetal-maternal hemorrhage volume, one can determine how many ampules to give.

❑❑   **What is the phenomenon of dosage with regard to antibody-antigen reactivity in transfusion medicine?**

This refers to the presence of stronger agglutination in a patient's serum reacting with homozygote RBCs compared to heterozygote RBCs for a particular antigen.

❑❑   **Which RBC antigen system is associated with susceptibility or lack of susceptibility to malaria?**

The Duffy system.  A patient with Fy (a-b-) is resistant to infection with Plasmodium vivax.  This phenotype is quite rare in the Caucasian population in the United States; however, it is the most common phenotype in African-Americans in the United States.  It is thought that the Duffy A and B antigens are located at the site of entry of the Plasmodium organism into the RBC.  Thus, it is protective to Africans living in endemic malarial regions in Africa to lack the Duffy antigens.

# BACTERIAL AND VIRAL DISEASE

□□ **What is the term used to describe reproduction in bacteria?**

Binary fission.

□□ **Do bacteria contain DNA or RNA?**

Both.

□□ **How do the cell walls of gram-positive bacteria differ from gram-negative bacteria?**

Gram-positive bacteria have a thick cell wall with abundant peptidoglycans and teichoic acids. In contrast, the gram-negative cell wall is thinner with much less peptidoglycans and no teichoic acids. The gram-negative cell wall does have a thick outer membrane which is composed of lipoprotein and lipopolysaccharide attached to the peptidoglycans.

□□ **What is the term used to describe bacteria that grow preferentially in an environment containing increased carbon dioxide?**

Microaerophilic.

□□ **What are the phases of growth in bacteria?**

Lag phase, logarithmic phase, stationary phase, and death phase.

□□ **What is the bacterial cell component that is found on gram-negative bacteria, is composed of protein, and plays a role in bacterial adherence?**

Pilus.

□□ **What does the term transformation refer to with regard to the transfer of genetic information in bacteria?**

This involves the uptake of free DNA by cells and is seen in both gam-positive and gram-negative organisms.

□□ **With regard to transfer of genetic information among bacteria, what does transduction refer to?**

This is the transfer of DNA present in the form of bacteriophages which, of course, are viruses that infect bacteria.

□□ **What does the term conjugation refer to?**

This is the transfer of genetic material between bacteria by sexual mating with the use of sex pili and a conjugative plasmid.

□□ **What are the two forms of toxins and how are they different?**

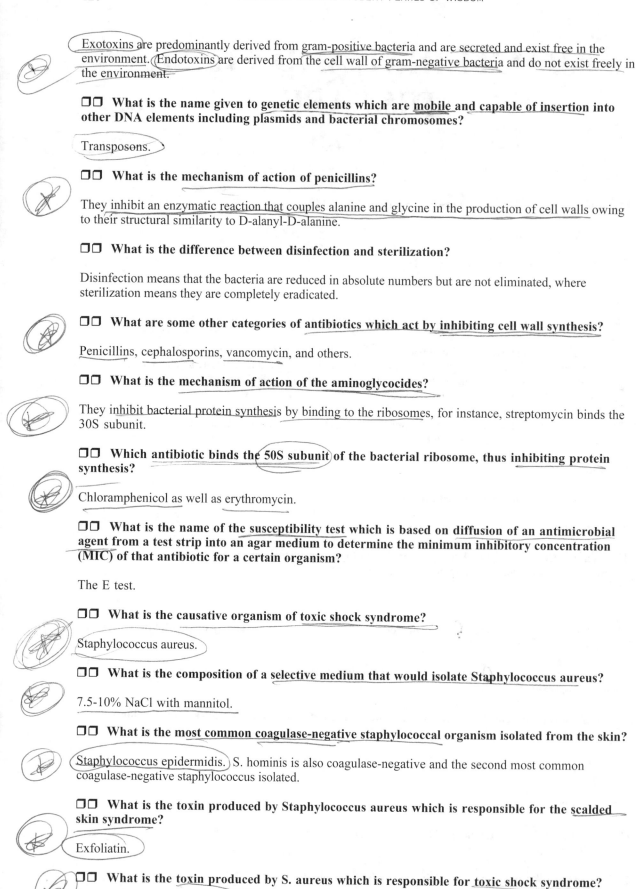

Exotoxins are predominantly derived from gram-positive bacteria and are secreted and exist free in the environment. Endotoxins are derived from the cell wall of gram-negative bacteria and do not exist freely in the environment.

☐☐  **What is the name given to genetic elements which are mobile and capable of insertion into other DNA elements including plasmids and bacterial chromosomes?**

Transposons.

☐☐  **What is the mechanism of action of penicillins?**

They inhibit an enzymatic reaction that couples alanine and glycine in the production of cell walls owing to their structural similarity to D-alanyl-D-alanine.

☐☐  **What is the difference between disinfection and sterilization?**

Disinfection means that the bacteria are reduced in absolute numbers but are not eliminated, where sterilization means they are completely eradicated.

☐☐  **What are some other categories of antibiotics which act by inhibiting cell wall synthesis?**

Penicillins, cephalosporins, vancomycin, and others.

☐☐  **What is the mechanism of action of the aminoglycocides?**

They inhibit bacterial protein synthesis by binding to the ribosomes, for instance, streptomycin binds the 30S subunit.

☐☐  **Which antibiotic binds the 50S subunit of the bacterial ribosome, thus inhibiting protein synthesis?**

Chloramphenicol as well as erythromycin.

☐☐  **What is the name of the susceptibility test which is based on diffusion of an antimicrobial agent from a test strip into an agar medium to determine the minimum inhibitory concentration (MIC) of that antibiotic for a certain organism?**

The E test.

☐☐  **What is the causative organism of toxic shock syndrome?**

Staphylococcus aureus.

☐☐  **What is the composition of a selective medium that would isolate Staphylococcus aureus?**

7.5-10% NaCl with mannitol.

☐☐  **What is the most common coagulase-negative staphylococcal organism isolated from the skin?**

Staphylococcus epidermidis. S. hominis is also coagulase-negative and the second most common coagulase-negative staphylococcus isolated.

☐☐  **What is the toxin produced by Staphylococcus aureus which is responsible for the scalded skin syndrome?**

Exfoliatin.

☐☐  **What is the toxin produced by S. aureus which is responsible for toxic shock syndrome?**

Toxic shock syndrome toxin (TSST-1).

❑❑ **What staphylococcal organism is an important cause of urinary tract infections in young, sexually active women?**

S. saprophyticus.

❑❑ **What substance is produced by S. aureus which makes it resistant to penicillin?**

Beta-lactamase.

❑❑ **What are the various types of hemolysis?**

Beta hemolysis - total red cell hemolysis.   Alpha hemolysis - partial red cell hemolysis causing "greening" of the agar.   Gamma hemolysis - lack of hemolysis.

❑❑ **In general, what is the typical catalase reaction of the most important streptococcal organisms?**

They are generally catalase negative.

❑❑ **What are the three schemes by which streptococci are classified?**

1. Based on their hemolysis pattern
2. The Lancefield classification which is based on the cell wall carbohydrate present
3. Based on physiologic action

❑❑ **What are some of the specific streptococcal organisms that are included in the viridans group?**

S. mitis, mutans, salivarius, and morbillorum.

❑❑ **Which Lancefield group with which type of hemolysis do the Streptococci which cause the majority of disease belong to?**

Lancefield group A and beta hemolysis, respectively.

❑❑ **Of the streptococcal organisms, which is bile-soluble and susceptible to optochin?**

Pneumococcus.

❑❑ **Enterococci and group D streptococci share several common test results, what are they?**

They both hydrolyze esculin in the presence of bile, grow in 6.5% NaCl, and exhibit hydrolysis of PYR.

❑❑ **Which Lancefield does a streptococcal organism belong to that exhibits PYR hydrolysis and susceptibility to bacitracin?**

Group A.

❑❑ **What  species is an alpha hemolytic streptococcal colony which is susceptible to optochin (P disk)?**

Streptococcus pneumoniae.

❑❑ **What filamentous organism is stained by the Fite or Putt modification of the acid-fast stain?**

Nocardia.

❑❑  Which streptococcal Lancefield group is the most common cause of the skin infection erysipelas?

Group A.

❑❑  Which genus is a facultatively anaerobic, non-sporeforming, gram-positive bacillus or coccobacillus that is susceptible to beta-lactam?

Corynebacterium.

❑❑  Which corynebacterium is known to produce a gray pseudomembrane at its initial site of infection on the tonsils and oropharynx?

C. diphtheriae.

❑❑  What is the preferred medium used to isolate C. diphtheriae?

Cystine-tellurite blood agar.

❑❑  What specific patient group is at risk for infection with C. jeikeium?

Patients with prosthetic devices.

❑❑  Which bacterium is an intracellular parasite, facultatively anaerobic, catalase and Voges-Proskauer positive, gram-positive, non-sporeforming, non-acid-fast that has a pleomorphic morphology and produces beta hemolysis?

Listeria monocytogenes.  Remember, this organism has a characteristic "tumbling motility" which is seen at room temperature and is lost as the temperature is elevated.

❑❑  Which organism is a catalase-negative, non-sporeforming, nonmotile, facultatively anaerobic, gram-positive bacillus, produces hydrogen sulfide (H2S) on triple sugar iron agar, and typically produces a local skin infection?

Erysipelothrix rhusiopathiae.

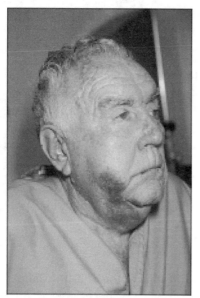

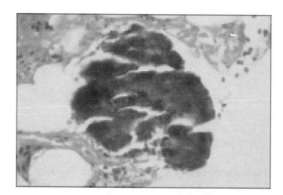

PATIENT WITH "LUMPY JAW"

❐❐ **Which genus is responsible for the infection shown above, sometimes referred to as "lumpy jaw"?**

Actinomyces.

❐❐ **Which organism is facultatively anaerobic, shows gram-variability, is coccobacillary, and is a common cause of nonspecific vaginitis?**

Gardnerella vaginalis.

❐❐ **What is the typical incubation period for symptomatology from "food poisoning" which is caused by Clostridium perfringens?**

7-15 hours producing severe diarrhea and abdominal pain. Nausea and vomiting are not typical and the symptoms typically end within 24 hours.

❐❐ **What is characteristic of the hemolysis pattern seen in cultures of C. perfringens?**

Double zone hemolysis on sheep blood agar.

❐❐ **What is the classic organism that causes pseduomembranous colitis?**

Clostridium difficile.

❐❐ **Which genus is characterized by a bacillary shape, spore formation, gram-positivity, catalase positivity, and varying from either strictly aerobic to facultatively anaerobic?**

The genus Bacillus.

❐❐ **Which member of the Bacillus genus is responsible for some cases of food poisoning?**

B. cereus.

❐❐ **What is the treatment for infection by B. anthracis (anthrax)?**

Penicillin.

❐❐ **Which organism is the classic cause of "gas gangrene"?**

Clostridium perfringens.

❐❐ **What is the name of the toxin produced by C. tetani which, among other things, results in trismus or "lock jaw"?**

A neurotoxin called tetanospasmin.

❐❐ **Which species of Nocardia is responsible for over 90% of Nocardial infection in humans?**

N. asteroides.

❐❐ **What is the antibiotic of choice for treatment of Nocardia infection?**

Sulfonamides.

❐❐ **Which organism is gram-negative, usually motile, has a flagellar antigen (H) and a capsular (Vi) antigen which serves a protective function, is associated with diarrhea and produces H2S?**

Salmonellae.

❏❏  **Where in the body is Salmonella frequently harbored in an asymptomatic chronic carrier?**

Gallbladder.

❏❏  **What is the illness caused by S. typhi, S. paratyphi A and, infrequently, other Salmonella species which include vague symptoms such as fever, myalgia, early constipation and subsequent diarrhea?**

Typhoid fever, treated by chloramphenicol.

❏❏  **In non-typhoid fever cases of general dehydration and diarrhea caused by Salmonella, what is the antibiotic of choice?**

None, treatment is supportive.

❏❏  **Compare the motility and H2S production of Shigella and Salmonella.**

Shigella is nonmotile and does not produce H2S, while Salmonella is motile and typically produces H2S.

❏❏  **Which species of Shigella causes the majority of disease in the United States?**

S. sonnei.

❏❏  **Describe the pathogenesis of Shigella infection.**

It is spread via the fecal-oral route.  The organism invades the colonic mucosa extending into the lamina propria.  It produces a lipopolysaccharide and a heat-labile Shigatoxin.

❏❏  **Which organism produces a toxin which is similar to the Shigatoxin?**

E. coli O157:H7 produces a similar toxin and is the most common association with hemolytic uremic syndrome although Shigella has an association as well.

❏❏  **What is the causative agent of rhinoscleroma?**

Klebsiella rhinoscleromatis.

❏❏  **What is the pathogenesis of cholera caused by vibrio?**

It stimulates the adenyl cyclase system of small intestinal mucosal cells with subsequent production of cyclic AMP resulting in dehydration via marked fluid loss.

❏❏  **Given that patients who are status post splenectomy are at an increased risk for infection by encapsulated organisms, what are some common organisms which may be a problem in splenectomy patients?**

Streptococcus pneumoniae, Klebsiella, and Haemophilus are three of the most common organisms.

❏❏  **What are some of the differences between the O and H antigens of the Salmonella species?**

The O antigens are somatic antigens, heat stable and typically elicit an IgM antibody response.  The H antigen is the flagellar antigen, it is not heat stable and elicits predominantly an IgG antibody response.

❏❏  **What is the typical culture medium growth pattern of organisms in the genus Proteus?**

They have marked motility and thus "swarm" on the growth medium.

❏❏  **What enzyme is produced by the members of Proteus?**

Urease.

❐❐ **What are some of the growth and physical characteristics of Pseudomonas?**

Gram-negative rods, motile (polar flagella), aerobic, catalase and oxidase positive.

❐❐ **Which organism can be diagnosed given the following characteristics: a grape-like odor, gram-negative rods, oxidase positive, growth at 42 degrees Celsius, alkaline slant/neutral butt reaction in triple sugar iron agar (TSIA) and the presence of one flagellum?**

Pseudomonas aeruginosa.

❐❐ **What is the characteristic gram staining pattern of Yersinia pestis?**

It is gram-negative with a bipolar-staining coccobacillary form.

❐❐ **How does one become infected with Yersinia pestis?**

Fleas, particularly Xenopsylla cheopis, transmit the bacterium and regurgitate it into the bloodstream of the host rodent. It can also infest humans should the rodent die.

❐❐ **What organism can cause a nonspecific enteritis, particularly limited to the terminal ileum, a regional mesenteric lymphadenitis and is sometimes misdiagnosed as an acute appendicitis?**

Yersinia enterocolitica or Y. pseudotuberculosis.

❐❐ **Which organism is associated with gastritis and development of gastric lymphoma of the mucosa-associated lymphoid tissue (MALT)?**

Helicobacter pylori.

❐❐ **Which gram-negative coccobacillary organism preferentially infects sheep, goats, and swine with subsequent infection of humans resulting in a characteristic diurnal fever?**

Brucella.

❐❐ **What is the drug of choice for treatment of Brucella?**

Tetracycline.

❐❐ **What are the two factors that help determine the species of Haemophilus that one is dealing with?**

The X factor (hemin or other porphyrins) and the V factor (NAD).

❐❐ **Of the major Haemophilus organisms, which two do not have a requirement for the V factor?**

H. ducreyi and H. aphrophilus.

❐❐ **What are the causative agents of a chancre, chancroid, lymphogranuloma venerum, and granuloma inguinale?**

Chancre - Treponema pallidum causing syphilis.
Chancroid - Haemophilus ducreyi
Lymphogranuloma venerum - Chlamydia trachomatis
Granuloma inguinale - Calymmatobacterium granulomatis

❑❑ **Name the organisms that are typically associated with being fastidious or difficult to culture.**

HACEK
    Haemophilus aphrophilus
    Haemophilus (formerly Actinobacillus) actinomycetemcomitans
    Cardiobacterium hominis
    Eikenella corrodens
    Kingella kingae

❑❑ **What is the causative organism of pertussis?**

Bordetella pertussis.

❑❑ **What antisera can cross react with B. pertussis in laboratory identification studies?**

Legionella.

❑❑ **What is unique about the rash seen in secondary syphilis?**

It is a macular rash which occurs all over the body including the palms and soles.

❑❑ **How frequently does primary syphilis (chancre) proceed to a secondary stage of syphilis?**

Only about 25% of the time.

❑❑ **What is the name of the granulomatous lesion seen in tertiary syphilis?**

Gumma. These are filled with organisms.

❑❑ **What is the vector of Lyme disease?**

The Ixodes tick transmits the causative agent which is Borrelia burgdorferi.

❑❑ **What is the causative agent of relapsing fever?**

Borrelia recurrentis which spreads via ticks and lice and is treated by tetracycline.

❑❑ **What disease is caused by infection with Leptospira interrogans?**

Leptospirosis which is characterized by fever and aseptic meningitis. Weil's disease is less common and is characterized by jaundice in addition to hepatorenal failure.

❑❑ **What is the term used to describe the characteristic pupillary findings in a patient with tertiary syphilis?**

Argyll-Robertson pupil.

❑❑ **When suspected, what method can one use to quickly and accurately identify Legionella pneumophila from culture?**

Direct fluorescent antigen.

❑❑ **What disease is classically transmitted via rabbits, although other rodents and insect bites can also be transmittors?**

Tularemia caused by Francisella tularensis.

❑❑ **What is the causative agent of cat-scratch disease?**

Bartonella henselae, which is a gram-negative rod and, of course, classically transmitted via a cat scratch.

❏❏ **In addition to being fastidious or difficult to grow, what do the organisms designated by the mnemonic HACEK have in common?**

They are all gram negative bacilli and can cause bacterial endocarditis.

❏❏ **Which anaerobic gram-negative bacterium shows a coccobacillary morphology and grows well in the presence of bile?**

Bacteroides fragilis.

❏❏ **Which of the main fastidious organisms sometimes produces a pit in the agar upon which it is grown?**

Eikenella.

❏❏ **What is the preferred medium for culture of Neisseria?**

They grow well in enriched chocolate agar and require extra $CO_2$.

❏❏ **What is the syndrome which comprises sepsis with bilateral hemorrhagic necrosis of the adrenal cortices?**

Waterhouse-Friderichsen syndrome. Classically, this is a result of Neisseria meningitidis; however, pneumococcal sepsis and infection with Haemophilus influenza have also been described as causative agents.

❏❏ **What is the anatomic site of the carrier state of Neisseria meningitidis?**

The nasopharynx.

❏❏ **What is the gram staining characteristic of N. gonorrheae?**

Gram-negative diplococcus.

❏❏ **What is the causative agent of Rocky Mountain Spotted Fever?**

Rickettsia rickettsii.

❏❏ **What is the infectious form of chlamydial disease which elicits its own phagocytosis, thereby allowing its further development?**

The elementary body. Once present within a cell, they transform into reticulate bodies, divide via binary fission, and transform once again into elementary bodies where they are again infectious and subsequently released for phagocytosis by other cells.

❏❏ **What is the causative agent of atypical pneumonia?**

Mycoplasma pneumoniae.

❏❏ **What is the treatment of choice for atypical pneumonia?**

Erythromycin or tetracycline.

❏❏ **What is the treatment of choice for infection with Legionella pneumophila (Legionnaire's disease)?**

Erythromycin.

❏❏  **Which of the chlamydial infections is spread via birds and results in a pneumonia?**

Psittacosis which is caused by C. psittaci.

❏❏  **Which mycobacterial organism is a photochromagen and characterized by a positive nitrate test?**

M. kansasii.

❏❏  **Which scotochromagen produces cervical lymphadenopathy in children?**

M. scrofulaceum.

❏❏  **Which proteus organism produces ornithine decarboxylase?**

P. morganii.

❏❏  **What is a Gohn lesion and a Gohn complex?**

A Gohn lesion is a primary focus of pulmonary infection by M. tuberculosis which occurs typically in the lower upper lobes or upper lower lobes of the lung.  A Gohn complex is a Gohn lesion with the addition of infection in regional tracheobronchial lymph nodes.

❏❏  **In the United States, which specific serotypes of Mycobacterium avium are typically found in patients with AIDS?**

Serotypes 4 and 8.

❏❏  **What is the causative agent of leprosy or Hansen's disease?**

Mycobacterium leprae.

❏❏  **Name a virus whose genome is composed of single-stranded DNA?**

Parvovirus which causes erythema infectiosum.

❏❏  **What is the only major virus whose genome is composed of double-stranded RNA?**

Rotavirus, serotypes 1-3, which is a common cause of diarrhea amongst children.

❏❏  **What is different about the genomes of hepatitis B compared to hepatitis A, C, and E?**

Hepatitis B is double-stranded DNA virus while the others are RNA viruses.

❏❏  **What family of viruses includes HTLV and HIV?**

Retroviridae.

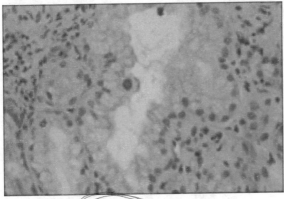

STOMACH WITH "OWL'S EYE" VIRAL INCLUSION

❑❑  **This gastric biopsy comes from a patient who is status post renal transplant.  What is your diagnosis?**

Cytomegalovirus  (CMV).

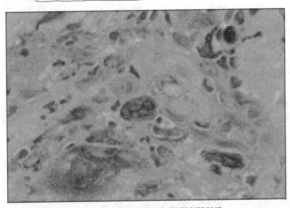

SKIN WITH MULTINUCLEATED VIRAL INCLUSIONS

❑❑  **This virus has a double-stranded DNA genome, what is your diagnosis?**

Herpes simplex virus (HSV).

❑❑  **Of the major viruses infecting humans, which is the smallest?**    *SS-DNA*

Parvoviridae.

❑❑  **What is the terminology used to describe a single-stranded RNA virus which can be translated directly to produce a protein without production of a second, intermediary strand?**

A positive-strand RNA virus.

❑❑  **In choosing a cell line for culture of influenza virus A and B as well as parainfluenza virus 1-3, which cell line would you choose?**

Primary monkey kidney (PMK).

❑❑  **Which virus has a double peak of infection, one in the fall and one in the spring?**

Parainfluenza 1 and 2.

❑❑  **Both influenza A and B and respiratory syncytial virus (RSV) peak in the winter, which peaks earlier?**

RSV.

❑❑  **Which virus is the principle causative agent of the so-called "hand, foot and mouth disease"?**

Coxsackie virus A16.

❑❑  **The causative agents for viral gastroenteritis differ in children and adults, which virus is one of the most common causes in adults but not children?**

Norwalk virus.

❑❑  **What is the shape of the infected cells in a culture of adenovirus?**

The cytopathic effect shows groups of round cells.

❑❑  **What is the likelihood of obtaining a positive result on a Tzanck preparation of a truly herpetic lesion?**

Although inexpensive and done quickly, the Tzanck preparation is not very sensitive as it detects herpes virus in positive cases only about 2/3 of the time.

❑❑  **In a patient who has a history of infection with Epstein-Barr virus, what would you expect the serology to show?**

IgG antibody to the viral capsid antigen (VCA), Epstein-Barr nuclear antigen (EBNA), and early antigen.

❑❑  **What is the viral cause of croup?**

Parainfluenza virus.

❑❑  **What would make a good panel of tests for respiratory illness-causing viruses during the winter for children with suspected upper respiratory infections?**

RSV, influenza virus A and B, and the various parainfluenza viruses.

❑❑  **What is the causative agent of exanthum subitum (roseola infantum)?**

Human herpes virus 6 (HHV 6).

❑❑  **Of the four Arboviruses that cause encephalitis in the United States, which has the highest morbidity and mortality?**

The eastern equine virus.  It is also the least common.

❑❑  **What is the mode of transmission of the parainfluenza viruses?**

They are spread via aerosolization.

❑❑  **What are the two surface antigens which define the various strains of influenza A?**

Hemagglutinin (H) and neuraminidase (N) antigens.

❑❑  **What is the terminology used to describe a change in the H or N antigen in influenza A?**

Antigenic shift.

❑❑  What is the causative agent of Fifth disease?

Parvovirus B19.

❑❑  What is the typical incubation period following infection with the influenza virus?

Two to three days.

❑❑  What is the classic appearance of a child with Fifth disease?

"Slapped-face" or erythematous cheeks.

❑❑  If a mother is infected with Parvovirus and it spreads across the placenta to the fetus, what may result?

Parvovirus can invade red cell precursors which, in an infant, can result in hydrops fetalis.

❑❑  What are the three structural components of the human herpesviruses?

The core (capsid surrounding DS DNA), tegument (beneath the envelope and outside the core), and the envelope.

❑❑  List the members of the human herpesviruses.

Herpes simplex virus (HSV) I and II, varicella-zoster virus (VZV), Epstein-Barr virus (EBV), cytomegalovirus (CMV), and human herpesvirus 6 (HHV-6), 7 (HHV-7) and 8 (HHV-8).

❑❑  What is the preferred anatomic location for infection with HSV-1 compared to HSV-2?

HSV-1 presents typically as vesicles on the face and oral mucosa. HSV-2 is the type which is associated with recurrent disease in the form of genital lesions. Either type can cause either oral lesions or genital lesions; however, HSV-1 tends to recur in the oral lesions and HSV-2 tends to recur in the genital lesions.

❑❑  What is the treatment for HSV?

Acyclovir.

❑❑  What part of the brain is classically involved in herpes encephalitis?

The temporal lobe.

❑❑  Which virus is associated with development of Burkitt's lymphoma?

EBV.

❑❑  What is the typical target for in situ hybridization to determine if there is a latent infection with EBV?

EBV encoded small RNAs (EBER).

❑❑  What is the site of latency for herpes simplex virus?

The dorsal root ganglia.

❑❑  Describe the viral inclusions seen in CMV.

They are both intranuclear and intracytoplasmic ("owl's eye").

❑❑  **What is the treatment for infection with CMV?**

Gancyclovir.

❑❑  **What is the causative agent of rubeola or measles?**

The measles virus, which is a single-stranded RNA virus belonging to the paramyxoviridae.

❑❑  **What is the term given to the giant cells sometimes seen in infection with measles virus?**

Warthin-Finkeldy giant cells.

❑❑  **What is the term given to the pathognomonic rash which is seen in the early cases of measles?**

Koplik's spots which are light lesions seen on the buccal mucosa.

❑❑  **How is measles spread?**

Aerosolization and secretions.

❑❑  **What family does the rubella virus belong to?**

Togaviridae, and it is a single-stranded RNA virus.

❑❑  **In the gastrointestinal tract, what is the most likely site of involvement by the measles virus?**

Appendix or the associated mesenteric lymph nodes.

❑❑  **What are some of the complications associated with congenital rubella infection?**

Nearly any organ can be affected in the infected infant; however, the major and classic complications include growth retardation, cataract formation, hearing loss, congenital heart disease, and meningoencephalitis.

❑❑  **In varicella or chicken pox, when is a patient considered infectious?**

Unfortunately, the disease can be spread two days prior to manifestation of a rash and the patient remains infectious until all skin lesions have crusted over.

❑❑  **How is erythema infectiosum or Fifth disease transmitted?**

Via aerosolized droplets in person to person contact.  The incubation period is from one to two weeks.

❑❑  **What time of the year is mumps most prevalent?**

Late winter to early spring.

❑❑  **In addition to parotitis seen in mumps, what are some other manifestations of this disease?**

Myocarditis, spontaneous abortion in pregnant women, orchitis in postpubertal males, hearing loss, meningitis, pancreatitis, arthritis, and encephalitis.

❑❑  **Which specific viruses of the polyomavirus genus cause disease in humans?**

The BK and JC viruses.

❑❑  **What are the diseases that are associated with JC and BK viruses?**

JC virus is the causative agent of progressive multifocal leukoencephalopathy (PML) and BK virus has an association with hemorrhagic cystitis.

❑❑   **Which serotypes of human papillomavirus (HPV) are associated with an increased risk of cervical carcinoma?**

16, 18, 31, 33, and 35; while types 6 and 11 are considered low risk serotypes.

❑❑   **Which serotype of HPV has been most commonly associated with endocervical adenocarcinoma?**

18.

❑❑   **Which type of HPV is associated with laryngeal carcinoma?**

Types 30 and 40.

❑❑   **What is the theoretical action of HPV such that it plays a role in dysplasia and development of carcinoma?**

Evidence shows that the early gene (E6) has a part in degradation of the p53 gene in high risk types of HPV.

❑❑   **Which influenza virus, A or B, causes a more severe disease?**

Influenza A.

❑❑   **What is the preferred collection method for diagnosing respiratory syncytial virus (RSV)?**

Via a nasal swab.

❑❑   **Which virus is the most common cause of the common cold?**

Rhinovirus.

❑❑   **What are the viral inclusions of rabies called?**

Negri bodies.

❑❑   **What is the most common causative agent of gastroenteritis in patients under two years of age?**

Rotavirus.

❑❑   **Which family of viruses causes eastern, western, and Venezuelan equine encephalitis?**

The Togaviridae family and, specifically, the Alphavirus genus.

❑❑   **If given the choice, would you rather have Eastern or Western equine encephalitis?**

I would choose Western, as the mortality is around 10% compared to 70% for Eastern equine encephalitis.

❑❑   **Which single virus causes all of the following: St. Louis encephalitis, dengue, tick-born encephalitis, and yellow fever?**

Flavivirus, also of the Togaviridae family.

❑❑   **What is the earliest histologic lesion seen in neurons in poliomyelitis?**

There is a loss of the cytoplasmic Nissl substance.

❑❑   **How is Coxsackie virus transmitted?**

Via the fecal-oral route.

❑❑   **What is the causative agent of hairy cell leukemia?**

Human T-cell leukemia virus (HTLV-II).

❑❑   **What is the difference between the oral polio (Sabin) and the intramuscular polio (Salk) vaccinations?**

The Sabin or oral polio is a live, attenuated virus while the Salk intramuscular vaccination is a killed virus.

# FUNGAL AND PARASITIC DISEASE

❑❑ **What is the causative agent of the superficial mycosis called tinea versicolor?**

Malassezia furfur.

❑❑ **What are some of the other diseases that are included in the general category of superficial mycoses?**

Black piedra, tinea nigra, tinea versicolor, white piedra, and dermatophytosis.

❑❑ **What does the term dimorphic mean in reference to fungi?**

This is a group of fungi that exhibit growth as a mold form or a non mold form, depending on their surroundings. That is, in the environment (at 25 degrees Celsius) they grow as hyphae or molds, while in tissue or in a laboratory (at 37 degrees Celsius) they grow as yeast or budding yeast, or spherules in the case of Coccidioides immitis.

❑❑ **If one wanted to demonstrate the capsule of a Cryptococcus neoformans organism, what stain would you use?**

One of the mucicarmines, India ink, or alcian blue.

❑❑ **What would you expect to see with a KOH preparation and on culture of Malassezia furfur?**

It gives a characteristic "spaghetti and meatballs" appearance on KOH preparation. Distinctively, by overlaying the surface of a culture agar with olive oil, M. furfur will grow exuberantly; whereas, it will not grow in the absence of the olive oil.

❑❑ **What are pseudohyphae?**

This is when a yeast undergoes asexual budding reproduction and the daughter cell (bud) does not completely detach from the parent cell. The pseudohypha, therefore, is always less than or equal to the size of the parent cell and shows a constriction where it is joined to the adjacent cell.

❑❑ **What are the genera of the causative agents of the superficial mycosis category of dermatophytosis?**

Epidermophyton, Microsporum, and Trichophyton which result in tinea capitis (infection of the scalp), tinea corporis (infection of the body), tinea cruris (infection of the groin), tinea pedis (infection of the feet), and tinea unguium (infection of the nails).

❑❑ **What are some of the diseases in the category of cutaneous and subcutaneous mycoses?**

Chromoblastomycosis, mycetoma, phaeohyphomycosis (subcutaneous and systemic), rhinosporidiosis, sporotrichosis, and zygomycosis.

❑❑ **What is the causative agent of sporotrichosis and how does one become infected?**

Sporothrix schenckii. This organism comes to reside in the host via traumatic implantation from a plant or the soil where the organism is found. The classic test question involves a gardener handling roses who gets stuck by one of the thorns and develops sporotrichosis ("drunk gardener").

❏❏ **What stain demonstrates the Cryptococcus neoformans capsule nicely by producing a negative image?**

India ink.

❏❏ **What is the characteristic hyphal branching pattern of Aspergillus?**

The hyphae show acute angle branching, frequently 45 degrees, with distinct septae.

❏❏ **Which species of Aspergillus are most likely to cause pulmonary infection and disseminated disease?**

A. fumigatus, A. flavus and less commonly, A. terreus.  A. niger is not typically associated with disseminated disease.

❏❏ **What is somewhat unique about the growth pattern of Aspergillus that aids in its ability to disseminate?**

It shows a propensity for vascular invasion, acting somewhat more like a tumor than an infection.

❏❏ **In a patient with a systemic mycosis, you isolate large, budding yeast characterized by broad-based buds and "double-contoured" walls.  What is your diagnosis?**

Blastomyces dermatidis.

❏❏ **What is the causative agent of thrush in infants?**

Candida albicans.

❏❏ **What is the fungal organism which is responsible for the disease that has been referred to in the past as San Joaquin Valley fever?**

Coccidioides immitis.

❏❏ **If one suspects a culture to be growing C. immitis, what special precautions would one take?**

The culture plate should be sealed with tape and great care should be taken to not keep the plate open to the air for extended periods of time nor should personnel breathe over the plate as it is easily spread.

❏❏ **Of the systemic mycoses, which is most likely to be seen in cytologic examination of cerebrospinal fluid?**

Cryptococcus neoformans.

❏❏ **What is the classic mode of spread of Cryptococcus neoformans?**

The fungus can be found in pigeon droppings and is then inhaled gaining entry into the human respiratory system.

❏❏ **Which fungal infection, found in South America, has the characteristic "mariner's wheel" morphology?**

Paracoccidioides brasiliensis.

❑❑  **How does Histoplasma capsulatum compare to Blastomycosis in the size of the yeast cells?**

Histoplasma is quite small measuring 2-4 microns, while Blastomycosis is quite large measuring 8-15 microns.

❑❑  **Geographically, where is Histoplasma capsulatum endemic?**

The Ohio River Valley.

❑❑  **Arrange the following organisms in order of increasing length of time for typical culture positivity: C. immitis, H. capsulatum, and B. dermatidis.**

C. immitis (less than a week), B. dermatidis (1-2 weeks), and H. capsulatum (2-several weeks).

❑❑  **What is the treatment of choice for paracoccidioidomycosis?**

Ketoconazole or amphotericin B.

❑❑  **What is a simple, inexpensive and rapid manner by which someone can confirm a suspicion of a cutaneous mycosis?**

By scraping the skin at the site of the lesion onto a slide, adding KOH and looking for the fungal elements under the microscope immediately.

❑❑  **A diabetic patient presents to you with poorly controlled diabetes and a fungal sinus infection, what is the most likely causative agent?**

Mucormycosis or zygomycosis.

❑❑  **What is the most common pathogen of the zygomycetes?**

Rhizopus.

❑❑  **Describe the culture characteristics of rhizopus.**

It is a very rapid growing organism which literally overgrows the dish within 2-3 days. The hyphae are initially white then turn dark gray or black as sporulation occurs. They have distinct root-type structures which are called rhizoids.

❑❑  **What are some of the organisms that have caused invasive fungal infection in immunocompromised hosts and are part of the zygomycetes?**

Rhizopus, Absidia, Rhizomucor, Mucor, and Cunninghamella.

❑❑  **Describe the hyphal characteristics of the zygomycetes.**

They are often described as ribbon-like in that they are broad, sometimes twisted and, when they branch, the branches are typically at right angles as opposed to the acute angle branching seen in Aspergillus.

❑❑  **Describe the rhizoids of the Mucor species.**

That's easy, they don't have any. Rhizomucor falls somewhere between Rhizopus and Mucor and has poorly developed rhizoids.

❑❑  **What is the most common mold isolated from either the sinuses or pulmonary parenchyma in patients with cystic fibrosis?**

Aspergillus fumigatus.

❑❑ In a patient with a subcutaneous mycosis, you isolate a slow-growing yeast form which has a "mouse-gray" colony color and small (3-5 microns) cigar-shaped yeast forms in the tissue. In addition, you see a group of the yeast surrounded by projections or rays of amorphous, pink material (asteroid body). What is your diagnosis?

Sporothrix shenckii.

❑❑ In most cases, how is histoplasmosis acquired?

Classically, the conidia are found in soil which contains bat or bird droppings and one inhales the conidia from the soil.

❑❑ What are some of the signs and symptoms of so-called "valley fever" caused by Coccidioidomycosis?

Skin lesions (erythema multiforme or erythema nodosum), upper respiratory signs such as cough and slight dyspnea, general malaise, and a low grade fever.

❑❑ What are some of the clinical signs and symptoms of disseminated Coccidioidomycosis?

It can cause osteomyelitis, arthritis, ulcerative skin lesions, and a meningitis.

❑❑ How common is Coccidioidomycosis in the southwestern United States?

Very, up to 90% of the people will be skin test positive in certain areas.

❑❑ What does the colony look like in a culture of Cryptococcus neoformans?

Remember, it has a thick capsule which can be demonstrated by negative staining with India ink, thus the colony is shiny and mucoid in appearance on culture media.

❑❑ What substance produced by Aspergillus flavus has an association with development of hepatocellular carcinoma?

Aflatoxins.

❑❑ What is the term used to describe the syndrome where one finds scattered hyphae consistent with Aspergillus species in the lung in association with excessive mucous production, numerous eosinophils with Charcot-Leyden crystals, granulomas, and bronchiolitis?

Allergic bronchopulmonary Aspergillosis.

❑❑ Compare the hyphae seen in Fusarium to Aspergillus species.

The hyphae themselves are quite similar, including similar size and septations. However, in Fusarium the branching is much more haphazard compared to Aspergillus and is quite frequently not acute angle, rather it is often closer to 90 degrees from the parent hyphae.

❑❑ What are some of the pathogenic species of the genus Fusarium?

F. moniliforme, F. oxysporum, F. solani and less frequently, F. macroforme and F. proliferatum.

❑❑ What is the treatment for Geotrichosis?

It has been treated in the past with oral potassium iodide and aerosolized nystatin. In addition, 5-fluorocytosine and the traditional amphotericin B have also been used.

❑❑ Describe the septation seen in the tissue phase of infection with the zygomycetes.

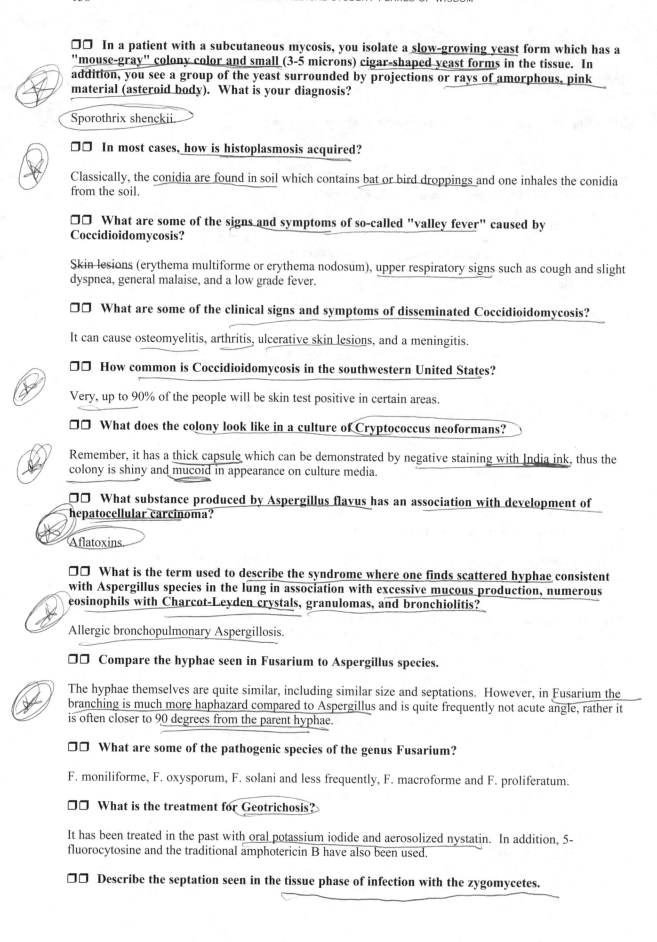

They are large, nonseptate hyphae and show a variable branching pattern generally perpendicular to the parent hyphae.

❑❑ **Which organism is most commonly the cause of the rhinocerebral mucormycosis seen in diabetics with diabetic ketoacidosis?**

Rhizopus oryzae.

❑❑ **A 32-year-old male with AIDS presents with diffuse, bilateral pulmonary infiltrates on chest x-ray and associated cough and dyspnea. What is the most likely diagnosis?**

Pneumocystis carinii.

❑❑ **Describe the cysts of Pneumocystis carinii.**

They are typically round and approximately 5 microns in diameter. Sometimes, they are somewhat collapsed and have a fold creating a line going down the middle. The terms "helmet-shaped" and "cup and saucer" appearance have been used. Often, there will be a small area of wall thickening creating a comma or exclamation point appearance.

❑❑ **What are some of the prophylactic treatments for Pneumocystis carinii?**

Trimethoprim-sulfamethoxazole (Bactrim) or aerosolized pentamadine.

❑❑ **You are told by the laboratory that a yeast has been isolated from a blood culture of a patient of yours who is immunosuppressed secondary to chemotherapy for an adenocarcinoma of the colon. You are told that the yeast has blastoconidia, chlamydoconidia, both true and pseudohyphae, and germ tube formation. What is your presumptive diagnosis?**

Candida albicans.

❑❑ **What color will the culture medium turn if you have a positive KNO$_3$ (potassium nitrate) assimilation test?**

Blue, while a negative test will turn immediately yellow. Candida albicans will give a negative test.

❑❑ **What would you expect to find should you have an isolated Cryptococcus on a simple urea agar plate?**

This should give a positive test resulting in a change of the media to a bright pink color.

❑❑ **A neonate in the intensive care unit is receiving a high lipid content formula via an intravenous catheter and develops a fungemia. The catheter is removed and cultured, what would you guess that the organism is?**

Malassezia furfur, remember that it requires long chain fatty acids for growth which can be provided from the lipid rich food being given through the catheter line.

❑❑ **What are the main pathogenic flagellates found in humans?**

Giardia lamblia, Trichomonas vaginalis, Trypanosoma brucei, T. cruzi, and Leishmania.

❑❑ **A patient presents with diarrhea and tells you of a recent backpacking trip to Colorado where he drank fresh water from the Colorado rivers. What organism do you suspect as a cause of his diarrhea?**

Giardia lamblia.

❑❑ **You suspect infection with G. lamblia, so you perform endoscopy and take biopsies. Which part of the GI tract should you biopsy to find the organism?**

Duodenum, where it will be found attached to the surface of the mucosal epithelium.

❑❑ **Histologically, describe the damage that occurs to the surface epithelium in infection with Giardia lamblia.**

There is typically no epithelial damage. The villi may show distortion and increased inflammation within the lamina propria; however, this is nonspecific and does not correlate with the degree of symptoms.

❑❑ **Describe the cyst stage in the life cycle of Trichomonas vaginalis.**

There is no cyst stage, the trophozoites are passed from one human host to the next typically during unprotected sexual intercourse.

❑❑ **What is the causative agent in African trypanosomiasis?**

Morphologically, the organisms in the Trypanosoma group are not distinguishable from one another by morphologic appearance. Thus, infection in animals is attributed to T. brucei while in humans it is attributed to T. gambiense (chronic form found in west Africa) or T. rhodesiensa (acute in east Africa).

❑❑ **Briefly describe the life cycle of the trypanosomes.**

They are spread via tsetse flies which bite a human, taking up the blood containing the trypomastigotes, where the flagellates then live and multiply in the fly intestine eventually making their way to the salivary glands of the fly. The next human is then bitten and the organisms in the salivary glands of the fly are passed into the blood of the next host.

❑❑ **What is another name for the disease of African trypanosomiasis?**

African sleeping sickness.

❑❑ **What is the causative agent of Chagas' disease?**

Trypanosoma cruzi.

❑❑ **What is the transmission vector of American trypanosomiasis or Chagas' disease?**

The "kissing" bug or reduviid.

❑❑ **What are some of the signs and symptoms seen in the chronic infection by T. cruzi, particularly in Brazil?**

Cardiac conduction system blocks, esophageal achalasia, megaesophagus, and megacolon.

❑❑ **What is the causative agent of kala azar?**

This is also referred to as visceral leishmaniasis and it is caused by Leishmania donovani (India), L. infantum (Mediterranean), and L. chagasi (Latin America).

❑❑ **What is the transmission vector for kala azar?**

The sand fly.

❑❑ **Briefly describe the life cycle of the Leishmania organisms.**

They are ingested as amastigotes by the sand fly where they are transformed into monomastigotes or flagellates. They are then regurgitated by the fly into the next host. In the human host, they are ingested by macrophages where they transform again into amastigotes, multiply, and eventually neutralize the lysosomal enzymes of the cell. They can cause massive splenomegaly.

❏❏ **Where in the gastrointestinal tract would you find Entamoeba histolytica?**

They tend to colonize the right colon and cecum.

❏❏ **Histologically what is the classic shape of the ulcer produced by E. histolytica?**

Flask-shaped.

❏❏ **Where in the liver is an amoebic abscess most likely to form?**

The right lobe, although those in the left lobe carry more serious potential complications as they may rupture into the pericardium.

❏❏ **How is Naegleria fowleri acquired?**

The patient acquires it by swimming in water contaminated with the organism. The organism then enters the nasal sinuses where it traverses the olfactory tracts through the cribiform plate to reach the brain where meningoencephalitis then develops.

❏❏ **What protozoa can cause keratitis and corneal ulceration in soft contact lens wearers?**

Acanthamoeba.

❏❏ **What is the manner of spread of Cryptosporidium?**

Fecal-oral.

❏❏ **If you were to look in a stool sample for Cryptosporidium, what stain would aid in your hunt?**

A modified acid fast stain such as the Kinyoun stain.

❏❏ **What cell type in the gastrointestinal tract harbors Isospora in infection with Isospora belli?**

They are found in the surface epithelial cells.

❏❏ **What type of reproduction does one find in human infection with Toxoplasma gondii?**

The parasite reproduces asexually in the tissues of humans and eventually produces cysts or bradyzoites.

❏❏ **In T. gondii infection in a cat, how is the organism passed on to others?**

Via the feces, which must mature (undergo sporulation) for several days in the environment prior to becoming infective.

❏❏ **How common is toxoplasmosis?**

In the United States, about half of the general population contains antibodies indicating previous infection. This number increases with older populations. Fortunately, these infections do not cause serious problems other than in immunocompromised hosts.

❏❏ **Although toxoplasmosis can infect nearly any organ, what are the two major clinically important organs involved?**

Brain and heart.

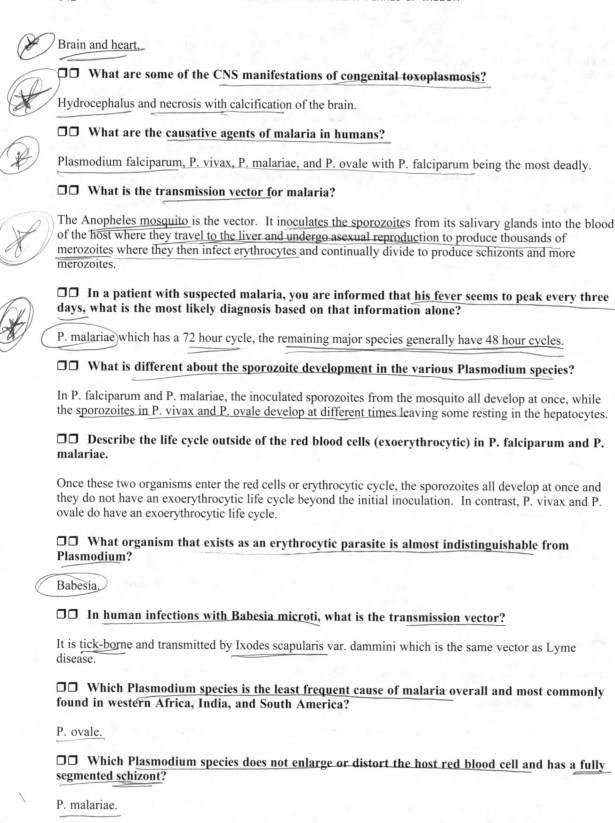

**□□  What are some of the CNS manifestations of congenital toxoplasmosis?**

Hydrocephalus and necrosis with calcification of the brain.

**□□  What are the causative agents of malaria in humans?**

Plasmodium falciparum, P. vivax, P. malariae, and P. ovale with P. falciparum being the most deadly.

**□□  What is the transmission vector for malaria?**

The Anopheles mosquito is the vector.  It inoculates the sporozoites from its salivary glands into the blood of the host where they travel to the liver and undergo asexual reproduction to produce thousands of merozoites where they then infect erythrocytes and continually divide to produce schizonts and more merozoites.

**□□  In a patient with suspected malaria, you are informed that his fever seems to peak every three days, what is the most likely diagnosis based on that information alone?**

P. malariae which has a 72 hour cycle, the remaining major species generally have 48 hour cycles.

**□□  What is different about the sporozoite development in the various Plasmodium species?**

In P. falciparum and P. malariae, the inoculated sporozoites from the mosquito all develop at once, while the sporozoites in P. vivax and P. ovale develop at different times leaving some resting in the hepatocytes.

**□□  Describe the life cycle outside of the red blood cells (exoerythrocytic) in P. falciparum and P. malariae.**

Once these two organisms enter the red cells or erythrocytic cycle, the sporozoites all develop at once and they do not have an exoerythrocytic life cycle beyond the initial inoculation.  In contrast, P. vivax and P. ovale do have an exoerythrocytic life cycle.

**□□  What organism that exists as an erythrocytic parasite is almost indistinguishable from Plasmodium?**

Babesia.

**□□  In human infections with Babesia microti, what is the transmission vector?**

It is tick-borne and transmitted by Ixodes scapularis var. dammini which is the same vector as Lyme disease.

**□□  Which Plasmodium species is the least frequent cause of malaria overall and most commonly found in western Africa, India, and South America?**

P. ovale.

**□□  Which Plasmodium species does not enlarge or distort the host red blood cell and has a fully segmented schizont?**

P. malariae.

**□□  What is the most commonly identified microsporon in humans where it is found to cause chronic diarrhea almost exclusively in patients with AIDS?**

Enterocytozoon bieneusi.

❏❏ What is the most prevalent cause of malaria?

P. vivax.

❏❏ Of the Plasmodium species causing malaria, which is most likely to result in nephrotic syndrome?

P. malariae.

❏❏ What effect does having Duffy negative blood type have on the rate of developing malaria?

Patients with Duffy negative blood are resistant to infection with P. vivax as the Duffy antigen is the receptor by which P. vivax invades the red blood cells as a merozoite.

❏❏ What is the relationship between the presence of hemoglobin S and infection with P. falciparum?

Patients with hemoglobin S (sickle cell trait) have protection from P. falciparum in that they suffer less severe disease.

❏❏ What is the name of the pigment produced by the trophozoites in malaria?

Hematin or hemozoin which is an iron-based pigment created from hemoglobin.

❏❏ In a patient with visceral Leishmaniasis, what would you expect the result of the Montenegro test to be?

Usually negative.

❏❏ Regarding the infected erythrocytes in malaria, what preference do the various Plasmodium species have for the age of the erythrocyte which they will infect?

P. falciparum has no preference and will infect any erythrocyte, P. malariae prefers older hosts, and P. vivax and P. ovale apparently enjoy associating with the young red blood cells.

❏❏ Regarding the size of the ring forms in the various Plasmodium species, which has the smallest ring forms in the red blood cells?

P. falciparum which are classically 1/5-1/6 the diameter of the red blood cell when young, while the other species are twice that.

❏❏ Which Plasmodium species is known for having "banana-shaped" gametocytes?

P. falciparum.

❏❏ What is the therapy for infection with Trichomonas vaginalis?

Metronidazole.

❏❏ Of the two forms of African trypanosomiasis or sleeping sickness, which exhibits the more rapid progression?

The Rhodesian form can progress to death within months, while the Gambian form may take several years.

❏❏ Of the intestinal flagellates, which is the only one that has two nuclei in the trophozoite form?

Giardia lamblia. The cyst form usually has four nuclei.

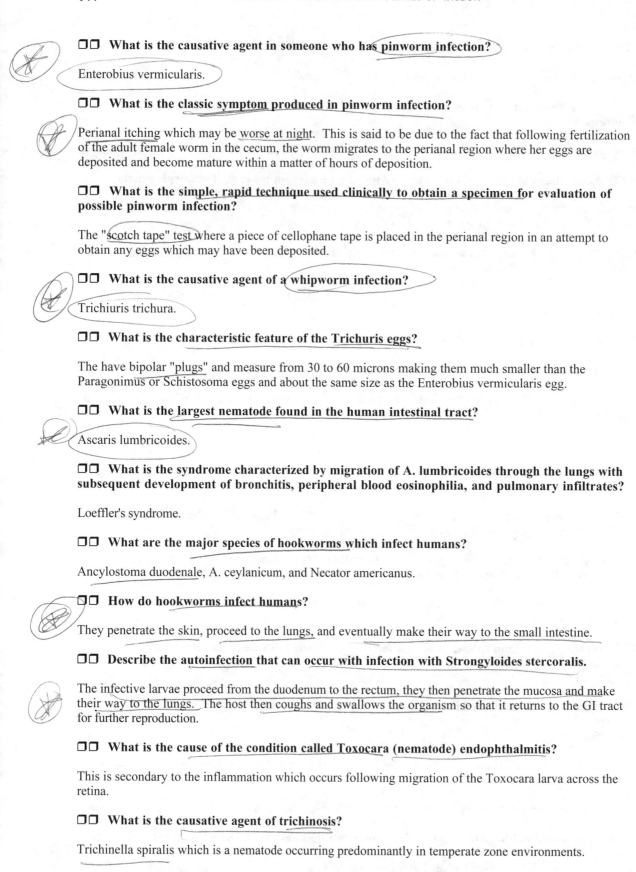

❏❏ **What is the causative agent in someone who has pinworm infection?**

Enterobius vermicularis.

❏❏ **What is the classic symptom produced in pinworm infection?**

Perianal itching which may be worse at night. This is said to be due to the fact that following fertilization of the adult female worm in the cecum, the worm migrates to the perianal region where her eggs are deposited and become mature within a matter of hours of deposition.

❏❏ **What is the simple, rapid technique used clinically to obtain a specimen for evaluation of possible pinworm infection?**

The "scotch tape" test where a piece of cellophane tape is placed in the perianal region in an attempt to obtain any eggs which may have been deposited.

❏❏ **What is the causative agent of a whipworm infection?**

Trichiuris trichura.

❏❏ **What is the characteristic feature of the Trichuris eggs?**

The have bipolar "plugs" and measure from 30 to 60 microns making them much smaller than the Paragonimus or Schistosoma eggs and about the same size as the Enterobius vermicularis egg.

❏❏ **What is the largest nematode found in the human intestinal tract?**

Ascaris lumbricoides.

❏❏ **What is the syndrome characterized by migration of A. lumbricoides through the lungs with subsequent development of bronchitis, peripheral blood eosinophilia, and pulmonary infiltrates?**

Loeffler's syndrome.

❏❏ **What are the major species of hookworms which infect humans?**

Ancylostoma duodenale, A. ceylanicum, and Necator americanus.

❏❏ **How do hookworms infect humans?**

They penetrate the skin, proceed to the lungs, and eventually make their way to the small intestine.

❏❏ **Describe the autoinfection that can occur with infection with Strongyloides stercoralis.**

The infective larvae proceed from the duodenum to the rectum, they then penetrate the mucosa and make their way to the lungs. The host then coughs and swallows the organism so that it returns to the GI tract for further reproduction.

❏❏ **What is the cause of the condition called Toxocara (nematode) endophthalmitis?**

This is secondary to the inflammation which occurs following migration of the Toxocara larva across the retina.

❏❏ **What is the causative agent of trichinosis?**

Trichinella spiralis which is a nematode occurring predominantly in temperate zone environments.

❑❑  In what tissue do the T. spiralis organisms harbor and subsequently become encapsulated in a dormant state?

Skeletal muscle. The adult nematode lays eggs in the small intestinal mucosa which then eventually reaches skeletal muscle, becomes encapsulated, and lies dormant.

❑❑  What are the two characteristic signs or symptoms which should raise the possibility of trichinosis?

Diffuse myositis or muscle aches and a peripheral blood eosinophilia.

❑❑  What is the typical muscle which is biopsied in an attempt to confirm a suspicion of trichinosis?

The deltoid muscle which, if there is an infection, should demonstrate larvae in varying stages of encapsulation with associated varying degrees of inflammatory response.

❑❑  In general, what is the life cycle of the filarial worms?

In the infected tissue, the adult worm produces offspring called microfilariae which enter the bloodstream and are then picked up by the vector arthropod where they then become infective larvae. The vector then transmits the infective larvae to the next host.

❑❑  What are the causative agents of elephantiasis?

This infection of the lymphatic system is caused by filarial worms of either Wuchereria or Brugia genera.

❑❑  What is the most common species of Wuchereria that causes elephantiasis?

W. bancrofti.

❑❑  If one wanted to demonstrate microfilariae in the blood of a patient with W. bancrofti infection, when would one draw the blood?

At night, between 10 p.m. and 2 a.m., as that is when the microfilariae circulate, otherwise they are dormant in the capillaries of the lungs during the day.

❑❑  What is the causative agent of river blindness or onchocerciasis?

Onchocerca volvulus.

❑❑  What is the transmission vector for O. volvulus?

The black fly (Simulium). In this case, the microfilariae are in the skin and cause nodules rather than circulating in the blood.

❑❑  Why is onchocerciasis referred to as "river blindness"?

Because microfilariae of O. volvulus have been found to migrate through the cornea causing a pronounced inflammatory response which can cause blindness. In addition, the black flies that transmit the disease are found along rivers, hence the name river blindness.

❑❑  What is the vector of Loa loa?

Flies of the genus Chrysops. In Loa loa, the microfilariae are most abundant in the blood at noon.

❑❑  Which of the filariae is characterized by a continuous migration under the epidermis and sometimes the ability to actually observe the parasite cross the conjunctiva?

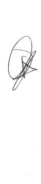

Loa loa.

❑❑  **What is the agent which is commonly referred to as the "dog heart worm"?**

Dirofilaria immitis.

❑❑  **If one were to see a D. immitis in the lung of a human, where in the lung would one expect to find it?**

They reside within branches of the pulmonary artery and can cause a distinct "coin lesion" resulting in surgical resection for evaluation.

❑❑  **Classically, how do humans become infected with Trichinella spiralis?**

By eating undercooked pork.

❑❑  **What is the common term for trematodes?**

Flatworms. They are transmitted via snails and are hermaphroditic.

❑❑  **What is the largest human trematode?**

Fasciolopsis buski, which is a parasite found in pigs measuring up to 8 cm in length.

❑❑  **Which trematodes can cause forms of choliangitis in humans?**

Fasciola hepatica, Clonorchis sinensis, Opisthorchis viverrini, and O. felines.

❑❑  **What is the genus of the pulmonary fluke or pulmonary trematode?**

Paragonimus, in humans the most common species is P. westermani.

❑❑  **In the life cycle of Paragonimus there are two intermediate hosts, what are they?**

First a snail, then a crustacean, most commonly a crayfish or a crab.

❑❑  **What is the characteristic feature of the egg of Paragonimus?**

The operculum is flattened and the opposite end is slightly thickened.  They measure 80-120 microns in length and have a fairly thick, brown shell.

❑❑  **What is the genus of the parasite commonly referred to as the blood fluke?**

Schistosoma.

❑❑  **What are the species of schistosomes which infect humans?**

S. mansoni, S. japonicum, and S. haematobium.

❑❑  **Which species of Schistosoma is found in the Nile River in Egypt and involves the bladder and includes an increased risk of squamous cell carcinoma of the bladder?**

S. haematobium.

❑❑  **How do you differentiate between the three main Schistosoma species eggs?**

S. mansoni has a large, lateral spine while S. haemotobium has a somewhat smaller terminal or end spine and S. japonicum features a very small, sometimes difficult to see lateral spine.  In addition, overall, S. japonicum is much smaller and more round than the other two species' eggs.

❏❏  **What is the pathologic finding in the liver in a case of schistomiasis?**

These patients develop hepatic fibrosis and subsequent portal hypertension.  Specifically, the fibrosis is portal in nature as the eggs are carried into the portal vein and elicit the fibrotic response.  Sometimes, this pattern of fibrosis is referred to as Symmer's or "pipestem fibrosis".

❏❏  **What is the common name for the general category for cestodes?**

Tapeworms.

❏❏  **What are the parts of the body in a tapeworm?**

The body is called the strobela, each segment making up the body is called a proglottid, the anterior end is the scolex and, internally, they have one or even two sets of male and female sex organs.

❏❏  **In which specific veins are S. mansoni and S. japonicum found in human hosts?**

S. mansoni is found in the inferior mesenteric vein and its branches while S. japonicum  is found in the superior mesenteric vein and its branches.

❏❏  **What is the name of the beef tapeworm?**

Taenia saginata.

❏❏  **What is the pork tapeworm?**

Taenia solium.

❏❏  **What is the fish tapeworm?**

Diphyllobothrium latum.

❏❏  **Which of the tapeworms can cause a megaloblastic anemia?**

Diphyllobothrium latum can and will absorb the vitamin B12 in the diet that the host normally would, resulting in a megaloblastic anemia.

❏❏  **What is the appearance of the scolex on Taenia saginata?**

It has four large suckers, and no hooks on the crown or rostellum.

❏❏  **What is the difference between the uteri in T. saginata and T. solium?**

T. saginata has 15-20 lateral branches of the uterus, while T. solium has less than 13 uterine lateral branches.

❏❏  **How can one tell the eggs of T. saginata and T. solium apart?**

You can't.

❏❏  **What is the term used to describe ingestion of T. solium eggs with development of larva which invade tissue (subcutaneous tissue, skeletal muscle, brain, and the eye) and encyst?**

Cysticercosis.

❏❏  **What is the causative agent of a hydatid cyst?**

Echinococcus granulosus.

❏❏  **Where is a unilocular hydatid cyst most commonly located in the human, accidental host?**

The liver (three quarters of the time) followed by the lungs and less frequently in muscles.

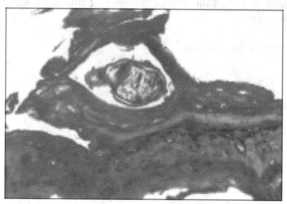

SKIN

❏❏  **What is the mite which burrows across the skin in the upper layers of the cornified layer as shown above?**

Sarcoptes scabiei (scabies).

❏❏  **If one wants to examine various arthropods to identify them, how should they be preserved?**

Lice, fleas, ticks, mites, maggots, grubs, caterpillars, spiders, and scorpions are best preserved in 70-80% ethanol while large larval forms should be placed in hot water prior to being placed in alcohol solution. The smaller arthropods like mites, fleas, and ticks may also be simply mounted whole on a slide immediately.

❏❏  **What are the most common bed bugs?**

Cimex lectularius and C. hemipterus.

❏❏  **What are the major species of fleas and what is the most prominent characteristic and anatomic feature of the organisms?**

The dog flea (C. tenocephalides canis), the cat flea (C. felis), and the human flea (Pulex irritans) each of which have large hind legs which explain their propensity for jumping incredible distances.

❏❏  **What are the major louse species?**

Pediculus capitis (the head louse), P. humanis (the body louse), and Phthirus pubis (the pubic louse). They deposit their eggs (nits) on hair or clothing.

❏❏  **What are the two species of mites which are found associated with the sebaceous glands on the face of all of us?**

Demodex folliculorum and D. brevis.

❏❏  **What is Lactrodectus mactans?**

This is the black widow spider.  The female spider has a leg span of up to 4 cm, is shiny black, and has an orange-red hour glass figure on the ventral abdomen.

☐☐  **What is the Loxosceles reclusa?**

This is the brown recluse spider which is smaller than the black widow at up to 2 cm in length, brown in color, and has a darker brown violin shaped figure on the dorsal thorax.  Although the bite may be initially painless, it eventually causes necrosis and sloughing of the skin in that area.

# CARDIOVASCULAR

**□□  What are the major types of arteries?**

Large elastic arteries, muscular arteries (distributing arteries), small arteries ( < 2 mm), and arterioles.

**□□  As one proceeds from a large elastic artery to an arteriole, what histologic changes occur?**

The media becomes smaller and the external elastic lamina is lost followed by the internal elastic lamina.

**□□  Which of the types of arteries is most responsible for changes in blood pressure by increasing or decreasing resistance?**

Arterioles.

**□□  What is the general term which encompasses vascular changes such as narrowing of the vascular lumina, thickening of arterial walls, and loss of arterial wall elasticity?**

Arteriosclerosis.

**□□  What is the term used to describe thickening and hyalinization of the walls of small arteries and arterioles?**

Arteriolosclerosis.

**□□  What is the histologic appearance of the atheroma or fibrofatty plaque seen in atherosclerosis?**

This is a plaque in the intima of a muscular artery consisting of a lipid, amorphous core and a fibrous "cap".

**□□  Specifically, which type of cholesterol is associated with an increased risk of development of atherosclerosis and which type is protective?**

Low density lipoprotein (LDL) and high density lipoprotein (HDL), respectively.

**□□  What is the major apoprotein comprising LDL?**

Apoprotein B100.

**□□  Which familial hyperlipidemia is associated with normal serum cholesterol, elevated VLDL, and moderate to severe hypertriglyceridemia?**

Type IV.

**□□  What are the most important risk factors in the development of atherosclerosis?**

Hyperlipidemia, hypertension, cigarette smoking, and diabetes mellitus.

**□□  What happens to the media in a muscular artery with significant atherosclerosis?**

It is compressed or thinned.

**□□  What is thought to be the effect of omega-3 fatty acids found in fish and fish oils on the risk of developing ischemic heart disease?**

These fatty acids seem to lower plasma LDL and increase plasma HDL. Although certain populations such as Greenland Eskimos have a high fat intake, they also have a high content of omega-3 fatty acids in their diet and yet a low incidence of ischemic heart disease.

❑❑  **Which vessels are most commonly involved with atherosclerotic plaques?**

The abdominal aorta at the origin of its branches, followed by the coronary arteries, popliteal arteries, descending thoracic aorta, internal carotid arteries, and the circle of Willis.

❑❑  **Besides the four major risk factors, what are some other risk factors for developing atherosclerosis that are of lesser importance?**

Lack of exercise, obesity, oral contraceptive use, hyperuricemia, high carbohydrate diet, and hyperhomocysteinemia.

❑❑  **What are some of the complications that develop in atherosclerotic plaques?**

Calcification, rupture or ulceration with release of microemboli, superimposed thrombus formation, hemorrhage into the plaque, and aneurysmal dilatation of the vessel.

❑❑  **What are the main causes of hypertension?**

The vast majority (95%) is idiopathic (essential hypertension) with the remaining cases secondary to renal disease or narrowing of the renal arteries by atherosclerosis.

❑❑  **Although there is some overlap, what are the large vessel and medium vessel vasculitides?**

The large vessel vasculitides include giant cell (temporal) arteritis and Takayasu's arteritis. The medium vessel vasculitides include polyarteritis nodosa and Kawasaki's disease.

❑❑  **Compare the typical patient age in giant cell arteritis and Takayasu's arteritis.**

Giant cell arteritis typically occurs in patients who are 50 or older while Takayasu's arteritis occurs in patients 15-50 years old.

❑❑  **What disease is found in more than half of the patients with giant cell (temporal) arteritis?**

Polymyalgia rheumatica.

❑❑  **What is the classic clinical picture in a patient with Takayasu's arteritis?**

They have markedly diminished pulses in the upper extremities, hence the designation "pulseless disease". The classic patient would be an Asian female less than 40 years old.

❑❑  **Is there a genetic predisposition to development of temporal arteritis?**

Yes, or I would not have asked. Many of the patients have the HLA DR4 haplotype.

❑❑  **Which vessels are classically involved in polyarteritis nodosa (PAN)?**

Visceral arteries and branches are involved in a segmental fashion.

❑❑  **What are the most serious potential complications of PAN?**

Myocardial infarction secondary to involvement of coronary arteries and/or ruptured aneurysm.

❑❑  **Compare the typical patient with PAN and Kawasaki's disease.**

PAN can occur at any age although most commonly middle-aged adults are affected and it is three times more common in males. Kawasaki is a condition of childhood with the majority of patients under 5 years of age, and it is more frequent in Asian children.

❑❑  **If you were to check the status of a patient's antineutrophil cytoplasmic autoantibody (ANCA) who has PAN, what would you expect it to be?**

If there is involvement of small vessels (microscopic polyangiitis), the ANCA is typically positive while patients with PAN and no small vessel involvement are typically negative.

❑❑  **More specifically, which type of ANCA would you expect in Wegener's granulomatosis compared to PAN?**

The cytoplasmic form of ANCA (C-ANCA) is found in patients with Wegener's and microscopic polyangiitis while the perinuclear ANCA (P-ANCA) is found in patients with PAN and not routinely in patients with Wegener's granulomatosis.

❑❑  **What are the signs and symptoms of Churg-Strauss syndrome?**

This is a disease of middle-aged adults, more commonly males, which includes asthma, peripheral blood eosinophilia, peripheral neuropathy, pulmonary infiltrates, pansinusitis, and hematuria.  If there is active vasculitis, most patients are P-ANCA positive.

❑❑  **What is another name for thromboangiitis obliterans?**

Buerger's disease.

❑❑  **Regarding Buerger's disease, what would be the classic patient description?**

A male, less than 40 with a strong cigarette smoking history who complains of claudication and Raynaud's phenomenon.

❑❑  **What is the pathogenesis of Henoch-Schonlein purpura?**

This is a vasculitis of the small vessels that shows IgA in immune deposits.

❑❑  **What is a saccular aneurysm?**

This is a dilatation of the vessel wall which is not circumferential.  A circumferential, gradual dilatation of a vessel is termed a fusiform aneurysm.

❑❑  **What is the most frequent etiology of aneurysms?**

Atherosclerosis.

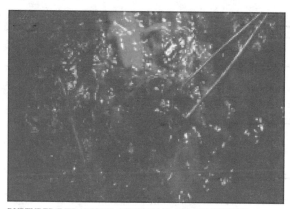

RUPTURED INFRARENAL ABDOMINAL AORTIC ANEURYSM

❑❑  **Where does one typically find atherosclerotic aneurysms?**

The abdominal aorta inferior to the renal arteries.  The example above shows a ruptured infrarenal aortic aneurysm at autopsy.

❏❏ **What is the annual risk of rupture for an abdominal aortic aneurysm measuring 5 cm or more?**

5-10%.

❏❏ **Where is a syphilitic aneurysm most likely to develop?**

The thoracic aorta, often involving the arch.

❏❏ **What is the colloquial term given to describe the characteristic intimal change seen in syphilitic aneurysms?**

"Tree-barking" which refers to the patchy, and uneven medial scarring with subsequent contraction of the scars. This causes a wrinkling or uneven surface appearance which simulates tree bark.

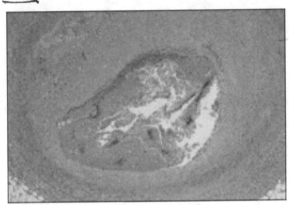

CORONARY ARTERY WITH ATHEROSCLEROSIS

❏❏ **What has occurred in this section of a coronary artery shown above?**

It has an acute occlusive thrombus overlying typical atherosclerosis.

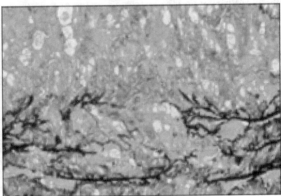

*(Photo courtesy of Stanley J. Radio, MD - University of Nebraska Medical Center)*

❏❏ **What would you suspect as the diagnosis based on the tissue section of the aorta shown above in this patient who had a thoracic aortic aneurysm at a young age and was extremely tall and thin?**

The section demonstrates marked loss of elastin, particularly in a single area. This area has an increased amount of ground substance or glycosaminoglycans consistent with the so-called "cystic medial necrosis" as seen in Marfan's syndrome.

❏❏ **What does one see morphologically and histologically in an aortic dissection?**

There is typically a tear in the intima of the vessel which extends into the tunica media. Hemorrhage then follows the tear into the media and compresses the vascular lumen. This can result in rupture and massive hemorrhage. The vessel does not typically exhibit pronounced dilatation.

## ❏❏ What is a varicose vein?

These are superficial veins, typically in the lower extremities, that are torturous and dilated secondary to a state of increased pressure for a variety of reasons. The valves in the veins become incompetent which produces venous stasis with possible complications including potentially stasis dermatitis.

## ❏❏ What vessels account for the development of thrombophlebitis?

Greater than 90% of the cases arise in the deep veins of the lower extremities. In addition, but much less commonly, the periprostatic venous plexus (males) and the pelvic veins (females) are the next most likely source.

## ❏❏ What does one see clinically in lymphangitis?

Classically, there are red streaks in the skin corresponding to the path of the lymphatics as well as associated regional lymphadenopathy.

## ❏❏ What is the name of the vascular lesion which is composed of large, dilated lymphatic spaces typically in the neck of children?

Cystic hygroma or cavernous lymphangioma.

## ❏❏ What are the two filaments which make up a sarcomere and produce muscle contraction?

Myosin (thick) and actin (thin).

## ❏❏ In general terms, what is the most common arrangement of vascular perfusion of the heart by the coronary arteries?

The left anterior descending (LAD) supplies most of the apex, the anterior left ventricle, and anterior 2/3 of the interventricular septum. The right coronary supplies the right ventricular free wall, the posterior 1/3 of the ventricular septum, and 1/2 of the posterior left ventricle. Whichever coronary artery is the originator of the posterior descending coronary artery is then assigned as dominant (most are right dominant).

## ❏❏ What are the cytologic features of cardiac hypertrophy?

The myocytes become increased in size with enlarged, hyperchromatic nuclei which sometimes assume a "boxcar" shape. Myofiber disarray is seen in cardiomyopathy.

## ❏❏ What are the primary clinical signs of left-sided congestive heart failure?

Pulmonary rales, often basal, cardiomegaly, an S3 gallop, and pulsus alternans.

## ❏❏ Why are hemosiderin laden macrophages sometimes referred to as "heart failure cells"?

The macrophages phagocytose transferrin from the fluid of pulmonary edema and hemoglobin from erythrocytes which leak from pulmonary capillaries. Thus, the presence of hemosiderin laden macrophages indicates that the patient has suffered from pulmonary edema or congestive heart failure at a prior time.

## ❏❏ What is the most frequent cause of pure right-sided heart failure?

Cor pulmonale.

## ❏❏ In pronounced right-sided heart failure of chronic nature, what is the classic pathologic finding in the liver?

The liver begins with passive congestion, eventually can develop centrilobular necrosis, and ultimately results in central fibrosis hence the term "cardiac sclerosis".

❏❏  **What is Prinzmetal's angina?**

This is also referred to as variant angina and is characterized by chest pain at rest and is thought to be due to coronary artery spasm.

❏❏  **What is the first histologic finding one can see in an acute myocardial infarction?**

Wavy fibers.

❏❏  **When can you often determine grossly that there has been a myocardial infarction?**

Not usually sooner than 12 and often not until 24 hours after the ischemic event.

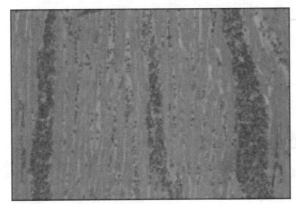

MYOCARDIAL INFARCTION

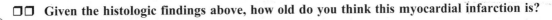

❏❏  **Given the histologic findings above, how old do you think this myocardial infarction is?**

Several hours to a day old.  There is coagulative necrosis with loss of nuclei, edema, and hemorrhage. However, the neutrophilic infiltrate is sparse and that typically peaks at two to three days.

❏❏  **Describe the gross changes that one finds as a myocardial infarction develops.**

Very early on, within hours, you will likely not see any change.  By 24 hours, the area of infarction will likely appear pale.  From 24-72 hours, the pallor continues with subsequent development of hyperemia. Gradually, the center of the lesion begins to turn yellow and becomes soft with persistence of the hyperemic rim of tissue over the course of the next several days.  By 10 days, the yellow appearance is most prominent and neovasculization begins manifesting as a red appearance on the border.  Over the course of the next several weeks, the area scars with development of white, fibrous tissue.

❏❏  **How common is sudden death following a myocardial infarction?**

Very, 20% of patients will be dead within two hours.

❏❏  **What is the most common site of cardiac rupture following myocardial infarction and when does it occur?**

The most likely time for rupture is four to up to seven days following the infarction.  The most common site is the left ventricular free wall, followed by the interventricular septum, and least commonly, papillary muscle rupture.

❏❏  **If one develops pericarditis following a myocardial infarction, when does it typically evolve?**

Within 24-72 hours following the infarct.  Of course, this typically occurs over the site of the infarction.

❏❏  What is the most common cause of death following myocardial infarction (MI)?

Ventricular fibrillation can occur within 48 hours of myocardial infarction, even if the infarction is quite small, and is the most common cause of death following MI.

❏❏  What is the most common cause of a focal, saccular aneurysm of the coronary arteries?

End stage involvement by polyarteritis nodosa, and Kawasaki's disease which shows diffuse involvement of the coronary arteries.

❏❏  What condition is most commonly associated with development of spontaneous dissection of a coronary artery?

Nearly half of the cases are found in women who are pregnant. The left anterior descending is four times more commonly involved than the right coronary artery.

❏❏  Classically, how much does a coronary artery lumen have to be narrowed to be "significant" as a cause of subsequent myocardial ischemia?

75% or greater.

❏❏  When does the level of CPK-MB peak following a myocardial infarction?

18 hours.

❏❏  What is the term used to describe dark, eosinophilic bands which appear across myocytes in ischemia and represent telescoped sarcomeres?

Contraction band necrosis.

❏❏  In the vast majority of cases, what is the mechanism of death in someone who suffers a sudden cardiac death (death within an hour of symptoms)?

An arrhythmia.

❏❏  What is the most prominent morphologic change seen in the heart in hypertensive heart disease?

Concentric left ventricular hypertrophy.

❏❏  What is cor pulmonale?

This is essentially a right-sided hypertensive heart disease. That is, the right ventricle becomes thickened as a direct result of pulmonary hypertension.

❏❏  What is the cause of acute cor pulmonale?

This is dilatation of the right ventricle which occurs as a result of massive or "saddle" pulmonary embolus.

❏❏  What is the most common cause of chronic cor pulmonale?

Chronic obstructive pulmonary disease (COPD).

❏❏  Of the various valve abnormalities, what is the most common?

Aortic stenosis.

❏❏  What happens to the levels of the LDH1 and LDH2 isoenzymes following myocardial infarction?

The normal ratio of LDH1 and LDH2, LDH2 > LDH1, reverses (LDH1 > LDH 2) owing to a disproportionate increase in LDH1.

☐☐  **What is the most common cause of death in hospitalized patients who have suffered an acute myocardial infarction?**

Cardiogenic shock as a result of a large infarction (greater than 40% of the left ventricle).

☐☐  **What is Dressler's syndrome?**

Pericardial effusion, fever, and pericarditis which develops from two weeks to months following an infarction.

☐☐  **What is the cause of Dressler's syndrome?**

No one knows.

☐☐  **What are some of the clinical signs and symptoms of malignant hypertension?**

Papilledema, retinal hemorrhage, encephalopathy, angina, and cardiac and/or renal failure.

☐☐  **Where is renin stored and what is the stimulus for its release?**

Renin is stored in the juxtaglomerular cells.  Its release is mediated by decreased pressure in the afferent arterioles, decreased sodium in the distal tubules, or direct sympathetic stimulation.                vasoconstriction

☐☐  **Where is atrial natriuritic factor stored?**

It is found in certain, specialized cells in the atria of the heart.

☐☐  **What is the most common cause of noncongenital (acquired) aortic stenosis?**

Old age or wear and tear resulting in fibronodular and sometimes calcific thickening of the valve. Rheumatic fever accounts for fewer than 10% of cases of acquired aortic stenosis.  In a bicuspid aortic valve, acquired stenosis occurs in patients in their 50s and 60s while tricuspid, otherwise normal aortic valves do not develop these changes typically until the patient is in his/her 70s or 80s.

☐☐  **What does the mitral valve look like in patients with aortic stenosis secondary to aging changes?**

Normal.  In contrast, patients with rheumatic fever typically have changes in their mitral valve in addition to their aortic valve.

☐☐  **How common is a congenitally bicuspid aortic valve?**

1-2% of the general population.

☐☐  **Who is most likely to develop mitral valve annular calcification?**

Elderly women.

☐☐  **How common is a "floppy" mitral valve resulting in mitral valve prolapse?**

It affects up to 10% of the population, by far most commonly in young women.

☐☐  **Besides connective tissue diseases like Marfan syndrome, what are some phenotypic changes seen in some patients with mitral valve prolapse?**

Some people have scoliosis; a straight, stiff back; and a high, arched palate.

❏❏ **What are the four main complications which occur in a very small number of patients with mitral valve prolapse?**

Infective endocarditis, mitral insufficiency, stroke or distal emboli, and arrhythmias which can cause sudden death in a small group of patients.

❏❏ **Which organism is associated with the development of rheumatic fever?**

Group A beta-hemolytic streptococci.

❏❏ **What are the major Jones criteria for diagnosing rheumatic fever?**

Carditis, polyarthritis, Sydenham's chorea, erythema marginatum, and subcutaneous nodules. In addition to evidence of a preceding group A streptococcal infection, one must have either two major Jones criteria or a major and two minor criteria to diagnose rheumatic fever.

❏❏ **A person with rheumatic fever may have elevated antibody titers to what substances produced by the streptococcus?**

Antibodies to streptolysin O (ASO) and hyaluronidase.

❏❏ **What are the minor manifestations of acute rheumatic fever according to the Jones criteria?**

Arthralgia, fever, elevated titers of acute phase reactants, and a prolonged PR interval on electrocardiogram.

❏❏ **Which part of the valve is typically involved in rheumatic fever?**

The entire valve, including the chordae tendineae, which serves as a clue to the changes seen in the valve being secondary to a post inflammatory process.

❏❏ **What age group most frequently develops acute rheumatic fever?**

Children age 6-15. It is very unusual in children less than 5 years old.

❏❏ **In acute rheumatic fever, where does one find Aschoff bodies?**

Anywhere in the heart, the pericardium, myocardium, or endocardium. They are composed of an area of necrosis surrounded by lymphocytes, macrophages, fewer plasma cells, and large activated histiocytes which are termed Anitschkow cells or Aschoff cells.

❏❏ **In a patient with a systolic ejection murmur and gastrointestinal hemorrhage, what is the most likely valvular abnormality?**

Calcific aortic stenosis has a fairly common association with gastrointestinal hemorrhage.

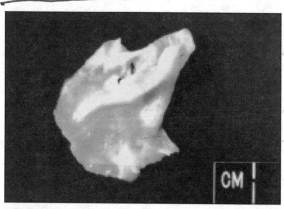

MITRAL VALVE WITH POST-INFLAMMATORY CHANGE

❏❏ **Based on the changes seen in the mitral valve leaflet shown above, what is the most likely etiology?**

Note the thickened, fused chordae tendineae, most consistent with post inflammatory change, with rheumatic fever being by far the most likely etiology.

❏❏ **What is the most common cause of acute aortic regurgitation?**

Infective endocarditis.

❏❏ **What is the most common location on a valve for the vegetations of rheumatic heart disease?**

These are traditionally characterized by small vegetations in a row along the line of closure of the valve leaflet.

❏❏ **Traditionally, what is the location of the vegetations seen in systemic lupus erythematosus?**

The lesions are typically found on the mitral and tricuspid valves and are small, nonbacterial and typically found on the under surface of the AV valve but may be found on either or both sides of the leaflets. This is referred to as Libman-Sacks endocarditis.

❏❏ **What is another term used to describe nonbacterial thrombotic endocarditis (NBTE)?**

Marantic endocarditis.

❏❏ **What particular type of carcinoma has a specific association with development of bland or marantic endocarditis?**

Mucinous adenocarcinoma, typically arising in either the pancreas, gastrointestinal tract, or ovary.

❏❏ **What organism is the most frequent cause of subacute infective endocarditis?**

Streptococci of the viridans group.

❏❏ **Which organism is the most common cause of acute infective endocarditis?**

Staphylococcus aureus.

❏❏ **Which cardiac valve is most commonly involved with Libman-Sacks endocarditis?**

The tricuspid valve followed by the mitral and pulmonic valves and, least frequently, the aortic valve.

❏❏ **What is the most common site of involvement of infective endocarditis in intravenous drug users?**

Remember, this is classically a right-sided endocarditis, with the tricuspid valve being the most frequent.

❏❏ **What are Osler's nodes and Janeway lesions?**

Osler's nodes are tender, erythematous punctate lesions found on the hands and feet while Janeway lesions are hemorrhagic, raised areas found on the palms and soles which are painless. Both lesions are found in sepsis related to infective endocarditis.

❏❏ **What are the most frequent organisms causing infective endocarditis of prosthetic valves?**

Staphylococcus epidermidis and S. aureus in the relatively early postoperative course while streptococci become more prominent later.

❏❏ **What are the three general categories of cardiomyopathy?**

Dilated, hypertrophic, and restrictive.

❏❏ **What type of cardiomyopathy does alcohol cause?**

Dilated.

❏❏ **What type of cardiomyopathy is sometimes seen in infants of diabetic mothers?**

Hypertrophic.

❏❏ **What specific chemotherapeutic agent is classically associated with potential development of a dilated cardiomyopathy?**

Adriamycin.

❏❏ **What are the three prominent histologic features seen in a hypertrophic cardiomyopathy?**

Prominent myocyte hypertrophy, interstitial fibrosis, and myofiber disarray characterized by haphazard arrangement of individual myocytes and small groups of myocytes.

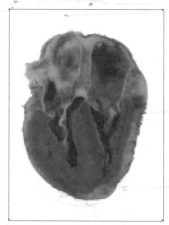

ASYMMETRIC HYPERTROPHY IN HYPERTROPHIC CARDIOMYOPATHY
*(Photo courtesy of Stanley J. Radio, MD - University of Nebraska Medical Center)*

❏❏ **In the majority of cases of hypertrophic cardiomyopathy as depicted above, how is the hypertrophy distributed amongst the ventricular septum, left ventricular free wall, and right ventricle?**

The vast majority of cases demonstrate asymmetric hypertrophy of the ventricular septum creating a ratio of the ventricular septum (VS) to the left ventricle (LV) of greater than 1.3:1.0. In a minority of cases the hypertrophy is evenly distributed between the VS and LV.

❏❏ **What type of cardiomyopathy is associated with Friedreich's ataxia?**

Hypertrophic.

❏❏ **Of the three general types of cardiomyopathy, which has the most prominent genetic or heritable pathogenesis?**

Hypertrophic cardiomyopathy is familial in approximately 50% of cases with an autosomal dominant pattern showing variable expression.

❏❏ **What is the frequency of sudden death in patients with hypertrophic cardiomyopathy?**

In adults, it is a 2-3% incidence per year, and you may double that for children.

❏❏ **In patients with a restrictive cardiomyopathy, what would you expect to see with regard to ventricular and atrial chamber size?**

The ventricles are typically normal or slightly enlarged while the atria classically exhibit bilateral dilatation.

❏❏  **In carcinoid syndrome, which side of the heart is typically involved?**

The right side shows the most prominent hypertrophy and the patients typically develop right-sided cardiac failure.

❏❏  **What are the most common etiologic agents of myocarditis?**

The vast majority of myocarditis is viral in origin and include Coxsackie virus A and B, ECHO, polio virus, and influenza A and B as the most common causative agents.

❏❏  **What is the most common protozoan infection of the heart?**

Trypanosoma cruzi in Chagas' disease. Some 80% of patients with Chagas' disease develop myocarditis.

❏❏  **What is the most common helminth infecting the heart?**

Trichinosis.

❏❏  **How common is myocarditis in patients with Lyme disease?**

Quite, nearly 70% of patients with Lyme disease develop myocarditis and may develop an AV block.

❏❏  **What dose of an anthracycline agent is necessary for a toxic myocardial injury?**

Typically, the dose is greater than 500 mg/square meter of body surface area.

❏❏  **What type of cardiomyopathy may develop as a consequence or manifestation of a patient's multiple myeloma?**

A restrictive cardiomyopathy secondary to amyloidosis.

❏❏  **What is the term used to describe the presence of 35 ml of serous fluid in the pericardial sack?**

Normal. There is normally 30-50 ml of clear fluid in the pericardium. If it is greater than that, then one has an effusion.

❏❏  **What are the major causes of acute serous pericarditis?**

These are typically noninfectious in nature and include rheumatic fever, systemic lupus erythematosus, scleroderma, some tumors, and uremia.

❏❏  **What are the most common cause of fibrinous and serofibrinous pericarditis?**

Acute myocardial infarction, Dressler's syndrome, uremia, chest radiotherapy, rheumatic fever, systemic lupus erythematosus, cardiac surgery, pneumonia or pleural infection, and trauma.

❏❏  **What is the characteristic clinical finding in some cases of fibrinous pericarditis?**

A distinct, loud pericardial friction rub on auscultation.

❏❏  **What are the most serious complications from pericarditis?**

Significant fluid accumulation in the pericardial sac can cause a tamponade and fibrous scarring as the pericarditis resolves. It can result in a restrictive pericarditis. In addition, adhesive mediastinopericarditis can develop when the pericardial sac is completely obliterated with resultant strict adherence to the surrounding mediastinal structures resulting in massive cardiac hypertrophy and dilatation.

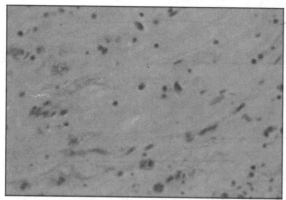

ATRIAL MYXOMA

❏❏  **What is the most common primary cardiac tumor?**

Benign myxoma (photo above) which occurs predominantly in middle aged females.

❏❏  **Anatomically, where are most myxomas located?**

They can occur anywhere including valves; however, 90% are located within the atria, and of those, 80% are located in the right atrium. Classically, they are found near the fossa ovalis.

❏❏  **How do myxomas often produce so-called constitutional symptoms?**

It is thought that the symptoms are secondary to production of interleukin-6 by the tumor which evokes an acute phase response.

❏❏  **What is the most common primary tumor of the heart found in infants and children?**

Rhabdomyoma. Over 90% of these tumors are multiple within a patient.

❏❏  **What are some of the differences between familial and nonfamilial cardiac myxomas?**

The familial cases are more often male (2:1), younger, and more often multifocal.  In contrast, nonfamilial cases are found in females three quarters of the time, have an average age twice that of in familial cases, and are frequently multicentric.

❏❏  **Embryologically, when does the cardiovascular system undergo its major development?**

From weeks 3-8.

❏❏  **By far, what is the most common cardiac malformation?**

Ventricular septal defect makes up about 1/4 of all cardiac malformations.

❏❏  **Which cardiac malformations demonstrate the greatest male preponderance?**

Both aortic atresia (hypoplastic left heart syndrome) and aortic stenosis feature a 3:1 male incidence.

❏❏  **What cardiac malformations are associated with maternal rubella infection occurring during the first trimester?**

Patent ductus arteriosus (PDA), pulmonary valvular and/or arterial stenosis, aortic stenosis, tetralogy of Fallot, and ventricular septal defect (VSD).

❏❏  **What is the most common congenital heart disease resulting in cyanosis?**

Tetralogy of Fallot which is composed of VSD, subpulmonary stenosis, overriding aorta, and right ventricular hypertrophy.

❏❏  **What is Eisenmenger's syndrome?**

This is the reversal of a left to right shunt secondary to pulmonary vascular changes resulting in an eventual right to left shunt and cyanosis.

❏❏  **How common is a patent foramen ovale?**

A small, slit-like patent foramen ovale occurs in about a third of the population;however, owing to pressure and its flap-like structure, it is usually nonfunctioning and asymptomatic.

❏❏  **Of the major types of atrial septal defects (ASD), what is the most common?**

The secundum-type accounts for some 90% of ASDs.

❏❏  **How common is coarctation of the aorta?**

It is approximately 5% of all cardiac malformations and is associated with a bicuspid aortic valve in half of the cases.  Transposition of the great vessels is slightly more common than coarctation of the aorta.

❏❏  **What is Epstein's anomaly?**

This abnormality involves a downward displacement of the tricuspid valve into the right ventricle with associated redundancy of the anterior leaflet of the valve with annular dilatation.  This results in varying degrees of regurgitation, subsequent right ventricular dilatation, and ultimately heart failure.

❏❏  **What is the utility of indomethicin in the treatment of patent ductus arteriosus?**

It can suppress prostaglandin E synthesis thus preventing its vasodilatory effects and allowing closure of the ductus.

❏❏  **What are the two classic types of coarctation of the aorta?**

The preductal and postductal forms.  Commonly, the preductal is referred to as the "infantile" form while the postductal is the "adult" form.  As suggested, the preductal form often manifests signs and symptoms very soon after birth while the postductal or adult form may not be diagnosed until adult life.

❏❏  **What is the radiographic change that can be seen in postductal coarctation of the aorta?**

In this form of coarctation of the aorta, collateral circulation between the precoarctation arteries and the postcoarctation arteries occurs in the intercostal and internal mammary arteries which become enlarged and can cause erosions or "notching" of the inferior aspects of the ribs which can be detected on chest x-ray.

# PULMONARY

❐❐ **What are the basic alveolar lining cells?**

Type I alveolar cells or type I pneumocytes. *90%*

❐❐ **What are the cells that produce the surfactant and serve a reparative function in the lung?**

Type II alveolar cells or type II pneumocytes.

❐❐ **How do alveolar macrophages traverse from one alveolar space to another?**

There are tiny holes in the septa which are called the pores of Kohn which allow for this transit.

❐❐ **What is the name of the nonciliated secretory cells which are interspersed in the bronchial lining and contain electron dense core granules?**

These are clara cells and their exact function in producing secretions is not agreed upon.

❐❐ **What are the five basic phases of embryonic lung development?**

Embryonal phase (weeks 4-6), pseudoglandular (weeks 7-16), canalicular (acinar) phase (weeks 17-27), sacular phase (weeks 28-35), and alveolar phase (weeks 36-delivery).

❐❐ **What is the most common type of tracheoesophageal fistula?**

This is the presence of esophageal atresia with an associated fistula from the trachea to the lower esophageal segment which comprises over 80% of the cases.

❐❐ **What is bronchial isomerism?**

This is a congenital bronchial anomaly in which a patient has bilateral right or left lungs. The condition is associated with several variants of polysplenia-asplenia syndromes and often has other abnormalities including gut malrotation.

❐❐ **What is a bronchogenic cyst?**

This is a cyst formed from an accessory lung bud from the foregut that gets separated from the bulk of the tracheobronchial tree during development resulting in a cyst lined by bronchial epithelium.

❐❐ **What is a bronchopulmonary sequestration?**

This is lung parenchyma that is not connected to the rest of the lung which obtains its blood supply from a systemic artery.

❐❐ **Of the two types of bronchopulmonary sequestration, which is most commonly associated with other anomalies such as pectus excavatum and is three times more common in males?**

Extralobar sequestration. The intralobar sequestration is nearly always found in one of the lower lobes (left lower lobe most commonly) and is characterized by symptoms of infection.

❐❐ **In obstructive atelectasis, if there is a mediastinal shift, which way does it go?**

Toward the involved lung.

◻◻ **With compressive atelectasis, in which direction does the mediastinum shift?**

Away from the involved lung.

◻◻ **What is the congenital anomaly which is marked by abnormal bronchiolar structures of varying sizes or location which has three variants?**

Congenital cystic adenomatoid malformation. Type I is composed of large cysts and accounts for half of the cases, type II has many small cysts and comprises 40% of the cases, while type III is more solid and the least frequent variant.

◻◻ **What is congenital emphysema and which part of the lung is normally affected?**

This is also termed, more correctly, congenital pulmonary overinflation and is characterized by overinflation of the pulmonary parenchyma due to obstruction of a bronchus. It most frequently involves a single lobe, and over 90% of the cases are the upper or middle lobe.

◻◻ **What is the pathologic correlate to the clinical term "adult respiratory distress syndrome" (ARDS)?**

Diffuse alveolar damage.

◻◻ **What are the so-called "heart failure cells"?**

These are hemosiderin-laden macrophages which occur as a result of engorgement of the alveolar capillaries with subsequent alveolar microhemorrhages.

◻◻ **In ARDS, where is the initial injury?**

The first insult occurs to the endothelium of the capillaries or, less commonly, the alveolar epithelium. This separation is somewhat arbitrary owing to the fact that both the capillaries and alveolar epithelium are eventually affected.

◻◻ **Roughly, what is the death rate in patients who develop ARDS?**

It is around 60% fatal.

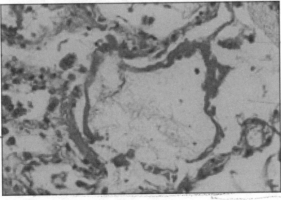

HYALINE MEMBRANE IN ARDS

◻◻ **Briefly, what are the stages of diffuse alveolar damage?**

Initially, there is an edematous stage with associated vascular congestion and fibrin deposition resulting in hyaline membrane formation (see above photo). Following that, the type II pneumocytes proliferate in an attempt to repair the damage resulting in intraalveolar fibrosis and eventual widening of the septa owing to an interstitial cell proliferation with collagen deposition.

❏❏ **What is the most common source of pulmonary emboli?**

The deep veins of the legs account for 90-95% of the cases.

❏❏ **How common is pulmonary embolus as a cause of death in hospitalized patients?**

Common, perhaps 10% of acute deaths in the hospital are attributable to pulmonary emboli.

❏❏ **Describe a typical pulmonary infarct.**

They are classically wedge-shaped, subpleural, hemorrhagic, and found in the lower lobes where there is the greatest amount of blood flow.

❏❏ **What is the pulmonary condition which is rather heterogeneous in nature and occurs in neonates who were premature and received oxygen and ventilation therapy for hyaline membrane disease?**

Bronchopulmonary dysplasia which may represent a continuing organization of diffuse alveolar damage.

❏❏ **What is the gross change that you see in pulmonary hypertension in the pulmonary vasculature?**

Yellow linear fatty streaks are seen in the vessel walls. Microscopically, there may be intimal proliferation, medial hypertrophy, extension of alveolar smooth muscle, and plexiform lesions.

❏❏ **In the vast majority of cases, what is the etiology of pulmonary interstitial air or pulmonary interstitial emphysema?**

Ventilator therapy for hyaline membrane disease or bronchopulmonary dysplasia.

❏❏ **What is the most common age for development of primary pulmonary hypertension?**

It is most common in the third to fifth decades of life.

❏❏ **What type of heart failure develops in longstanding primary pulmonary hypertension?**

Cor pulmonale.

❏❏ **What is the five year survival rate in primary pulmonary hypertension?**

About 35%.

❏❏ **What is pulmonary veno-occlusive disease (PVOD)?**

This is the fibrous obliteration of small veins in the lungs occasionally with thromboses. It is a rare cause of pulmonary hypertension, occurs in younger patients, has no significant sex predilection, and the etiology is unknown.

❏❏ **What are some clinical entities which are disorders characterized by obstructive airway disease?**

Chronic bronchitis, bronchiectasis, asthma, bronchiolitis, and emphysema.

❏❏ **What are the two manners in which one may develop expiratory air flow obstruction?**

This can be a product of either loss of the airway's elasticity/ability to recoil or from a physical or anatomic narrowing of the airway.

❑❑ **By definition, what are the criteria for the diagnosis for chronic bronchitis?**

Cough with sputum production on the majority of days, at least three months a year for greater than or equal to two successive years. Of course, there can be no other underlying disease to account for these changes.

❑❑ **What happens to the mucus gland to wall thickness ratio in a bronchus of a patient with chronic bronchitis?**

It increases, that is, the mucus glands increase in size, although this correlates better with the degree of sputum production and the history of cigarette smoking than with the degree of measured airway obstruction.

❑❑ **What are the most common organisms associated with exacerbations of chronic bronchitis?**

Haemophilus influenzae, Streptococcus pneumoniae, and Branhamella catarrhalis.

❑❑ **What are some of the anatomic and histologic changes which are seen in the small airways of smokers?**

There is narrowing of the bronchioles; they undergo goblet cell metaplasia; there is airway mucus plugging; the smooth muscle in the airways increases in thickness; and there is associated inflammation and fibrosis. In addition, in the larger airways, there is squamous metaplasia.

❑❑ **What is emphysema?**

This is a form of chronic obstructive pulmonary disease clearly associated with smoking that is typified by abnormal and permanent increase in the size of air spaces distal to the terminal bronchiole with associated alveolar wall destruction. air trapping

❑❑ **In general, what degree of emphysema is necessary to produce clinical symptoms?**

Greater than 20% of parenchymal involvement.

❑❑ **What are the four types of emphysema?**

Centriacinar (central lobular), panacinar, paraseptal, and irregular.

❑❑ **Of the four types of emphysema listed above, which is the most common?**

Irregular emphysema is almost always found in association with scarring and, with meticulous inspection, most lungs examined at autopsy will be found to have some degree of irregular emphysema.

❑❑ **What is the most severely affected site of panacinar emphysema within the lungs?**

Typically, although both upper and lower lobes are involved, the bases tend to have the worst lesions.

❑❑ **Where does one typically find centriacinar emphysema?**

The upper lobe is the most common site and typically most severely involved.

❑❑ **What is the most common cause of spontaneous pneumothorax in young patients?**

Spontaneous rupture of apical bullae.

168

❑❑  **What is thought to be the cause of the septal destruction seen in emphysema?**

Proteolytic enzymes.  Smokers have higher levels of elastase as smoke stimulates its release from neutrophils which are also present in greater numbers due to the effects of smoking.  In addition, smoking also increases the activity of elastolytic proteases in macrophages and ultimately results in the inhibition of alpha-1-antitrypsin.

❑❑  **What is the action of alpha-1-antitrypsin?**

It inhibits proteases, most significantly elastase.

❑❑  **What type of emphysema is associated with alpha-1-antitrypsin deficiency?**

Panacinar with a lower lobe preference.

❑❑  **If one wanted to demonstrate the alpha-1-antitrypsin protein accumulation in hepatocytes secondary to alpha-1-antitrypsin deficiency, what tissue stain would one perform?**

These globules are resistant to diastase digestion with a PAS stain, thus PAS with diastase is the stain of choice.

❑❑  **What is senile emphysema?**

It is not emphysema at all, rather  it is simply a reference to the enlarged, overdistended air sacs seen in lungs with aging.  There is no true alveolar destruction.

LUNG

❑❑  **Based on the image above and a history of silica exposure, what is your diagnosis?**

Alveolar proteinosis.  Most cases are of unknown cause although sometimes there is a silica exposure history.

❑❑  **What are some of the causes of intrinsic asthma?**

Aspirin, infections, stress, exercise, cold air, and inhaled irritants.

❑❑  **In patients with asthma triggered by aspirin, what other clinical findings would you expect?**

They have nasal polyps and recurrent rhinitis.

❑❑  **What is a Curshman spiral?**

These are characteristic mucus plugs which contain bronchial epithelium arranged in a spiral formation and are seen in patients with asthma.

❐❐ **What is the name given to the collections of a crystalloid material derived from eosinophil membrane protein which is sometimes seen in patients with asthma?**

Charcot-Leyden crystals.

❐❐ **What is Kartagener's syndrome?**

This syndrome results in bronchiectasis, sinusitis, and situs inversus with the two former components secondary to defective ciliary motility owing to absent or irregular dynein arms. It is inherited in an autosomal recessive fashion.

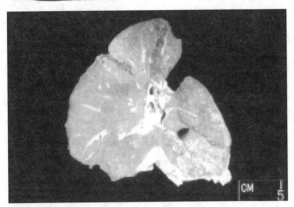

LOBAR PNEUMONIA

❐❐ **What is the most common cause of lobar pneumonia?**

Approximately 90% are caused by Streptococcus pneumoniae (usually types I, II, III, and VII).

❐❐ **What is the major causative organism of so-called atypical pneumonia?**

Mycoplasma pneumoniae.

❐❐ **What lobe of the lung is classically involved in aspiration pneumonia?**

Right lower lobe.

❐❐ **What is the organism which can cause an epiglottitis-tracheitis that can result in massive airway obstruction in children?**

Haemophilus influenzae.

❐❐ **Of the gram-negative organisms causing pneumonia in adults, which has the highest mortality?**

Pseudomonas aeruginosa which has a mortality rate that can be greater than 80%.

❐❐ **What are the two clinical syndromes caused by Legionella pneumonophila?**

So-called Pontiac fever which is a febrile illness with a relatively short incubation time and very little mortality. The other clinical scenario is pneumonia which is less common but features a longer course with a 25% mortality.

❐❐ **Describe the gram stain of the Legionellae organism.**

It typically does not stain well with a gram's stain. Rather, you must use something like the Dieterle stain, or better yet, frozen tissue can be used to apply a fluorescent antibody method.

❑❑  **In pulmonary abscesses caused by anaerobic organisms, what is the most frequent mechanism of the infection?**

Aspiration.

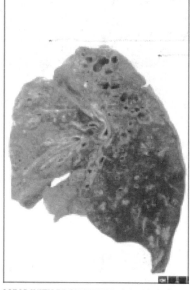

LUNG WITH BRONCHIECTASIS AND MUCUS PLUGGING
*(Photo courtesy of Julie Breiner, M.D., University of Nebraska Medical Center)*

❑❑  **This autosomal recessive disorder in children often results in treatment by lung transplantation.  What is your diagnosis?**

Cystic fibrosis.

❑❑  **Of the various types of pulmonary fibrosis, which predominantly feature a diffuse distribution?**

Acute interstitial pneumonia (Hamman-Rich syndrome) and desquamative interstitial pneumonia (DIP).  In contrast, idiopathic organizing pneumonia (bronchiolitis obliterans-organizing pneumonia or BOOP), crytpogenic organizing pneumonitis (COP), usual interstitial pneumonia (UIP), and nonspecific interstitial pneumonia (cellular interstitial pneumonia or CIP) are patchy in their distribution.

❑❑  **In UIP, what is the most common etiology?**

Unknown, 40% have a prodrome viral-like illness and 20% have a collagen vascular disorder.

❑❑  **Of the major forms of pulmonary fibrosis, which characteristically has a heterogeneous appearance in that there may be areas of more end stage change adjacent to active inflammatory change?**

UIP.

❑❑  **Describe the prognosis of UIP.**

While indolent, it is progressive and has a poor survival with a median survival of about five years.  Fewer than 1 in 5 patients respond to therapy with steroids.

❑❑  **Describe the radiographic appearance of the chest in cases of UIP and DIP.**

DIP features a "ground glass" infiltrate in the bases, or the chest may actually be normal radiographically. UIP shows diffuse bilateral interstitial infiltrates which are worse in the lower lungs; however, this is not diagnostic.

**❑❑ What is the prognosis of DIP compared to UIP?**

DIP is much better although it can progress to "honeycomb lung". Histologically, the lesions of DIP are homogeneous without the presence of fibrosis and active inflammation simultaneously as in UIP.

**❑❑ What is the causative agent in most cases of allergic bronchopulmonary mycosis which typically occurs in atopic individuals?**

Aspergillus fumigatis or one of the other Aspergillus species.

**❑❑ What are the most likely causative agents of "farmer's lung"?**

Micropolyspora faeni and Thermoactinomyces viridis from moldy hay.

**❑❑ What is the causative agent of maple bark stripper's disease?**

Cryptostroma corticale.

**❑❑ What is the causative agent of woodworker's lung?**

Species of Alternaria.

**❑❑ With regard to the pneumoconioses, what size of particle represents the greatest hazard by virtue of its ability to reach the air sacs and terminal airways?**

Those that are less than 5 microns in diameter.

**❑❑ In a typical hypersensitivity pneumonitis (extrinsic allergic alveolitis), when do the symptoms begin following exposure to the causative antigen?**

In a matter of hours. The symptoms, which may include cough, shortness of breath, and fever, occur quite abruptly. Classically, this occurs within 4-8 hours of exposure to the inciting agent.

**❑❑ What is simple coal worker's pneumoconiosis?**

This is a pneumoconiosis as a result of exposure to coal dust which is characterized by the presence of "coal macules" and "coal nodules". The macules are tiny pigmented foci consisting of carbon-laden macrophages in the lung, particularly the upper lobes. The nodules are pigmented and feature excess collagen deposition. These lesions are found primarily around respiratory bronchioles.

**❑❑ What is Caplan's syndrome?**

This is the presence of rheumatoid arthritis and a pneumoconiosis resulting in nodular pulmonary lesions that resemble rheumatoid nodules with central necrosis and surrounding histiocytes.

**❑❑ What part of the lung is typically initially involved in cases of silicosis?**

Upper lobes.

**❑❑ What is the association, if any, of silicosis with the development of lung cancer?**

Unknown, there does not appear to be definitive evidence in humans that it is carcinogenic at this time.

❑❑ **What is the radiographic feature of hilar lymph nodes that would be strong evidence for silicosis?**

So-called "egg shell" calcification.

❑❑ **What does the presence of asbestos bodies in the lung indicate?**

This is an indication of exposure to asbestos; however, this is certainly not diagnostic of the condition of asbestosis.

❑❑ **How does an asbestos body differ from a ferruginous body?**

A ferruginous body is simply the accumulation of iron on foreign material in the lung other than asbestos fibers. Histologically, the asbestos bodies feature a clear core representing the asbestos fiber as opposed to the general category of ferruginous bodies which have a dark core.

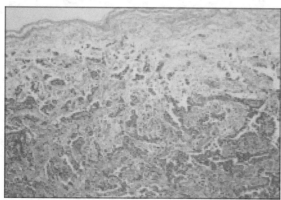

MALIGNANT MESOTHELIOMA

❑❑ **What are the four basic pleural diseases that can develop in patients exposed to asbestos?**

Benign pleural plaques, visceral pleural thickening, pleural effusions, and malignant mesothelioma.

❑❑ **What effect does cigarette smoking have on potential development of mesothelioma?**

None.

❑❑ **What is the risk, compared to the general population, of development of mesothelioma amongst workers who are exposed to asbestos?**

Greater than 1,000 times that of the general population.

❑❑ **What exposure associated pneumoconiosis closely mimics the findings in sarcoidosis?**

Beryllosis.

❑❑ **How common is pulmonary or hilar lymph node involvement in patients with sarcoidosis?**

90% of patients with sarcoidosis will have pulmonary involvement or bilateral hilar lymphadenopathy. This is the most consistent finding in sarcoidosis.

❑❑ **Compare the prevalence of sarcoidosis amongst African-Americans and Asians.**

Blacks are 10 times more likely to have sarcoidosis than whites and Asians almost never have it.

❑❑ **What is the classical histologic finding of pulmonary sarcoidosis?**

Multiple noncaseating granulomas with relatively few surrounding lymphocytes ("naked" granulomas) which are characteristically found along bronchovascular bundles. Central necrosis is rare but can occur.

❑❑ **The presence of Schaumann bodies and asteroid bodies are two histologic features which, although not pathognomonic, are characteristic of what condition?**

Sarcoidosis.

❑❑ **What are the three main categories of pulmonary hemorrhage syndromes?**

1. Goodpasture's syndrome
2. Hemosiderosis
3. Various vasculitides (hypersensitivity angiitis, lupus, and Wegener's granulomatosis)

❑❑ **What are the general characteristics of a patient with Goodpasture's syndrome?**

They are more commonly male and age 10-29. The most common cause of death is uremia.

*Kidney lung*

❑❑ **What is the therapy for Goodpasture's syndrome?**

Plasma exchange and immunosuppression.

❑❑ **What are the various manners in which rheumatoid arthritis can involve the lung?**

Pleural effusion, chronic pleuritis, diffuse interstitial pneumonia with fibrosis, intraparenchymal rheumatoid nodules, vasculitis, pulmonary hypertension, and rheumatoid nodules with pneumoconiosis (Caplan's syndrome).

❑❑ **What is the most common pulmonary manifestation of systemic lupus erythematosus (SLE)?**

Pleurisy occurs in about 1/3 of the patients with or without associated effusion.

❑❑ **Does scleroderma ever involve the lung?**

Of course, or I would not have asked. Following involvement of the skin, kidney and gastrointestinal tract, the lung is the next most common manifestation. In fact, the pulmonary involvement by scleroderma now is the number one cause of death in this disease.

❑❑ **Of the pulmonary hemorrhage syndromes, which is associated with the presence of HLA-DRw2 haplotype in the majority of patients?**

Goodpasture's syndrome.

❑❑ **What is the classic ultrastructural finding in the Langerhans cell seen in Langerhans histiocytosis?**

The presence of Birbeck granules.

❑❑ **What effect does cigarette smoking have on the presence of Langerhans cells in the lungs in patients without the diagnosis of Langerhans cell histiocytosis?**

They are increased.

❑❑ **What are the three different forms of pulmonary amyloidosis?**

Tracheobronchial involvement, nodular parenchymal involvement, or diffuse interstitial septal involvement.

❒❒  If one suspects amyloidosis, what stains can be performed on the pulmonary parenchyma to confirm that diagnosis?

Several stains including Congo red, thioflavin T or S.

❒❒  What is the basic difference in treatment between small cell carcinomas of the lung and non small cell carcinoma?

Non small cells are primarily treated surgically (of course only if resectable) while small cell carcinomas are not typically resected.

❒❒  What are the two most common forms of lung cancer?

Squamous cell carcinoma and adenocarcinoma each account for 1/3 of the cases.

❒❒  What are some of the known risk factors or etiologies of bronchogenic carcinoma?

Cigarette smoking, various industrial exposures (including radiation, asbestos, and beryllium), air pollution (including indoor radon gas), various genetic influences and possibly scars in the lung.

❒❒  In general, of the various types of lung cancer, which are most closely associated with smoking?

Squamous cell carcinoma and small cell carcinoma.

❒❒  In a female nonsmoker, what type of lung cancer is she most likely to develop?

Adenocarcinoma.

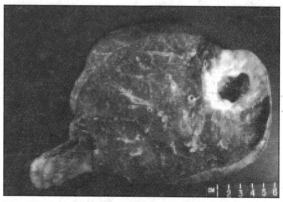

LUNG WITH PERIPHERAL TUMOR
*(Photo is courtesy of Julie Breiner, M.D., University of Nebraska Medical Center)*

❒❒  In contrast to squamous cell carcinomas of the lung, where do adenocarcinomas tend to arise?

Peripherally.

❒❒  What type of interstitial pneumonia is associated with a possible progression to lymphoma?

Lymphoid interstitial pneumonia (LIP).

❒❒  What is the association of a transudative pleural effusion in association with an ovarian fibroma called?

Meigs' syndrome.

❑❑  **What is the most common pulmonary hamartoma?**

Cartilaginous tissue with invaginations which are lined by respiratory-type epithelium.

❑❑  **What is the most frequent type of lung cancer in Japan?**

Adenocarcinoma.

❑❑  **What is the most common type of lymphoma involving the lung?**

Lymphoma typically involves the lung in a secondary fashion; however, primary lymphoma of the lung typically arises from the mucosa associated lymphoid tissue (MALT).

❑❑  **What are the three basic types of mesothelioma?**

Epithelial, sarcomatoid, and biphasic.

❑❑  **What is the most common benign tumor of the lung?**

Hamartoma.

❑❑  **What is the most common site of bronchioloalveolar carcinoma, peripheral or central?**

Peripheral, almost always.

❑❑  **Similarly, where do most bronchial carcinoids arise?**

They are typically centrally located.  About 1 in 5 arise as peripheral masses and are often associated with a spindle cell morphology.

❑❑  **What benign pulmonary tumor is characterized by a well circumscribed mass composed of cells with clear cytoplasm which are filled with glycogen and can be mistaken for metastatic renal cell carcinoma?**

Benign clear cell tumor ("sugar tumor").

❑❑  **What two types of pulmonary carcinomas are associated with potential development of paraneoplastic syndromes?**

Small cell carcinoma and squamous cell carcinoma.

❑❑  **What is the term given to a bronchogenic carcinoma arising in an apical location with involvement of C1, T1, and T2 with subsequent motor and sensory loss in addition to Horner's syndrome (ptosis, myosis, and anhydrosis)?**

Pancoast's tumor.

❑❑  **What type of interstitial pneumonia can occur in association with Sjogren's syndrome?**

Lymphoid interstitial pneumonia (LIP).

# MEDIASTINUM

☐☐ **What are some of the cystic lesions that can occur in the mediastinum?**

Parathyroid cysts, thymic cysts, bronchogenic cysts, pericardial cysts, enteric cysts, "cystic hygromas" or lymphangioma, cystic meningoceles, cystic teratoma, and cystic thymoma.

☐☐ **What is the differential diagnosis of a mass in the superior mediastinum?**

Lymphoma, thymoma, thyroid lesions, and parathyroid lesions.

☐☐ **What is the differential diagnosis of an anterior mediastinal mass?**

Thymoma, teratoma, lymphoma, thyroid lesions, and parathyroid lesions.

☐☐ **What is the differential diagnosis of a posterior mediastinal mass?**

Neurogenic tumors including schwannoma, lymphoma, and gastroenteric hernia.

☐☐ **What is the differential diagnosis of a mass in the middle mediastinum?**

Bronchogenic cyst, pericardial cyst, and lymphoma.

☐☐ **Which compartment of the mediastinum is most typically involved with acute mediastinitis?**

The middle mediastinum.  This typically requires surgical drainage.

☐☐ **What is the most frequent site of chronic mediastinitis?**

The anterior mediastinum.

☐☐ **What is the histologic picture seen in chronic fibrosing mediastinitis?**

It is typically consists of an ill-defined firm mass with dense fibrosis and sometimes granulomatous inflammation.

☐☐ **When there is granulomatous inflammation in a picture of chronic mediastinitis secondary to infection, what is the most common etiologic agent?**

Histoplasma capsulatum.

☐☐ **You are given information that a patient has a cystic lesion in the middle mediastinum which histologically contains cartilage and a columnar epithelial lining.  What is your diagnosis?**

Bronchogenic cyst.

☐☐ **In addition to chronic mediastinitis, what else should one consider when faced with a picture of mediastinal fibrosis and granulomatous inflammation?**

Seminoma and Hodgkin's disease.

☐☐ **Where in the mediastinum would you expect to find a seminoma?**

Anterior mediastinum.

❑❑  **In general terms, what is the most common lesion of the middle mediastinum?**

Benign cysts are by far most common; however, lymphoma may also arise here.

❑❑  **What are the two main types of thymic cysts?**

Unilocular with a thin wall and multilocular with a thick wall.  Unilocular cysts usually contain serous fluid while multilocular cysts have more turbid or even hemorrhagic cyst contents.

❑❑  **What is the most common type of lining seen in thymic cysts?**

A "squamoid" lining which is flattened and bland in unilocular cysts while it can be more exuberant and mixed with columnar appearing epithelium in multilocular cysts.

❑❑  **What type of epithelium typically lines a bronchogenic cyst?**

Respiratory epithelium which, of course, is defined as pseudostratified columnar epithelium which is often ciliated.

❑❑  **Describe the lining of pericardial cysts.**

It is typically a monolayer of mesothelium.

❑❑  **What age group typically is found to have enteric mediastinal cysts?**

These are typically found in patients in the first or second decade of life and for all intents and purposes are restricted to the posterior mediastinum.

❑❑  **What is thought to be the mechanism of rupture in enteric cysts?**

Enteric cysts are lined by an epithelial lining that can range from squamous to pseudostratified columnar and those that are gastroesophageal in nature have at least foci of gastric mucosa complete with chief and parietal cells which can produce acid and lead to rupture.

❑❑  **What is the name of the triad of a mediastinal paraganglioma, gastric stromal tumor, and pulmonary chondroma?**

Carney's triad.

❑❑  **In children, what type of lymphoma most commonly involves the mediastinum?**

Lymphoblastic lymphoma.

❑❑  **In adults, what type of lymphoma most frequently involves the mediastinum?**

Nodular sclerosis or mixed cellularity type of Hodgkin's disease.

❑❑  **What age patient is most likely to present with a cystic hygroma?**

Children.

❑❑  **What is the most common neoplasm found in the mediastinum?**

Thymoma.

❑❑  **What is the most common benign germ cell neoplasm occurring in the mediastinum?**

Mature (cystic) teratoma.

☐☐ **What is the accepted definition of an immature teratoma?**

The presence of immature neuroepithelial elements are necessary in order to confidently diagnose an immature teratoma.

☐☐ **What lymphoid neoplasm is found frequently as a solitary mass in the mediastinum and has a hyaline vascular form and a plasma cell variant?**

Angiofollicular hyperplasia (Castleman's disease).

☐☐ **Describe the typical patient with a gastroenteric cyst in the mediastinum.**

More than half the patients are less than one year old, it is more common in males, and they often have associated vertebral anomalies.

☐☐ **What is the most common primary sarcoma of the mediastinum?**

Leiomyosarcoma.

☐☐ **Among mediastinal tumors, how common are neurogenic tumors?**

Quite, they range from 20-40% of mediastinal tumors and typically are found in the posterior compartment.

☐☐ **A tumor of the mediastinum demonstrates Antoni A areas (cellular), Verocay bodies, and Antoni B areas (myxoid), what is it and where would you find it?**

This is a description of a neurilemoma or schwannoma which is the most frequent neurogenic tumor in the mediastinum and, as with all neurogenic tumors in the mediastinum, is found almost exclusively in the posterior compartment.

☐☐ **You identify a neurofibroma in the posterior mediastinum that exhibits a plexiform pattern of growth. What diagnosis does this patient carry?**

Neurofibromatosis or von Recklinghausen's disease.

☐☐ **What are some malignancies which can commonly involve the mediastinum either via direct extension or via metastatic spread?**

Esophageal carcinoma and bronchogenic carcinoma can spread directly to the mediastinum and many tumors including germ cell tumors, melanoma, breast, and renal carcinomas can metastasize to the mediastinum.

☐☐ **What is probably the most important predictor of behavior of a thymoma?**

Its local extent and growth.

☐☐ **What happens to the thymus in an infant in the neonatal intensive care unit with hyaline membrane disease?**

Any type of stress causes involution of the thymus. This is reversible initially; however, eventually it is not and the thymus involutes prematurely.

☐☐ **Describe the appearance of the thymus in DiGeorge's syndrome.**

It is grossly absent as are the parathyroid glands in conjunction with cardiovascular anomalies, abnormal facial appearance, and a cleft palate.

❑❑  **What is the most common abnormality seen in the thymus of patients with myasthenia gravis?**

Lymphofollicular thymitis occurs in over half of patients.

❑❑   **In addition to lymphofollicular thymitis, what other thymic changes are seen in patients with myasthenia gravis?**

In addition to a thymitis with diffuse infiltration of the medulla by B cells, atrophy and, rarely, thymolipoma and thymic hyperplasia can also be seen.

# HEAD AND NECK

❑❑  **What is white sponge nevus?**

These lesions are composed of large white plaques in the oral mucosa which have prominent intraepithelial edema in the malpighian layer and are inherited in an autosomal dominant fashion.

❑❑  **What is Fordyce's disease?**

This is abnormal sebaceous glands that occur in the oral cavity.

❑❑  **Other than the lymph nodes, what is another common site of biopsy in the head and neck to confirm a diagnosis of sarcoidosis?**

Lower lip.

❑❑  **What is Melkersson-Rosenthal syndrome?**

The triad of facial edema and a fissured tongue in a patient with paralysis.

❑❑  **Which herpes virus causes herpetic gingivostomatitis?**

Herpes simplex virus type 1 (HSV-1).

❑❑  **What painful condition of the oral cavity is characterized by a shallow ulceration of the oral mucosa with an associated fibrinopurulent exudate?**

Aphthous stomatitis.

❑❑  **What antiepileptic drug is classically associated with gingival hyperplasia?**

Phenytoin.

❑❑  **What is a ranula?**

This is a cyst found in the floor of the mouth near the frenulum which may be either a remnant branchial cleft cyst or a type of retention cyst.

❑❑  **What common benign tumor of the tongue contains abundant lysosomes within the tumor cells ultrastructurally?**

Granular cell tumor.

❑❑  **What is the term given to a mass occurring on the gums (more commonly mandible than maxilla) which contains a mixed inflammatory infiltrate including multinucleated giant cells?**

Epulis.

❑❑  **What descriptive term is given to describe a raised, white patch that occurs in mucous membranes, more commonly in men?**

Leukoplakia.

❏❏ What term describes a cyst occurring on the lips that histologically has pools of mucus with admixed inflammation?

Mucocele.

❏❏ List some lesions of the oral cavity which are associated with human papillomavirus (HPV).

Squamous papillomas, condylomas, and verrucae.

❏❏ What is the most common cause of viral sialadenitis?

Mumps.

❏❏ What are the components of Mikulicz's syndrome?

Xerostomia secondary to salivary and lacrimal gland inflammation and enlargement secondary to any number of diseases.

❏❏ What is the most common benign neoplasm of salivary glands?

Pleomorphic adenoma.

❏❏ What is the most common malignant neoplasm of salivary glands?

Mucoepidermoid carcinoma.

❏❏ Where do most salivary gland tumors arise?

The parotid gland accounts for up to 80% of the tumors.

❏❏ Is a tumor arising in the parotid gland most likely to be benign or malignant?

Benign, only about 15% are malignant.

❏❏ Is a tumor most likely to be benign or malignant when it arises in the minor salivary glands?

Malignant, greater than 50% of the time.

❏❏ What is the average age that a patient presents with a benign salivary gland tumor?

Between the fifth and seventh decade of life.

❏❏ What are the characteristic histologic findings in a mixed tumor (pleomorphic adenoma)?

A mixed content of both epithelial and mesenchymal components.

❏❏ What percentage of parotid gland tumors are pleomorphic adenomas?

Up to 70%.

❏❏ What are the typical patient demographics in pleomorphic adenoma?

Women are four times more commonly affected than men with a mean age of approximately 40 years.

❏❏ Is a pleomorphic adenoma more likely to arise in the superficial or deep lobe of the parotid gland?

Almost 90% are in the superficial lobe.

❏❏  **What is the biologic behavior of pleomorphic adenoma?**

Adequate excision, not simple enucleation, is sufficient.  Although the tumors often appear  well circumscribed, simple enucleation will result in a higher incidence of local recurrence.

❏❏  **Which of the minor salivary glands is most likely to contain a pleomorphic adenoma?**

The minor salivary glands of the palate.

❏❏  **Which of the salivary gland tumors is almost entirely restricted to the parotid gland?**

Warthin's tumor (papillary cystadenoma lymphomatosum).

❏❏  **Of the salivary gland tumors, which is most likely to be bilateral?**

Warthin's tumor (10% of the time).

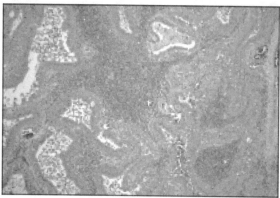

WARTHIN'S TUMOR

❏❏  **Is Warthin's tumor more common in men or women?**

Five times more common in males.

❏❏  **Ultrastructurally, what are the oncocytic cells in Warthin's tumor filled with?**

Mitochondria.

❏❏  **If a Warthin's tumor were to occur in a minor salivary gland, where is the most common site?**

Lower lip.

❏❏  **A history of exposure to what therapeutic agent is obtained in approximately 20% of patients with oncocytoma?**

Radiation therapy or occupational exposure to radiation.

❏❏  **How common is oncocytoma?**

Less than 1% of all salivary gland tumors.

❏❏  **What is oral hairy leukoplakia?**

This is a lesion of the mouth particularly in HIV+ male homosexuals but also other immunodeficient patients which shows hyperkeratosis or parakeratosis, acanthosis, often yeast and budding yeast consistent with Candida species, degeneration of keratinocytes in the spiny layer and superficial inflammation. It is thought to be induced by EBV.

❑❑   What is the Plummer-Vinson syndrome?

This is the presence of iron-deficiency anemia, glossitis, and esophageal dysphasia.

❑❑   What is the term used to describe a benign, protuberant nodule that can appear on the gingiva of a patient who has dentures?

Fibroma or irritation fibroma.

❑❑   How frequently does leukoplakia in the oral cavity progress to squamous cell carcinoma in situ or invasive carcinoma?

It is quite variable; however, perhaps about 5% of the time.

❑❑   What is the Pierre-Robin syndrome?

Cleft palate, micrognathia (hypoplastic mandible), microglossia with a posterior position, and abnormalities of the larynx.

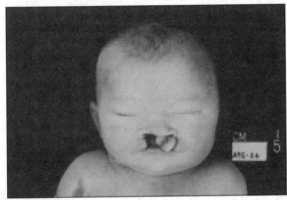

CLEFT LIP AND PALATE

❑❑   How common is cleft lip and/or palate?

It varies among ethnic groups; however, a cleft occurs in about 1 in 800 Caucasians, 1 in 2500 African-Americans, and as many as 1 in 250 native Americans. It is more common in males and occurs greater on the left than the right.

❑❑   What is the most common malignant tumor of the oral cavity?

Squamous cell carcinoma.

❑❑   What are the greatest risk factors for a development of squamous cell carcinoma of the head and neck?

Alcohol and tobacco use.

❑❑   What are the terms which describe exostoses or benign bony growths which can occur on the palate or the lingual mandible?

Torus palatinus and torus mandibularis, respectively.

❏❏ **What is another name for acute necrotizing ulcerative gingivitis (ANUG)?**

It is also referred to as Vincent's disease and appears to be related to stress, tobacco use, and Down's syndrome with resultant infection by various organisms including Borrelia vincenti or Bacteroides intermedius. It is characterized by gingival necrosis occurring initially between the teeth and extending to encompass the entire gingiva subsequently requiring surgical debridement.

❏❏ **What is the most common site of squamous cell carcinoma in the oral cavity?**

Lip.

❏❏ **How frequent is focal, conventional squamous cell carcinoma in verrucous carcinoma and how do these tumors behave?**

About 20% of verrucous carcinomas will have foci of typical squamous cell carcinoma and these tumors then recur at a greater rate than normal, pure verrucous carcinoma which is characteristically indolent.

❏❏ **What is the benign tumor which is composed of seromucinous salivary gland-type tissue admixed with normal appearing sebaceous glands?**

Salivary gland choristoma.

❏❏ **What is the most common type of salivary gland carcinoma in the palate?**

Adenoid cystic carcinoma followed by polymorphous low grade adenocarcinoma.

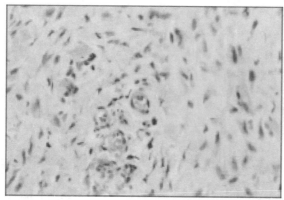

NASAL MASS

❏❏ **A 15-year-old boy presented with nasal obstruction and the polypoid mass shown above was resected and bled extensively. What is your diagnosis?**

Juvenile nasopharyngeal angiofibroma.

❏❏ **What malignant tumor of the nasopharynx is very common among Asian populations, has a bimodal incidence curve, and a strong association with EBV?**

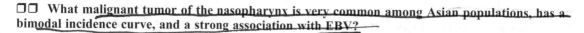

Nasopharyngeal carcinoma.

❏❏ **What are the two peaks of occurrence for nasopharyngeal carcinoma?**

Ages 15-25 and 60-69.

❏❏  **What is the most common presentation of a patient with nasopharyngeal carcinoma?**

Cervical lymphadenopathy.

NASAL MASS OF NEUROGLIAL TISSUE

❏❏  **This soft, polypoid nasal mass was resected from a young child and histologically looked like brain tissue.  What is your diagnosis?**

Glial heterotopia (nasal glioma).

❏❏  **What is the five year survival for olfactory neuroblastoma?**

Approximately 50%.

❏❏  **What is the major treatment of nasopharyngeal carcinoma?**

Radiotherapy.  They are classically difficult to delineate clinically and multiple biopsies must be taken in order to outline its extent.

❏❏  **What is the causative organism of acute epiglottitis which can occur in children?**

Haemophilus influenzae type B.

❏❏  **What is the malignant potential of a "singer's nodule"?**

Essentially none.  These typically occur on the anterior true vocal cord.

❏❏  **Which form of papilloma on a vocal cord, adult or juvenile, has a stronger association with HPV?**

The juvenile, multiple papillomatosis form has a very strong association with HPV of the "benign types" including 6 and 11.  In contrast, the adult, solitary papilloma has no such correlation.

❏❏  **In a patient with pharyngeal squamous cell carcinoma, would you guess that the patient is male or female?**

Greater than 95% of patients are male.

❏❏  **Compare the prognosis of verrucous carcinoma to conventional squamous cell carcinoma.**

Verrucous carcinomas almost never metastasize, in contrast to squamous cell carcinoma.  Verrucous carcinoma has a strong association with HPV and typically should not be radiated as radiation can cause transformation to a higher grade tumor.

□□  What is the general term given to cysts which arise secondary to abnormalities in tooth development?

Odontogenic.

□□  What is the most common epithelial odontogenic tumor?

Adamantinoma or ameloblastoma.

□□  What is the most common age for development of ameloblastoma?

20s to 40s without a gender preference.

□□  What is the term given to describe a tumor which is odontogenic and contains parts of dentin, enamel, and cementum?

Odontoma, which is divided into complex, compound, and ameloblastic.

□□  What is the lesion of the ear typically seen in children which is composed of inflammatory cells and abundant degenerative keratin debris?

Cholesteatoma.

□□  What is otosclerosis?

This is the production and deposition of bone within the middle ear cavity and on the rim of the promontory window.  It is inherited with variable penetrance as an autosomal dominant trait.

□□  What is the most common lining of a branchial cyst?

Pseudostratified columnar epithelium with an associated mononuclear cell inflammatory response which can even form reactive follicles.

□□  Histologically, how does one differentiate between the parotid glands, submandibular glands, and sublingual glands?

The parotid glands are composed of serous acini only, while the sublingual glands are composed of mucinous acini only, and the submandibular glands have a mixture of the two.

□□  Where is a patient most likely to develop sialolithiasis or stones in the ducts of the major salivary glands?

The submandibular gland accounts for about 80% of cases, followed by the parotid and only rarely (1%) do stones occur in the sublingual glands.

□□  What is the lining of a thyroglossal duct cyst composed of?

It can either be squamous epithelium or pseudostratified columnar epithelium or a mixture of both.

□□  What is the most common etiologic agent of acute suppurative sialadenitis?

Staphylococcus aureus.

□□  A triad of xerostomia (dry mouth), xerophthalmia (dry eyes), and arthritis is the classic triad of what syndrome?

Sjogren's syndrome, which is nine times more common in women, usually postmenopausal.

❏❏ **What is the sicca syndrome?**

The combination of dry eyes and dry mouth which is seen in Sjogren's syndrome. Patients with Sjogren's also frequently have autoimmune diseases including rheumatoid arthritis and systemic lupus erythematosus.

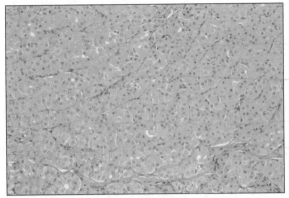

SALIVARY GLAND TUMOR WITH ABUNDANT EOSINOPHILIC CYTOPLASM

❏❏ **The tumor shown above has bland, uniform nuclei, abundant pink cytoplasm and is shown ultrastructurally to be composed of tumor cells filled with abundant mitochondria. What is your diagnosis?**

Oncocytoma.

❏❏ **In a patient who presents with bilateral salivary gland tumors, what is your best diagnosis?**

Warthin's tumor.

❏❏ **Which salivary gland tumor is characterized by prominent perineural invasion, infiltrative borders, and a slow but relentless biologic course?**

Adenoid cystic carcinoma.

❏❏ **Describe the most common patient characteristics and tumor location for acinic cell carcinoma.**

These tumors make up about 2% of salivary gland tumors and will classically occur in a male in his 20s presenting with a mass in his parotid gland.

❏❏ **How common are oral ulcers in patients with Behcet's syndrome?**

90% of patients.

# GASTROINTESTINAL TRACT

□□ **How common is isolated esophageal atresia and tracheoesophageal fistula?**

These occur every 2-4,000 births; however, only half of the time is it an isolated lesion. The rest are associated with other congenital anomalies.

□□ **What is the most common type of esophageal atresia/tracheoesophageal fistula?**

Most commonly, the proximal esophagus ends in a blind pouch and the distal esophagus is the site of a tracheoesophageal fistula. This form accounts for almost 90% of the cases.

□□ **What is a Schatzki's ring?**

Schatzki's rings are constrictions of the esophagus which are found near the gastroesophageal junction that may simply represent an exuberant lower esophageal sphincter.

□□ **A patient develops an adenocarcinoma of the lower 1/3 of the esophagus. Where would you expect the lymph node metastases to occur?**

Aortic and celiac axis lymph nodes. The upper 1/3 of the esophagus drains to the cervical lymph nodes and the middle 1/3 drains into the paratracheal and paraesophageal lymph nodes.

□□ **Describe the typical patient and symptomatology in congenital pyloric stenosis.**

Classically, the patient is a first born male who develops projectile vomiting and a palpable abdominal mass at two to three weeks of age.

□□ **Where is heterotopic gastric mucosa in the esophagus most likely to arise?**

In the posterior cricoid region.

□□ **What are the two major types of esophageal diverticula?**

Pulsion (example Zenker's or cervical) and traction diverticula.

□□ **What is achalasia?**

This is a disorder typically of the lower esophagus whereby the myenteric plexus is nearly completely absent resulting in stricture formation and proximal dilatation.

□□ **What infectious agent and disease present a nearly identical clinical and pathologic scenario as achalasia?**

Chagas' disease caused by Trypanosoma cruzi.

□□ **What type of tumor are patients with achalasia more prone to?**

These patients rarely develop squamous cell carcinoma of the esophagus; however, this risk is much greater than the general population.

□□ **What is the most common type of hiatal hernia?**

The sliding type accounts for about 90% of cases while the "rolling" type accounts for the remainder.

❑❑  **In general terms, what is the definition of Barrett's esophagus?**

This is a metaplasia of the esophagus resulting in transformation of the squamous epithelium to columnar epithelium.  Varying opinions regarding the diagnosis of Barrett's esophagus exist; however, there is no debate as to the increased risk of development of adenocarcinoma in the specialized or intestinal type of metaplasia.

❑❑  **How frequent is columnar epithelial metaplasia in cases of reflux esophagitis?**

About 1 in 10 cases of reflux esophagitis will also have columnar epithelial metaplasia.

❑❑  **What is the most common tumor type of the esophagus?**

Squamous cell carcinoma.

❑❑  **What are some risk factors for development of squamous cell carcinoma of the esophagus?**

Smoking, alcohol, history of lye stricture, achalasia, previous radiation, diverticula (rarely), Plummer-Vinson's syndrome, and tylosis (rarely).

❑❑  **Anatomically, where is squamous cell carcinoma most likely to arise in the esophagus?**

It is unusual in the upper 1/3 and occurs most commonly in the middle and lower esophagus.

❑❑  **What is the most common treatment for esophageal carcinoma?**

It depends on the location.  In the lower 1/3 of the esophagus, surgical resection is the most important method with radiation therapy being very commonplace in esophageal carcinomas of the upper part of the esophagus.

❑❑  **How frequently is the esophagus involved in progressive systemic sclerosis (scleroderma)?**

About 80% of patients have some esophageal abnormality including obstruction or reflux.

❑❑  **What is the term given to the longitudinal, linear mucosal tears in the lower esophagus/proximal stomach which typically occur following excessive, continuous vomiting?**

Mallory-Weiss tears.

❑❑  **What general condition results often times in esophageal varices?**

Portal hypertension, most frequently secondary to cirrhosis of the liver. Nearly half the patients die during the first episode of variceal bleeding and most of the survivors can look forward to more bleeding in the upcoming year.

❑❑  **Describe the demographics of the typical patient who develops squamous cell carcinoma of the esophagus.**

A black male greater than 50 years old with a tumor in the mid or lower esophagus.  Interestingly, whites have a higher incidence of adenocarcinoma arising in Barrett's esophagus.

❑❑  **What are the main non-mucin secreting cells in the stomach and where would you find them?**

The parietal cells produce hydrochloric acid and intrinsic factor and are found predominantly in the body or corpus.  The chief cells are also found in the corpus and are the producers of pepsinogen.  The G cells or gastrin secreting cells are found in the antrum.

❏❏  **What is the most common heterotopic tissue found in the stomach?**

Pancreas.  Most are found in the submucosa of the distal stomach, antrum or pylorus.

❏❏  **What organism is associated with development of gastritis and even lymphoma of the mucosa associated lymphoid tissue (MALT)?**

Helicobacter pylori.

❏❏  **What effect does intestinal metaplasia of the gastric mucosa have on the number of Helicobacter pylori organisms present?**

They are typically not found in areas of intestinal metaplasia.

❏❏  **What are the terms given to gastric ulcers occurring from extensive thermal or burn injury and increased intracranial pressure secondary to central nervous system trauma?**

Curling's ulcer and Cushing's ulcer, respectively.

❏❏  **What is the most common location for a peptic ulcer?**

The first part of the duodenum.

❏❏  **Who is more likely to develop peptic ulcers, men or women?**

Men are more than twice as likely to develop peptic ulcers.

❏❏  **Where in the stomach is the most common location for chronic peptic ulcer disease?**

The lesser curvature.

❏❏  **What are some factors associated with development of gastric ulcers?**

Cirrhosis due to alcohol abuse, cigarette smoking, high dose steroid use, "type A" personality, stress, NSAID use, Helicobacter pylori infection, and Zollinger-Ellison syndrome, among other things.

❏❏  **What are some of the complications that occur with gastric ulcers?**

Hemorrhage, perforation, gastric outlet obstruction, pain unresponsive to therapy.

❏❏  **What is a bezoar?**

These are foreign bodies in the stomach, most commonly composed of hair (trichobezoar).

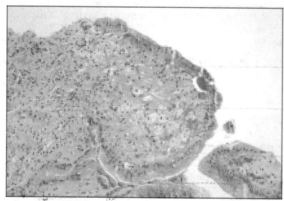

STOMACH BIOPSY

❏❏   **The benign histiocytic lesion shown above typically appears yellow endoscopically and contains intracellular lipid material.  What is your diagnosis?**

Xanthoma or xanthelasma.

❏❏   **What are three forms of hypertrophic gastropathy characterized by enlarged rugal folds?**

Menetrier's disease, hypertrophic-hypersecretory gastropathy, and gastric gland hyperplasia in Zollinger-Ellison syndrome.

❏❏   **Describe the typical patient with Menetrier's disease?**

A man (3:1 over females) ranging in age from the fourth to sixth decade of life who presents with weight loss, abdominal pain, and occasionally peripheral edema.

❏❏   **Are the majority of gastric polyps neoplastic or non-neoplastic?**

The vast majority are non-neoplastic (greater than 90%).

❏❏   **What is the most common setting in which one finds a hyperplastic or inflammatory gastric polyp?**

Chronic gastritis.

❏❏   **What is the most common location of an adenomatous gastric polyp?**

The antrum.

❏❏   **How common are gastric polyps in familial colonic polyposis and Gardener's syndrome?**

There are gastric polyps of some type (adenomatous, hyperplastic or regenerative, or fundic gland type) in more than half of the patients.

❏❏   **Where do the gastrinomas typically arise in a patient with Zollinger-Ellison syndrome?**

Most occur in the pancreas or duodenum.

❏❏   **What is the pattern of inheritance of autoimmune gastritis associated with pernicious anemia?**

It is autosomal dominant with incomplete penetrance.  Patients of northern European ancestry are at increased risk.

❏❏   **What type of gastritis is associated with an increased incidence of gastric carcinoid?**

Autoimmune gastritis.

❏❏   **What is the most common malignant tumor arising in the stomach?**

Adenocarcinoma accounts for the vast majority of tumors (greater than 90%), followed by lymphoma and carcinoids.

❏❏   **Describe the five year survival for gastric carcinoma.**

It is dismal, approximately 10%.

❏❏   **What are some features of the stomach which are associated with predisposition to development of gastric carcinoma?**

The presence of adenomatous polyps, history of partial gastrectomy (increased reflux), chronic atrophic gastritis and, of course, infection with Helicobacter pylori.

□□  **What is the most common location for gastric carcinoma?**

The anterior lesser curvature near the pylorus.

□□  **What is the term given to describe a gastric carcinoma with metastases to the ovaries?**

Krukenberg tumor.

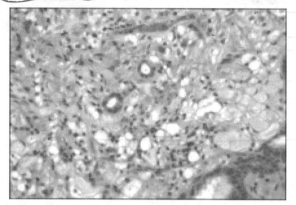

STOMACH WITH SIGNET RING CELL CARCINOMA

□□  **What does the term "linits plastica" refer to in gastric carcinoma?**

Adenocarcinoma of the stomach can be divided into the intestinal type (50%) and diffuse type (33%) with combinations of the two comprising the remainder of cases.  The classic linitis plastica is the most characteristic type of diffuse gastric carcinoma and is characterized by an infiltrating signet ring cell carcinoma (see above figure).

□□  **What would you expect to find ultrastructurally in the tumor cells of a carcinoid tumor?**

Dense core secretory granules.

□□  **Of the various sites of lymphoma in the gastrointestinal tract, which is the most common site of origin of primary lymphoma?**

The stomach accounts for about half of the cases.

□□  **Of the various sites for gastrointestinal stromal tumor (GIST), which is the most common site of origin?**

The stomach accounts for about half of all the cases.

□□  **With regard to gastrointestinal stromal tumors, what are the two most important predictors of tumor behavior?**

Size and mitotic rate.

□□  **What is the most common site of origin of a carcinoid tumor?**

Appendix.

□□  **What is the most common location for heterotopic pancreas?**

Duodenum.

**□□   What are some congenital anomalies associated with persistence of the vitelline or omphalomesenteric duct?**

Persistent fibrous cord (from umbilicus to the bowel wall), enteroumbilical fistula, or Meckel's diverticulum.

**□□   What is a Meckel's diverticulum?**

This is a congenital anomaly which results from persistence of the proximal vitelline duct; is found within 90 cm of the ileocecal valve on the antimesenteric border and is usually lined by small intestinal mucosa; however, pancreatic tissue, gastric, duodenal, or colonic mucosa may also be found.

**□□   What is the "rule of 2s" as it refers to Meckel's diverticulum?**

Meckel's diverticulum is found within two feet of the ileocecal valve, is two inches long, causes symptoms in 2% of cases, and is found in 2% of the population.

**□□   What are some of the complications that can develop from Meckel's diverticulum?**

Perforation, ulceration, hemorrhage, intussusception, obstruction, tumors, and vesicodiverticular fistula.

**□□   What is Hirschsprung's disease?**

This is typically found in the large intestine but can occasionally involve the small intestine as well.  It is characterized by a loss of both the submucosal (Meissner's) and myenteric (Auerbach's) plexuses with resultant nerve trunk hyperplasia, and functional obstruction with secondary proximal dilatation.  The disease always affects the rectum and exhibits varying degrees of involvement of the remaining colon and rarely will extend to the small intestine.

**□□   Is Hirschsprung's disease more common in males or females?**

It varies, males are four times more likely to have a short segment of affected colon while patients with long segments are more frequently female. In addition, 10% of Hirschsprung's disease is found in patients with trisomy 21 (Down's syndrome).

**□□   What are some synonyms for celiac disease?**

Celiac sprue, gluten-sensitive enteropathy, or nontropical sprue.

**□□   What is the main histologic finding in patients with gluten-sensitive enteropathy?**

Markedly blunted villi and an increased number of plasma cells within the lamina propria.

**□□   In patients with celiac sprue, what circulating antibodies are present?**

These patients have antibodies against gliadin which is a glycoprotein found in gluten.  These patients must follow a diet that is devoid of gluten products such as wheat and barley.

**□□   What are some rare but possible complications of celiac disease?**

These patients have a slightly increased risk of development of malignancy, most commonly lymphomas which seem to have a higher than expected frequency of T-cell phenotype, carcinoma, and chronic nonspecific ulcerative duodenojejunoileitis.

**□□   What is the characteristic histologic finding in patients with disaccharidase deficiency including, most commonly, lactase deficiency?**

Normal small bowel mucosa.

**❑❑  What is the causative agent of Whipple's disease?**

Tropheryma whippelii.  These patients have diarrhea, malabsorption and biopsy of the small bowel (predominantly jejunum and ileum) shows distorted villi with dilated lacteals and expansion of the lamina propria by macrophages which are "stuffed" with organisms.

**❑❑  What is microvillous inclusion disease?**

This is a condition characterized by absence of surface villi and, ultrastructurally, microvillous inclusions are found within the cytoplasm of the enterocytes.  These infants, without small bowel transplantation, typically die before reaching the age of two.  This is an autosomal recessive condition.

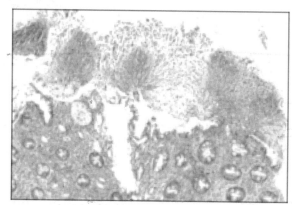

PSEUDOMEMBRANOUS COLITIS

**❑❑  What is the typical causative agent of pseudomembranous colitis as shown above in this colonic biopsy?**

Pseudomembranous colitis is classically caused by a toxin produced by Clostridium difficile.

**❑❑  How is abetalipoproteinemia inherited?**

Autosomal recessive.

**❑❑  What is the most common etiology of intussusception in an adult?**

Intussusception is when the small bowel "telescopes" on itself.  In adults, there is typically an intraluminal tumor mass which serves as a point of traction and origin of the intussusception.  In contrast, infants and children typically have no associated abnormality and it appears to occur spontaneously.

**❑❑  What condition of the large intestine typically occurs in premature infants, can be associated with umbilical artery catheterization and results in abdominal distention, loss of bowel sounds, bloody stools, and the presence of submucosal cysts?**

Neonatal necrotizing enterocolitis.

**❑❑  What is the most common location of adenocarcinoma of the small bowel?**

Duodenum.

**❑❑  In the small intestine, what is the most common site of a carcinoid tumor?**

Ileum.

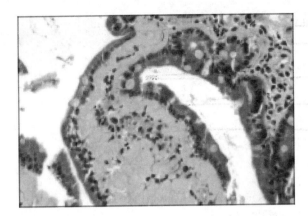

❏❏  What is the glassy eosinophilic material in this small bowel biopsy which is positive with a Congo red stain (thioflavin T or S could have also been used)?

Amyloid.

❏❏  What are some of the classic symptoms characterizing carcinoid syndrome which may occur in association with carcinoid tumors of the small intestine?

Palpitations, watery diarrhea, irregular hypertension, facial and anterior chest wall cyanosis, cutaneous flushing, abdominal pain, and wheezing.

❏❏  What two substances are elevated in the blood and urine in patients with the classic carcinoid syndrome?

*serotonin*          *when mets to liver*

5-hydroxytryptamine (5-HT) and 5-hydroxyindoleacetic acid (5-HIAA).

❏❏  In general terms, what is the five year survival rate for non appendiceal carcinoids?

It is around 90%. Even with liver metastases from a small bowel carcinoid, the five year survival is still around 50%. Widespread, multiple metastatic lesions carries a poor prognosis.

❏❏  What is Torkelson syndrome?

This is an autosomal dominant condition found in people of Mennonite descent in Canada which is associated with diarrhea and dehydration in young childhood and can be deadly. These patients sometimes show evidence of a common variable immunodeficiency. Histologically, the changes are not specific and include blunting of the villi, edema, and focal acute inflammation.

❏❏  How frequently is the appendix involved in Crohn's disease?

1 in 4 cases.

❏❏  What is the term given to the replacement of the lumen of the appendix by fibrous tissue, particularly in the distal tip?

Fibrous obliteration.

❏❏  What happens to the lymphoid tissue that is normally present in the appendix as one ages?

It gradually disappears, and eventually may be essentially absent with associated fibrous obliteration.

❏❏  What is the most common cause of acute appendicitis?

Typically there is luminal obstruction with resultant ischemia and bacterial infection. The luminal obstruction is caused by a fecalith in the majority of cases.

❑❑   **What are the classic clinical features associated with acute appendicitis?**

Right lower quadrant pain, anorexia, fever, nausea, vomiting, and leukocytosis.

❑❑   **What is a common pinworm that can be associated with acute appendicitis, or more commonly, may be an incidental finding in the appendix?**

Enterobius vermicularis, which is found in about 3% of appendectomy specimens in the United States.

❑❑   **You are given an appendix removed for acute appendicitis and histlogically notice the presence of Warthin-Finkeldey cells. What is your diagnosis?**

These cells occur in the prodromal stage of measles infection in the appendix. The patient will likely develop a typical measles rash shortly.

❑❑   **What is a mucocele in the appendix?**

This generic term is associated with a great deal of confusion but probably is best thought of as a descriptive term describing a dilated appendix filled with thick mucin. There are a variety of causes including retention cysts, mucinous cystadenomas, and mucinous cystadenocarcinoma.

❑❑   **What is pseudomyxoma peritonei?**

This is the presence of abundant pools of mucin within the peritoneum. Histologically, one would see bland-appearing glandular epithelium in the middle of large pools of mucin.

❑❑   **What is the most common primary tumor of the appendix?**

Carcinoid tumor.

❑❑   **In patients with Hirschsprung's disease, what would you expect the acetylcholinesterase activity to be?**

It is markedly increased.

❑❑   **Are most diverticula acquired or congenital?**

Acquired, they either lack a muscularis propria or it is greatly attenuated. In contrast, congenital diverticula (such as Meckel's diverticulum) have all three layers of the intestinal wall.

❑❑   **What part of the colon is the most commonly involved site of diverticulosis?**

Sigmoid.

❑❑   **What are the main complication of diverticulosis?**

Hemorrhage, perforation, and diverticulitis.

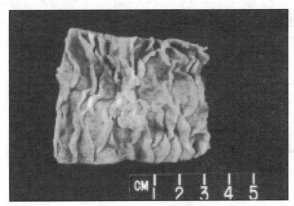

COLON

❑❑  **What is the term given to describe the presence of numerous gas filled submucosal cysts creating polypoid projections as shown in the picture above?**

Pneumatosis intestinalis.  In children, it is associated with necrotizing enterocolitis and in adults there is usually an associated gastrointestinal disorder or chronic obstructive pulmonary disease.

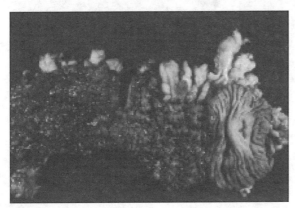

ASCENDING COLON AND CECUM

❑❑  **The findings shown above in this segment of the right colon and cecum, were uniformly present from the anus to the cecum as shown.  What is your best diagnosis?**

This is massive pseudopolyp formation as seen in ulcerative colitis.

❑❑  **What is the most common age of development of ulcerative colitis?**

Between the ages of 20 and 30, and there is a second much smaller peak in the eighth and ninth decades of life.

❑❑  **Between ulcerative colitis and Crohn's disease, which is characterized by transmural inflammation, skip lesions, and "creeping fat"?**

Crohn's disease.

❑❑  **Between ulcerative colitis and Crohn's disease, which is most likely to develop carcinoma?**

Ulcerative colitis has a greater risk and a quicker progression.

❑❑  **How commonly is the ileum involved in ulcerative colitis?**

So-called "backwash" ileitis occurs in about 10% of patients.

❑❑  **How frequently is the ileum involved in Crohn's disease?**

About 75% of the time.

❑❑  **Of ulcerative colitis and Crohn's disease, which is characterized by transmural inflammation and the presence of granulomas?**

Crohn's disease.

❑❑  **Of ulcerative colitis and Crohn's disease, which is more likely to develop strictures and fistulas?**

Crohn's disease.

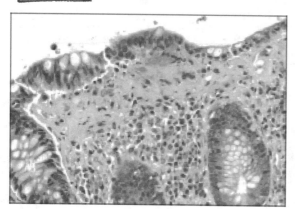

COLON BIOPSY

❑❑  **What is the term given to describe the type of colitis which is characterized by thickening of the subepithelial collagen band under the surface epithelium and clinically is typically seen in older females with watery diarrhea?**

Collagenous colitis (see photo above).

❑❑  **What is the term given to describe the colitis characterized by increased numbers of intraepithelial lymphocytes which is characteristically seen in middle aged women?**

Lymphocytic or microscopic colitis.

❑❑  **What is the arbitrary thickness which the subepithelial collagen band must reach to qualify as collagenous colitis?**

The normal collagen band measures up to 7 microns and collagenous colitis is said to occur when it reaches 10 microns or greater. Again, this is much more common in women.

❑❑  **What are some of the microscopic features of mucosal prolapse syndrome or solitary rectal ulcer syndrome?**

In about 10% of cases, the ulcers are not solitary at all but are multiple. In addition, the dilatation and irregular branching of the crypts can create a villiform appearance. The goblet cells are often mucin depleted and the lamina propria exhibits fibrosis and vascular congestion.

❑❑  **What is typhlitis?**

This is a colitis which is restricted to (or predominantly found in) the cecum.

❑❑   **What condition can develop with excessive use of certain types of laxatives and imparts a brown-black color to the mucosa?**

Melanosis coli.

❑❑   **What is the most common polyp seen in children?**

Juvenile or retention polyps; however, 1/3 of the cases occur in adults.

❑❑   **What is the most common site for development of an arteriovenous malformation in the large intestine?**

The vast majority are in the cecum and ascending colon.

❑❑   **How common are hemorrhoids?**

Half of people over 50 have them and the incidence increases with age.

❑❑   **What is the term given to the benign, non-neoplastic polyp characterized by surface glands and crypts featuring serrated glandular lumina?**

Hyperplastic polyps.

❑❑   **What is the most common site for a juvenile or retention polyp?**

Rectum.

RIGHT HEMICOLECTOMY WITH A VILLOUS ADENOMA CONTAINING HIGH GRADE DYSPLASIA
*(Photo courtesy of Julie Breiner, MD - University of Nebraska Medical Center)*

❑❑   **Which type of adenomatous polyp, like the one shown above, has the highest incidence of development of carcinoma?**

Villous adenomas.

❑❑   **In what fashion is the Peutz-Jeghers syndrome inherited?**

Autosomal dominant.

❑❑   **What is the syndrome that is characterized by multiple hamartomatous polyps of the gastrointestinal tract, and abnormal pigmentation of mucosa and skin?**

I just gave you a huge hint in the previous question - Peutz-Jeghers syndrome.

❑❑   **What is the malignant potential of the hamartomatous gastrointestinal polyps seen in Peutz-Jeghers syndrome?**

These patients are at an increased risk for developing carcinoma; however, this is not related to the polyps, rather there is an increased incidence of malignancy in other organs such as the breast or pancreas.

❏❏ **What are the three types of adenomatous polyps of the colon?**

Tubular, villous, and tubulovillous.

❏❏ **What are the main factors which determine the risk of malignancy developing in an adenomatous polyp?**

Size, architecture (greatest in sessile villous adenomas), presence of high grade dysplasia, and rate of growth.

❏❏ **What is the most common type of adenomatous polyp?**

Tubular adenoma.

❏❏ **What chromosome is the gene for familial polyposis located on?**

Chromosome 5q21.

❏❏ **How is familial polyposis inherited?**

Autosomal dominant.

❏❏ **How many polyps are necessary to diagnose familial polyposis?**

At least 100.

❏❏ **If untreated, how often will patients with familial polyposis develop adenocarcinoma of the colon?**

Essentially 100% of the time.

❏❏ **What is Turcot's syndrome?**

This is the combination of adenomatous polyposis of the colon and associated tumors of the central nervous system, typically gliomas.

❏❏ **Is there a gender preference for adenocarcinoma of the colon?**

Only in the rectum, there it is twice as common in males.

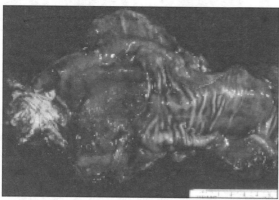

RECTAL CARCINOMA

❑❑  **On average, would the patient with the tumor shown above be male or female?**

I just told you, males have twice the incidence of rectal cancer compared to women.

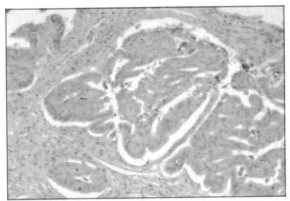

INVASIVE ADENOCARCINOMA IN MUSCULARIS PROPRIA

❑❑  **What is the approximate five year survival for a patient with an Astler-Coller stage B2 carcinoma of the colon?**

A B2 tumor is characterized by penetration through the muscularis propria without involvement of regional lymph nodes and is associated with an approximate 50% five year survival. Stage A is limited to the mucosa, B1 into the muscularis propria without penetration or involved nodes, B2 described above, C1 penetration into the muscularis propria but not through it with positive lymph nodes, C2 penetration by tumor through the muscularis propria with associated involved lymph nodes, and D represents distant metastatic spread.

❑❑  **What is the most common location for colon carcinomas?**

About 2/3 are located distally (sigmoid or further distal). However, there seems to be an increasing incidence of more proximal tumors so this may change.

❑❑  **In general, how do right-sided colon cancers differ from left-sided colon cancers?**

The left-sided lesions are classically circumferential forming a "napkin ring" and are associated with bowel obstruction while the right-sided tumors are more exophytic and polypoid and do not typically obstruct.

❑❑  **What is another name for hereditary non polyposis colorectal cancer syndrome?**

Lynch syndrome.

❑❑  **Where in the colon do most carcinomas in the Lynch syndrome occur?**

They are typically right-sided.

❑❑  **What are the components of Torre-Muir syndrome?**

Colorectal carcinoma with multiple sebaceous tumors and keratoacanthomas.

❑❑  **How is Cowden's syndrome inherited?**

It is autosomal dominant, and it is characterized by the presence of oral mucosal papillomas, trichilemmomas of the face, and acral hyperkeratosis with about a third of the patients having intestinal polyposis.

❏❏  **What is the syndrome characterized by numerous gastrointestinal polyps and abnormalities of the nails termed onychodystrophy?**

Cronkhite-Canada syndrome.

❏❏  **What are the two major watershed areas of the large colon which often result in ischemic bowel disease?**

The splenic flexure which is the watershed for the superior and inferior mesenteric arteries and the rectum representing the watershed for the inferior mesenteric and hypogastric arteries.

❏❏  **What is the line in the anus which marks the transition from squamous to non squamous mucosa?**

The dentate or pectinate line.

❏❏  **Within the anus, what is the most common site of origin of an anal fistula?**

The dentate line.

❏❏  **Is there a sex predilection for carcinomas arising in the anus?**

Yes, women are two to four times more commonly afflicted with anal carcinomas than men.

# LIVER AND BILIARY TRACT

☐☐ **What is the major blood supply to the liver?**

The portal vein supplies the majority of the hepatic blood while the hepatic artery accounts for the rest.

☐☐ **What is the term given to the space or potential space that exists between the sinusoidal endothelial lining cells and the underlying hepatocytes?**

The space of Disse.

☐☐ **What cell in the liver functions as a storage vehicle as well as metabolizing vitamin A and aiding in the production of collagen?**

The Ito cells or perisinusoidal lipocytes.

☐☐ **What general pattern of necrosis would one expect to see in ischemic injury in the liver?**

Central lobular necrosis as the pericentral region of the lobule or zone 3 of the acinus is farthest from the blood supply.

☐☐ **What zone of the liver acinus is characteristically involved in acetaminophen toxicity?**

Zone 3.

☐☐ **What is a Dane particle?**

This is the complete hepatitis B virus virion which includes the surface antigen, core antigen, DNA polymerase, and the e antigen.

☐☐ **When does the hepatitis B surface antigen appear in the blood?**

It first appears approximately six weeks following infection and is gone by 12 weeks. One is considered a carrier of hepatitis B if the surface antigen is detectable for greater than six months.

☐☐ **How frequently does chronic hepatitis develop in hepatitis A infection?**

Neither hepatitis A nor E infection are associated with chronic hepatitis.

☐☐ **Which hepatitis virus infection is associated with the greatest incidence of chronic hepatitis and cirrhosis?**

Hepatitis C is associated with chronic hepatitis in half the cases and proceeds to cirrhosis in up to 1 in 5 cases. Not surprisingly, it also has the highest carrier state.

☐☐ **Which hepatitis virus has the greatest association with development of hepatocellular carcinoma?**

Hepatitis B.

☐☐ **Which of the hepatitis viruses is a DNA virus?**

Hepatitis B.

❑❑  **What is the most common cause of post transfusion hepatitis?**

Hepatitis C causes the vast majority of post transfusion hepatitis.

❑❑  **What is the difference between the pattern of necrosis in acute viral hepatitis B and acute viral hepatitis A infection?**

Acute hepatitis B infection typically causes necrosis of zone 3 while acute hepatitis A is characteristically a zone 1 pattern of necrosis.

❑❑  **What are some drugs which can be associated with massive hepatic necrosis?**

Isoniazid, halothane, methyldopa, propylthiouracil, diphenylhydantoin, phenelzine, ticrynafen, among others.

❑❑  **What is the most common cause of cirrhosis in the western world?**

Alcoholic liver disease resulting in cirrhosis accounts for up to 70% of cases of cirrhosis.  It is followed in frequency by viral hepatitis and biliary tract diseases.

In about 10% of cases, the etiology remains a mystery (cryptogenic cirrhosis).

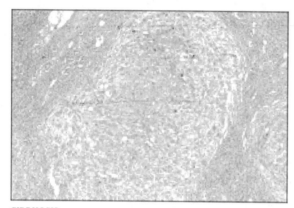

CIRRHOSIS

❑❑  **What type of collagen is deposited to an excessive degree in cases of cirrhosis?**

Types I and III.

❑❑  **What cell is thought to be the producer of the excess collagen seen in cirrhosis?**

The Ito cell.

❑❑  **What zone of the acinus do certain mushrooms cause necrosis in?**

Zone 1.

❑❑  **What are the four major clinical manifestations of portal hypertension?**

Ascites, splenomegaly, abnormal portosystemic venous shunts such as esophageal varices and, occasionally, encephalopathy.

❑❑  **What are the major sites of development of portosystemic shunts in instances of portal hypertension?**

Esophageal varices, rectum (hemorrhoids), retroperitoneum, hepatic falciform ligament (umbilical striae).

❑❑  **Where is the majority of bilirubin derived from?**

Most bilirubin is derived from the normal, daily breakdown of old red blood cells as bilirubin is the end product of heme degradation.

❑❑  **At what level of bilirubin does jaundice become clinically evident?**

When bilirubin exceeds 2.0-2.5 mg/dl.

❑❑  **What form of bilirubin (conjugated or unconjugated) is tightly bound to albumin, insoluble, and can cause kernicterus in the newborn?**

The unconjugated form of bilirubin.  It cannot be excreted in urine while the conjugated form can.

❑❑  **The presence of noncaseating granulomas with a "fibrin ring" pattern in the center should raise the diagnostic possibility of what type of hepatitis?**

That is the classic lesion seen in Q-fever hepatitis which, as you remember, is caused by Coxiella burnetii.  Sometimes, this is referred to as a "doughnut" granuloma.

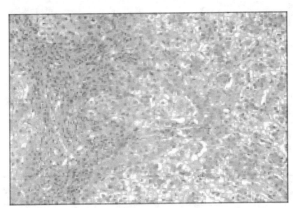

ALCOHOLIC LIVER

❑❑  **This liver comes from a patient who had intracytoplasmic eosinophilic structures within the hepatocytes that stained positive with ubiquitin in addition to the changes shown above.  What is your best diagnosis?**

This figure depicts sclerosing hyaline necrosis among other changes like steatosis that are classically seen in alcoholic liver disease.  Mallory's hyaline is the eosinophilic inclusion that stains with ubiquitin.

❑❑  **What type of cirrhosis is classically associated with alcoholic liver disease?**

Micronodular.

❑❑  **Are Mallory bodies pathognomonic for alcoholic hepatitis?**

Of course not, or I would not have asked.  They can be seen in many diseases including Wilson's, primary biliary cirrhosis (PBC), amiodarone toxicity, and other things.

❑❑  **The presence of sclerosing hyaline necrosis, neutrophils surrounding degenerating hepatocytes with Mallory bodies, and some degree of micro- and macrovesicular steatosis is associated with what type of liver disease?**

Alcoholic hepatitis.

❑❑ **What type of steatosis is associated with Reye's syndrome, valproic acid toxicity, and acute fatty liver of pregnancy?**

Microvesicular steatosis.

❑❑ **What are the two items which must be commented on in the pathology report on when making the diagnosis of chronic hepatitis on a liver biopsy?**

Degree of activity (grade) and degree of fibrosis (stage) and, of course, etiology if possible.

❑❑ **The presence of a portal area with a lymphoid aggregate, or even a follicle with a germinal center, in a biopsy showing chronic hepatitis is most suggestive of which type of viral hepatitis?**

Hepatitis C.

AUTOIMMUNE HEPATITIS

❑❑ **Classically, what is the most characteristic inflammatory cell in the infiltrate of autoimmune hepatitis?**

Plasma cells.

❑❑ **Of the various agents of viral hepatitis, which has the longest incubation period?**

Hepatitis B. The incubation period can range up to 180 days with hepatitis C being the next longest at 150 days.

❑❑ **In the liver, what is the term given to the presence of multiple large blood-filled spaces which lack an endothelial lining?**

Peliosis hepatis.

❑❑ **What is the most common etiology of peliosis hepatis?**

Treatment with anabolic or androgenic steroids. Less commonly, tamoxifen, history of use of Thorotrast, and elevated levels of vitamin A can result in peliosis hepatis.

❑❑ **What is the term used to describe the extension of portal inflammation in the form of lymphocytes beyond the limiting plate resulting in surrounding and destroying individual cells or small groups of hepatocytes?**

So-called piecemeal necrosis or interface hepatitis.

❑❑ **What are some other indications in addition to hepatitis B infection, which can produce so-called "ground-glass" cells?**

Certain drugs including phenobarbital, cyanamide, diphenylhydantoin, chlorpromazine, Lafora's disease, type IV glycogenosis, and hepatocellular carcinoma.

❑❑ **What produces the characteristic ground glass change in the cytoplasm of hepatocytes in hepatitis B infection?**

The change seen histologically is the presence of actual hepatitis B surface antigen particles filling the cytoplasm of the infected cells.

❑❑ **A young female presents with hepatitis, is found to have the HLA B8 haplotype, has liver and kidney microsome antibodies (LKM), and elevated levels of serum immunoglobulin G. What is the most likely diagnosis?**

Autoimmune hepatitis.

❑❑ **What specific mushroom is associated with liver toxicity and even fulminant hepatic failure?**

Amanita phalloides.

❑❑ **What type of hyperbilirubinemia, conjugated or unconjugated, is seen in both Dubin-Johnson and Rotor's syndrome?**

Conjugated.

❑❑ **What are the three major types of hereditary unconjugated hyperbilirubinemias?**

Crigler-Najjar syndrome types I and II and Gilbert's syndrome.

❑❑ **What zone of the acinar model is first to be involved by cholestasis?**

Zone 3, less frequently zone 2.

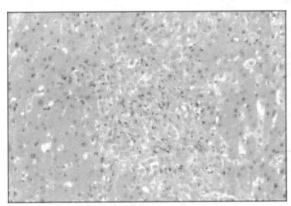

LIVER WITH CHOLESTASIS AND ACUTE PORTAL INFLAMMATION
*(Photo courtesy of Stanley J. Radio, MD - University of Nebraska Medical Center)*

❑❑ **In the biopsy shown above, there is bile duct proliferation, portal edema, hepatocellular and canalicular cholestasis, and scattered portal neutrophils. What is the most likely etiology of these changes?**

Biliary tract obstruction.

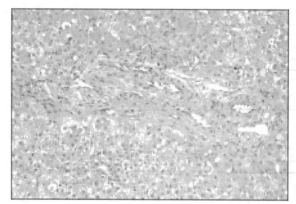

ALAGILLE'S SYNDROME

❏❏  **What is the most noteworthy histologic finding in Alagille's syndrome?** -

There is a marked reduction of the original intrahepatic bile ducts.

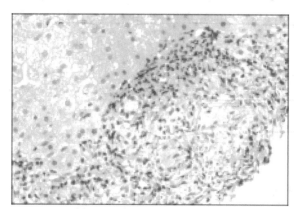

LIVER WITH A PORTAL GRANULOMA

❏❏  **A 45-year-old female presents with fatigue, pruritus, elevated liver function tests, and an elevated titer of antimitochondrial antibody (AMA). What is your diagnosis until proven otherwise?**

Primary biliary cirrhosis, in this case demonstrating a portal granuloma.

❏❏  **What are the typical histologic features of PBC?**

There is destruction of small bile ducts with a portal lymphoplasmacytic infiltrate with lymphoid follicles and even granulomas.  Of course, the bile ducts are absent from half or more of the portal areas in most biopsies of PBC.

❏❏  **A patient presents with abnormal liver function tests and undergoes endoscopic retrograde cholangiography (ERCP) which shows a pattern of "beading" or areas of stricture followed by dilatation of the bile ducts. What is your best diagnosis?**

Primary sclerosing cholangitis (PSC).

❏❏  **What is the classic finding in the portal areas of patients with PSC?**

They have a typical periductal fibrosis or sclerosis resulting in a so-called "onion skin" pattern.

❏❏  **What antibody titer may be elevated in patients with PSC?**

The perinuclear antineutrophil cytoplasmic antibodies (p-ANCA).

❏❏ **Histologically and grossly, how can one differentiate between Dubin-Johnson and Rotor's syndromes?**

Dubin-Johnson is characterized by a black discoloration of the parenchyma seen both grossly and histologically. Histologically, the pigment is contained within the hepatocytes in zones 2 and 3. In contrast, Rotor's syndrome is devoid of pigment and histologically, the liver may be normal.

❏❏ **What is the inheritance pattern of Dubin-Johnson syndrome and Rotor's syndrome?**

Autosomal recessive.

❏❏ **Which enzyme is deficient or abnormal in Gilbert's syndrome?**

Glucuronyl transferase.

❏❏ **What is the difference in the enzyme activity at fault in Crigler-Najjar syndrome types 1 and 2?**

In type 1 there is absent bilirubin glucuronyl transferase while in type 2, it is deficient. In either case, the symptoms are more severe than those seen in Gilbert's syndrome.

❏❏ **On what chromosome does the defect responsible for Wilson's disease lie?**

Chromosome 13.

❏❏ **Which type of hyperbilirubinemia, conjugated or unconjugated, is typically associated with cholestasis in a liver biopsy?**

Conjugated hyperbilirubinemia.

❏❏ **Where is a solitary, unilocular cyst of the liver typically found?**

They are twice as common in the right lobe.

❏❏ **What is the inheritance of the two types of Crigler-Najjar syndrome?**

Type 1 is autosomal recessive and type 2 is autosomal dominant with incomplete penetrance.

❏❏ **In viral hepatitis, in which of the liver function test parameters would you expect to find the greatest elevation?**

The AST and ALT are much more elevated than are the alkaline phosphatase or GGT.

❏❏ **What is the term given to the individually necrotic hepatocytes that are sometimes seen in viral hepatitis and other toxic liver injuries?**

Councilman bodies.

❏❏ **What is the earliest and most common finding in liver biopsies of alcoholics?**

Steatosis.

❏❏ **How is genetic hemochromatosis inherited?**

Autosomal recessive.

❏❏ **How common is hepatocellular carcinoma in patients with hemochromatosis and cirrhosis?**

Up to 20% of patients will develop hepatocellular carcinoma in that setting.

❑❑  **You see a patient who has Kayser-Fleischer rings. What is your diagnosis?**

These are copper deposits in Descemet's membrane in the cornea which are pathognomonic of Wilson's disease.

❑❑  **What is the treatment of choice for patients with Wilson's disease?**

D-penicillamine is a chelator of copper which induces excretion of copper in the urine.

❑❑  **In a patient with Wilson's disease, what would you expect the serum ceruloplasmin and urinary copper to be?**

Decreased serum ceruloplasmin and increased urinary excretion of copper.

❑❑  **Where would one expect to find the PAS+, diastase-resistant globules in a non-cirrhotic liver with alpha1-antitrypsin deficiency?**

Periportal hepatocytes.

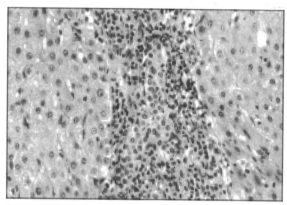

ORTHOTOPIC LIVER TRANSPLANT WITH MILD ACUTE (CELLULAR) REJECTION

❑❑  **What type of lymphocytes are shown here attacking this duct in a case of acute (cellular) rejection of a liver allograft?**

T lymphocytes.

❑❑  **What are some of the etiologies of granulomas occurring in the liver?**

Sarcoidosis, primary biliary cirrhosis, berylliosis, Brucellosis, drug injury, and polymyalgia rheumatica.

❑❑  **What is the most common parasitic disease involving the liver which often produces a granulomatous response?**

Schistosomiasis.

❑❑  **What are some of the clinical features of hepatic failure in males?**

Owing to decreased breakdown of estrogens, patients develop hypogonadism and gynecomastia. In addition, they develop various telangiectasias of the skin and palmar erythema from vasodilatation. Regardless of sex, ascites and coagulation disorders are very common.

❑❑  **In general terms, what is the normal cause of portal vein thrombosis?**

This usually occurs in the setting of some other condition and is secondary to that condition. Etiologies include protein C deficiency, myeloproliferative disorders, cirrhosis, tumor invasion, nodular regenerative hyperplasia, pyelophlebitis and, rarely, oral contraceptives.

**❏❏  In hepatic amyloidosis, where is the amyloid deposited?**

It can either occur in the vessel walls or it can also involve the parenchyma, specifically in the space of Disse with compression of the underlying hepatocytes.

**❏❏  What does a characteristic "nutmeg" appearance of the liver indicate?**

Chronic passive congestion, typically from chronic heart failure.

**❏❏  What are the two major categories of venous outflow tract obstruction in the liver?**

1.  Budd-Chiari syndrome or hepatic vein thrombosis
2.  Venoocclusive disease.

**❏❏  What are some of the causes of Budd-Chiari syndrome?**

About half the cases are idiopathic and the remainder are associated with various states of hypercoagulability including presence of a cardiolipin antibody, deficiency of protein C or antithrombin III, pregnancy, oral contraceptives, myeloproliferative disorders, and paroxysmal nocturnal hemoglobinuria. In addition, fibrous webs of the inferior vena cava, tumor impingement on the veins, and hepatic abscesses or cysts may also cause it.

**❏❏  What are some causes of venoocclusive disease?**

Ingestion of pyrrolizidine alkaloids, radiation, various cancer chemotherapies, urethane, azathioprine, dacarbazine, and hypervitaminosis A.

**❏❏  What is the difference in typical patient age in the Budd-Chiari syndrome and venoocclusive disease (VOD)?**

Budd-Chiari is older, 20-39 year olds. Venoocclusive disease is typically found in younger patients, 18 months to 3 years. Clearly, however, the patients that develop VOD secondary to various chemotherapy agents are often older.

**❏❏  What is the term give to describe the pattern of central lobular fibrosis seen in the liver in chronic, marked congestive heart failure?**

Cardiac sclerosis or "cardiac cirrhosis".

**❏❏  What are the three basic morphologic types of cirrhosis?**

Micronodular (0.3 cm or less), macronodular (greater than 0.3 cm), and mixed micro and macronodular.

**❏❏  In general, what are some conditions that are associated with a micronodular cirrhosis?**

Alcoholic liver disease, primary biliary cirrhosis, hemochromatosis, non alcoholic steatohepatitis (NASH), Indian childhood cirrhosis, galactosemia, and glycogenosis type IV.

**❏❏  In general, what are some conditions that are associated with a macronodular cirrhosis?**

Viral hepatitis, alpha-1-antitrypsin deficiency, hereditary tyrosinemia, Wilson's disease, and some drug injury.

**❏❏  What is Caroli's disease?**

This is a condition of congenital intrahepatic cystic dilatations of bile ducts. The lumens of the cystic dilatations can be filled with mucin, bile, or pus if infected.

☐☐ **What is Caroli's syndrome?**

This is Caroli's disease found in association with congenital hepatic fibrosis.

☐☐ **What is the inheritance pattern of Caroli's disease?**

Autosomal recessive.

☐☐ **What are the main clinical manifestations of congenital hepatic fibrosis?**

In general, patients present with hepatosplenomegaly or bleeding esophageal varices due to portal hypertension. Cholangitis can also be a presenting condition.

CONGENITAL HEPATIC FIBROSIS

☐☐ **What syndrome is characterized by the histologic features of congenital hepatic fibrosis in addition to pancreatic cysts and dysplastic changes in the pancreas, liver, and kidneys?**

Ivemark's syndrome.

☐☐ **What syndrome is characterized by features similar to congenital hepatic fibrosis plus an association with with encephalocele, polydactyly, and cystic kidneys?**

Meckel's syndrome.

☐☐ **What are two hepatic complications associated with autosomal dominant polycystic kidney disease?**

Infection of the liver cysts is the main complication and cholangiocarcinoma is the second most common complication.

☐☐ **What is a von Meyenburg's complex?**

This is a collection of abnormally dilated bile ducts in a background of fibrous stroma.

☐☐ **Where are most hydatid cysts located in the liver?**

Right lobe.

☐☐ **What is a mesenchymal hamartoma of the liver?**

This is a tumor which can be quite large, develops in children (average age less than 2), is more common in males, and is characterized by a loose, connective tissue stroma with admixed bile ducts and vascular structures. A translocation involving chromosome 19q18.4 has been described.

❑❑ Which benign tumor of the liver is associated strongly with the use of oral contraceptives?

Hepatocellular adenoma.

❑❑ Which is most likely to hemorrhage or rupture, focal nodular hyperplasia or hepatocellular adenoma?

Hepatocellular adenoma. Focal nodular hyperplasia very rarely does.

❑❑ A single 5 cm in diameter mass in an otherwise normal liver is characterized by a central, stellate scar. What is your diagnosis?

Focal nodular hyperplasia.

❑❑ Which lesion of the liver is associated with numerous conditions including rheumatoid arthritis, CREST syndrome and other autoimmune diseases, occurs in adults, and is sometimes confused with cirrhosis?

Nodular regenerative hyperplasia (nodular transformation).

❑❑ Describe the typical patient and clinical presentation of someone with a bile duct cystadenoma.

These occur in women in the fourth and fifth decades of life. They are usually found in the right lobe of the liver (just like the solitary cyst) and often cause abdominal pain owing to the large size. Serum levels of CA19-9 are often elevated.

❑❑ What tumor of the liver has been shown to occur in patients with Fanconi's anemia who are taking anabolic steroids?

Hepatocellular adenoma.

❑❑ What tumor of the liver has been reported to occur with increased frequency in patients with familial diabetes mellitus and type I glycogen storage disease?

Hepatocellular adenoma.

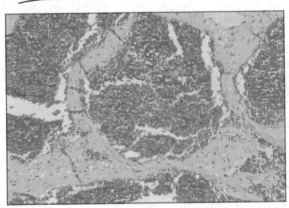

LIVER WITH VASCULAR LESION

❑❑  **What is the most common benign tumor occurring in the liver?**

Hemangioma (see above photo).

❑❑  **What is the most common presenting symptom of patients with angiomyolipoma of the liver?**

None, they are typically asymptomatic and are found during the course of radiographic studies for some other reason.

❑❑  **What is the most common location of cholangiocarcinoma?**

The right lobe of the liver, although 1/3 of cholangiocarcinomas are multifocal.  Remember, if you have to guess, most things are more common in the right lobe of the liver.

❑❑  **What is the relationship of serum alphafetoprotein to cholangiocarcinoma?**

The vast majority have no increase in serum AFP.

❑❑  **What is the relationship of serum alphafetoprotein to patients with hepatocellular carcinoma?**

About 1/2 of the patients with hepatocellular carcinoma have an elevated AFP; however, cirrhosis and viral hepatitis can both cause an elevated AFP as well.  In those cases, it is usually less elevated than in hepatocellular carcinoma (less than 1,000 ng/ml).

❑❑  **What is the incidence of production of bile by the tumor in cholangiocarcinoma and hepatocellular carcinoma?**

Cholangiocarcinoma does not produce bile; although, the compressed liver at the edges of the tumor may.  In contrast, a minority of cases of hepatocellular carcinoma do produce bile which can be tremendously helpful in making the diagnosis.  Unfortunately, this only occurs in about 10-30% of the cases.

❑❑  **In general, which is most suggestive of hepatocellular carcinoma, detection of elevated serum AFP or immunoperoxidase reactivity for AFP in tissue sections?**

The serum AFP.  The reported sensitivity of AFP in tissue sections varies widely and it can be detected in adenocarcinomas of other origins.

❑❑  **Which histologic type of hepatocellular carcinoma occurs in young adults or adolescents?**

Fibrolamellar.

❑❑  **Other than young age at diagnosis, how else does fibrolamellar carcinoma differ from the other variants of hepatocellular carcinoma?**

It does not have a male preponderance, nor is it associated with cirrhosis, hepatitis B, or alcohol abuse.  It has a much better prognosis and is not associated with elevated serum AFP.  Interestingly, in contrast to many of the other things we have discussed, it is more common in the left lobe of the liver.

❑❑  **What is the most common primary hepatic malignancy in children?**

Hepatoblastoma.

❑❑  **What is the most common age, sex, and location of tumor in a patient with hepatoblastoma?**

A 2-year-old male with a well circumscribed mass in the right lobe of the liver.

❑❑  **What is the relationship of hepatoblastoma and serum AFP?**

AFP is elevated in about 90% of cases, which is more frequent than in hepatocellular carcinoma.

❏❏  **What are the two histologic components of hepatoblastoma?**

They consist of an epithelial component comprising embryonal-type cells and fetal cells within a mesenchymal stroma. Extramedullary hematopoiesis is almost always present.

❏❏  **What is the gross appearance of an epithelioid hemangioendothelioma of the liver?**

They are typically multicentric, involve both lobes of the liver, are firm and white-tan. Angiosarcoma can also be multifocal.

❏❏  **Describe the typical patient who develops epithelioid hemangioendothelioma.**

It is more common in females with an average age of 50. The presenting symptoms are nonspecific and include pain and jaundice.

❏❏  **What is the prognosis for epithelioid hemangioendothelioma?**

Although the tumor grows slowly, it has a five year survival of around 30%. Liver transplantation has been used to prolong survival.

❏❏  **What tumor has been associated with previous exposure to Thorotrast and workers exposed to vinyl chloride monomer?**

Angiosarcoma.

❏❏  **What is the latent period for development of angiosarcoma of the liver following Thorotrast?**

15-20 years. Thorotrast is no longer used as a contrast medium in radiology.

❏❏  **In acute graft versus host disease involving the liver, what liver function tests are typically elevated?**

The alkaline phosphatase and bilirubin both go up, while the transaminases may very well be only slightly elevated.

❏❏  **Can chronic graft versus host disease occur in the absence of previous acute graft versus host disease?**

Yes, in 1/4 of the cases.

❏❏  **In bone marrow transplant patients who develop chronic graft versus host disease, how frequently is the liver involved?**

90% of the time.

❏❏  **What is the most common type of viral hepatitis in drug addicts?**

It is probably evenly distributed between hepatitis B and hepatitis C.

❏❏  **What is the most common cause of fulminant hepatitis?**

Hepatitis B.

❏❏  **What substance binds to and detoxifies acetaminophen in the liver and is overwhelmed and unable to keep up in cases of acetaminophen overdose?**

Glutathione. → *Acetominophen detox.*

□□ **What are the serologic markers of hepatitis B infection that occur during the so-called "window period" which is the time following disappearance of hepatitis B surface antigen and the appearance of hepatitis B surface antibody?**

Anti-hepatitis B core antigen and anti-hepatitis B e antigen.

□□ **What other virus is necessary in association with the hepatitis delta protein antigen for hepatitis D virus infection?**

Hepatitis B virus is necessary simultaneously for effective replication.

□□ **What is the etiologic agent of the viral hepatitis seen in immunocompromised hosts which is characterized by hepatocytes with intranuclear and intracytoplasmic viral inclusions?**

Cytomegalovirus (CMV).

□□ **What parasitic infection results in so-called "pipestem fibrosis"?**

Schistosomiasis.

□□ **What are the characteristic ultrastructural changes seen in Reye's syndrome?**

The mitochondria become enlarged and variable in size with disrupted cristae and electron lucency of the matrices.

□□ **Describe the clinical presentation of a patient with Reye's syndrome.**

It classically involves children (less than 9) who are treated with aspirin for a viral illness and develop vomiting, irritability, and hepatomegaly some 5 days later. About 1/4 of the patients progress to very serious illness with coma, progressive liver failure, and convulsions.

□□ **What is the therapy for Reye's syndrome?**

It is entirely supportive in nature.

□□ **What are the components of the HELLP syndrome?**

Hemolysis, elevated liver enzymes, and low platelets.

□□ **What is the primary treatment of acute fatty liver of pregnancy?**

Termination of the pregnancy.

□□ **What is the classic triad of hemochromatosis?**

Cirrhosis, diabetes mellitus, and skin pigmentation.    *"Bronze diabetes"*

□□ **What is the characteristic "tremor" of the hands seen in patients with hepatic encephalopathy?**

Asterixis.

□□ **What area of the brain is classically involved and damaged in Wilson's disease?**

The basal ganglia, particularly the putamen of the lenticular nucleus. Hence, the alternative designation "hepatolenticular degeneration".

❑❑  **What happens to the steatosis in alcoholics when they quit drinking alcohol for an extended period of time?**

It resolves.

❑❑  **How common is a hepatic infarction?**

They are quite rare as the liver has a dual blood supply and therefore can support itself in the face of fairly significant vascular obstruction.

❑❑  **What is the term given to a subcapsular, wedge-shaped lesion in the liver characterized  by sinusoidal dilatation from obstructed intrahepatic portal veins?**

"Zahn infarct".

❑❑  **Which of the major coagulation factors is not produced in the liver?**

Von Willebrand's factor.

❑❑  **What is the normal amount of hepatic iron concentration compared to that seen in patients with hemochromatosis?**

Normally, there is less than 1,000 micrograms of iron per gram of liver; however, in hemochromatosis, patients have over 10,000 micrograms of iron per gram of liver.  When this reaches greater than 20,000, hepatic fibrosis and cirrhosis develop.

❑❑  **What is the most common cause of death in patients with long-standing hereditary hemochromatosis?**

Hepatocellular carcinoma.

❑❑  **Where is alpha-1-antitrypsin produced?**

Hepatocytes predominantly and, to a lesser degree, in macrophages.

❑❑  **What percent of patients with alpha-1-antitrypsin deficiency characterized by a PiZZ phenotype have demonstrable liver disease?**

Less than 20%; however, 100% will have PAS+, diastase-resistant globules within the cytoplasm of hepatocytes.

❑❑  **How frequently do patients with primary sclerosing cholangitis have concomitant ulcerative colitis?**

70% of the time; however, patients with ulcerative colitis have concomitant primary sclerosing cholangitis in less than 5% of cases.

❑❑  **What is the most common complication of amebiasis?**

Hepatic abscess.

❑❑  **What histologic pattern of hepatoblastoma carries the best prognosis?**

Those that have a pure fetal pattern have the best prognosis while those with a pure anaplastic pattern, resembling neuroblastoma, have the worst.

❏❏  **What quantity of acetaminophen is generally ingested to cause significant acetaminophen toxicity in the liver?**

Greater than 15 grams.

❏❏  **What are Rokitansky-Aschoff sinuses?**

These are herniations of gallbladder mucosa through the muscular wall of the gallbladder which occur in instances of chronic cholecystitis and cholelithiasis.

❏❏  **What are the classic "F's" describing patients at risk for cholelithiasis?**

"Fat, female, forty, fertile" - certainly not a politically correct memory assistance device!

❏❏  **What are the two main risk factors for development of cholelithiasis?**

Obesity and a high fat calorie diet.

❏❏  **What is the most common type of gallstone in the United States?**

Cholesterol stone.

❏❏  **What are some of the components of pigment gallstones?**

Calcium salts including calcium bilirubinate, mucin glycoprotein, and cholesterol monohydrate crystals.

❏❏  **What are the two types of pigment stones?**

Black and brown. Black stones are found usually in elderly patients without other disease and are associated with "sterile bile". Brown stones are associated with bacteria or parasites in the bile and are rarely found in the United States.

❏❏  **Which type of gallstones, pigment or cholesterol, are associated with radioopacity more frequently?**

More than half of black pigment stones are radiopaque, while less than 20% of cholesterol stones are.

❏❏  **Which type of gallstone is more frequently associated with hemolytic anemia?**

Pigment stones.

❏❏  **What is the most common cause of acute calculus cholecystitis?**

In more than 90% of cases acute calculus cholecystitis occurs as a result of impaction of a gallstone in the cystic duct or neck of the gallbladder.

❏❏  **What does the finding of so-called "strawberry" mucosa of the gallbladder indicate?**

Cholesterolosis

❏❏  **What is the association of cholesterolosis with development of cholelithiasis?**

None.

❏❏  **What is the most common tumor of the gallbladder?**

Adenocarcinoma.

❏❏ **What is choledocholithiasis?**

These are calculi of the gallbladder which exist in the common bile duct. Most frequently, they are stones from the gallbladder that enter the common duct via the cystic duct.

❏❏ **What is the most common cause of death from liver disease in infants and children?**

Extrahepatic biliary atresia.

❏❏ **In patients with extrahepatic biliary atresia, what form of bilirubin constitutes their hyperbilirubinemia?**

It is conjugated or direct bilirubin.

❏❏ **What is cholangitis?**

This is a bacterial infection of the bile ducts. It is often referred to as ascending cholangitis when it involves the bile ducts within the liver. It often results from anything causing obstruction of bile flow.

❏❏ **What are the most common bacteria that serve as the etiologic agents of cholangitis?**

Gram-negative rods like E. coli, Klebsiella, Enterobacter, and others.        *Salmonella ?*

❏❏ **What is a choledochal cyst?**

This is a congenital anomaly characterized by a dilatation of the common bile duct. It is more common in females (4:1) and sometimes occurs in conjunction with Caroli's disease.

❏❏ **What is the prognosis for adenocarcinoma of the gallbladder?**

Dismal, it has almost 0% survival at five years even with surgery.

❏❏ **Where is adenocarcinoma of the gallbladder most likely to arise?**

Fundus and neck.

❏❏ **What is the name given to the tumor which originates from the common bile duct at the junction of the cystic duct and the right and left hepatic ducts?**

Klatskin tumor.

❏❏ **What is the lesion of the gallbladder which is characterized by crypts amidst hyperplastic muscularis?**

Adenomyosis and, when localized to the fundus, it is called an adenomyoma although it is not a true neoplasm.

# PANCREAS

☐☐ **What is the term given to describe a congenital malformation of the pancreas in which it encircles the duodenum and may, rarely, cause obstruction?**

Annular pancreas.

☐☐ **What is pancreas divisum?**

This is a congenital abnormality whereby the pancreas either anatomically or functionally exists as two, separate, functioning organs with persistence of the accessory duct (duct of Santorini) which drains separately into the duodenum in addition to the normal main pancreatic duct (duct of Wirsung).

☐☐ **What are the most common sites of heterotopic (ectopic) pancreas?**

Stomach, duodenum, and jejunum.

☐☐ **What is the inheritance pattern of familial pancreatitis?**

It is an autosomal dominant inheritance with limited penetrance. It is much less common than cystic fibrosis and is, as the name suggests, characterized by bouts of acute pancreatitis beginning at a young age. Eventually, these patients develop chronic pancreatitis and have an increased risk of pancreatic carcinoma.

☐☐ **What happens to the amount of adipose tissue in the pancreas as a person ages?**

The number of adipocytes increases and the acinar cell mass decreases. This is similar to the changes seen in the parathyroid glands.

☐☐ **What is a cystic ductal complex in the pancreas?**

This is a group of simple cysts that are lined by a single layer of variable epithelium with underlying fibrous walls. The lumen may or may not contain secretions.

☐☐ **What is the risk of development of carcinoma in areas of squamous metaplasia of ductal epithelium?**

There is no increased risk.

☐☐ **What is the most common benign change found in ductal epithelium of the pancreas?**

Non-papillary ductal hyperplasia which has an association with obstruction and chronic pancreatitis.

☐☐ **What is the association of non-papillary ductal hyperplasia and papillary ductal hyperplasia with pancreatic carcinoma?**

There is no association with non-papillary ductal hyperplasia. Papillary ductal hyperplasia is found at an increased rate compared to controls in patients with pancreatic carcinoma.

☐☐ **Which hormone, produced in the duodenum, is responsible for stimulation of water and bicarbonate secretion by the duct cells of the pancreas?**

Secretin.

❑❑   Which hormone, produced in the duodenum, is responsible for secretion of various zymogens by the acinar cells of the pancreas?

Cholecystokinin.

❑❑   What is the most common congenital disorder of the pancreas?

Pancreas divisum.

❑❑   What are the most common clinical associations of acute pancreatitis?

Alcoholism and cholelithiasis.

❑❑   In addition to cholelithiasis and alcoholism, what are some other major causes of pancreatitis?

Trauma, hyperlipidemia (including hereditary hyperlipidemias), viruses (mumps, Coxsackie, cytomegalovirus), parasites (Ascaris lumbricoides, Clonorchis sinensis), ischemia, drugs (such as thiazide diuretics, pentamidine, estrogens, azathioprine, furosemide, and others), hyperparathyroidism, hypercalcemia in general, and up to 1 in 5 cases are idiopathic.

❑❑   Describe the typical patient with pancreatitis.

If the etiology is related to alcohol, it is most commonly a male. In contrast, if the etiology is cholelithiasis, it is more commonly a female. In either case, the patients are typically middle-aged.

❑❑   What are Turner's and Cullen's signs?

Each are signs of acute (hemorrhagic) pancreatitis. The discoloration which occurs around the umbilicus is termed Cullen's sign and similar appearing discoloration in the loin is termed Turner's sign.

❑❑   What are some of the clinical signs of acute pancreatitis?

Mid epigastric pain radiating to the back, nausea, vomiting, and occasionally fever.

❑❑   What are the two main enzyme levels one can follow in the serum and urine to diagnose pancreatitis?

Amylase and lipase.

❑❑   What is the histologic appearance of acute pancreatitis?

Initially, there may be edema followed by liquefactive necrosis of the acini, necrosis of blood vessels with associated hemorrhage, fat necrosis, infiltration by neutrophils, and focal dystrophic calcification.

❑❑   What are some of the systemic signs of acute pancreatitis?

Peripheral blood leukocytosis, hemolysis, disseminated intravascular coagulation (DIC), adult respiratory distress syndrome (ARDS) and, ultimately, shock.

❑❑   Which enzyme, amylase or lipase, is the first to rise in acute pancreatitis?

Serum amylase rises within the first day and at about 72 hours, the lipase also begins to rise.

❑❑   What specific electrolyte disturbance imparts a very grave prognosis in pancreatitis?

Hypocalcemia, which is a result of calcium precipitation in the areas of fat necrosis.

❑❑ **In addition to the systemic signs of shock, ARDS and renal failure, what are some of the other major complications of acute pancreatitis?**

Abscess formation, pseudocyst formation, and obstruction of the duodenum.

❑❑ **What is the recurrence rate of patients who develop acute pancreatitis?**

More than half will have a recurrence within two years of the first episode of acute pancreatitis.

❑❑ **When does a pancreatic pseudocyst typically form: days, weeks, or months?**

It typically takes at least four weeks for fibrous tissue to form and develop a pseudocyst. The contents are typically sterile and, if they become infected, may form an abscess and carry a significant risk of sepsis.

❑❑ **In a patient with chronic pancreatitis, when would you expect to see symptoms of pancreatic insufficiency such as malabsorption and steatorrhea?**

Destruction of about 90% of the pancreas is required before these symptoms become apparent.

❑❑ **Describe the appearance of the islets of Langerhans in patients with chronic pancreatitis.**

While the acini are destroyed and replaced by fibrous tissue, the islets are typically spared.

❑❑ **Is there an increased risk of developing pancreatic carcinoma in patients with chronic pancreatitis?**

Yes.

❑❑ **Describe the lining of a pancreatic pseudocyst.**

They lack an epithelial lining and are composed of a fibrous wall only.

❑❑ **What is the disease characterized by hemangiomas in the retina and cerebellum in association with pancreatic, hepatic, and renal cysts?**

von Hippel-Lindau disease.

❑❑ **What is the major etiology of pancreatic pseudocysts in children?**

Trauma.

❑❑ **What is the primary etiology of pancreatic pseudocysts in adults?**

Chronic pancreatitis.

❑❑ **What is the difference between a retention cyst and a pancreatic pseudocyst?**

Retention cysts are true cysts characterized by a flattened epithelial lining, and they occur as a result of obstruction of a large pancreatic duct. As stated above, pancreatic cysts lack an epithelial lining (hence the term "pseudocyst") and are a result of chronic pancreatitis or trauma.

❑❑ **What is the average survival of patients with pancreatic carcinoma?**

Less than 12 months.

❑❑ **What histologic component of the pancreas is the originator of the vast majority of pancreatic adenocarcinomas?**

The pancreatic ducts account for about 90% of cases.

❑❑ **What is the most clear etiologic factor imparting an increased risk of developing pancreatic adenocarcinoma?**

Cigarette smoking.

❑❑ **Demographically, what gender, race, and age is most likely to develop pancreatic carcinoma?**

African-American males in the sixth to eighth decades of life. It is also more common in diabetics.

❑❑ **Anatomically, what part of the pancreas is most likely to harbor a pancreatic carcinoma?**

Lesions in the head of the pancreas account for more than half of cases. The remainder of cases are almost equally divided between the body, tail, and diffuse involvement of the pancreas precluding determination of the precise origin.

❑❑ **What is Trousseau's sign?**

This is a migratory thrombophlebitis which occurs in about 10% of patients with pancreatic carcinoma and occasionally in other malignancies.

❑❑ **What are the most common signs and symptoms of pancreatic carcinoma?**

Patients complain of a vague abdominal pain, back pain, and occasionally vomiting. Weight loss and other constitutional symptoms may occur. More than half of the patients have jaundice.

❑❑ **What is Courvoisier's sign?**

This is the presence of painless jaundice in a setting of a palpable gallbladder.

❑❑ **What is the average survival of patients with typical ductal adenocarcinoma compared to acinar cell carcinoma?**

Acinar cell carcinoma appears to have a longer survival and better prognosis than typical ductal adenocarcinoma.

❑❑ **At what age does a patient typically develop pancreatoblastoma?**

This is the most common tumor of childhood with a mean age of around three; however, it can occur in adults as well with a mean age of about 30 in the adult population.

❑❑ **What are the most common sites of spread of pancreatic carcinoma?**

They tend to metastasize to regional lymph nodes as well as the liver, lungs, peritoneum, and pleura.

❑❑ **What exposure-related substances are associated with development of ductal adenocarcinoma of the pancreas?**

Workers exposed to beta-naphthylamine and benzidine have an increased incidence of pancreatic cancer.

❑❑ **How common is extrapancreatic spread of ductal adenocarcinoma at the time of initial presentation?**

Extremely common, over 80% of patients have extrapancreatic spread.

❑❑ **What is nesidioblastosis?**

This is the admixture of islets of Langerhans with pancreatic ducts. This is sometimes referred to as ductulo-insular complexes, and they can be either focal or diffuse.

❑❑ **What is the mortality rate of acute pancreatitis?**

Up to 20%.

❑❑ **What type of fluid is found in pancreatic pseudocysts?**

They are filled with pancreatic enzymes, particularly high contents of amylase are found.

❑❑ **Compare the age of patients with serous cystadenoma to those with mucinous cystic tumors of the pancreas.**

Serous cystadenomas tend to occur in older patients while mucinous lesions are found in younger patients.

❑❑ **What is the typical appearance of the lining epithelium in mucinous cystadenomas?**

The lining is a columnar-type epithelium which often covers true papillae.

❑❑ **Where in the pancreas is a mucinous cystadenoma typically found?**

Body or tail.

❑❑ **Is there a sex predilection in mucinous cystadenomas of the pancreas?**

Yes, they are more common in women.

❑❑ **Compare the prognosis of a mucinous cystadenocarcinoma to that of typical ductal adenocarcinoma of the pancreas.**

Mucinous cystadenocarcinoma has a better survival.

❑❑ **What anatomic part of the pancreas typically harbors intraductal epithelial proliferations?**

Most are found in the head of the pancreas and in middle-aged to elderly males.

❑❑ **What is the most common cystic lesion of the pancreas?**

Pseudocyst.

❑❑ **In contrast to pseudocysts, what does the fluid of cystic tumors typically contain?**

They are typically low in pancreatic enzymes but have high levels of carcinoembryonic antigen.

❑❑ **Where are microcystic adenomas typically found within the pancreas?**

They are evenly distributed throughout.

❑❑ **What are the various cell types of the islets of Langerhans and what do they secrete?**

Alpha cells - glucagon
Beta cells - insulin
Delta cells - somatostatin
Pancreatic polypeptide cells (PP) - pancreatic polypeptide

❑❑ **What is the most common cell type in the islets of Langerhans?**

Beta cells comprise about 70% of the population, followed by alpha cells and delta cells.

❑❑  **What is the source of vasoactive intestinal polypeptide (VIP) in the pancreas?**

The D1 cells.

❑❑  **What are the two principle types of diabetes mellitus?**

Type I/juvenile-onset/insulin dependent and type II/adult-onset/non-insulin dependent.

❑❑  **What is the most common type of diabetes mellitus?**

Type II accounts for about 80% of cases.

❑❑  **Which type of diabetes mellitus is characterized by a profound loss or absence of beta cells?**

Type I.

❑❑  **Where is the gene responsible for insulin-dependent diabetes mellitus (type I) thought to reside?**

On the short arm of chromosome 6, which is near the HLA-DR and DQ clusters.

❑❑  **What HLA antigen types are associated with an increased risk of developing type I DM?**

HLA-DR3, HLA-DR4, or the heterozygote HLA-DR3/DR4.

❑❑  **In monozygotic twins, which type of diabetes has the greater concordance rate?**

By far, type II.  In type II DM, it is well over 90% while in type I DM, the concordance rate is around 50%.

❑❑  **Compare the typical patient with type I DM and type II DM.**

Type I is typically an adolescent patient who is thin and has a sudden onset of symptoms.  In contrast, Type II is classically found in patients older than 40, often much older, who are obese and have a very gradual onset of symptoms.

❑❑  **Which type of diabetes is associated with an increased incidence of various autoimmune disorders such as Hashimoto's thyroiditis?**

Type I.

❑❑  **Which type of diabetes is characterized by the presence of various autoantibodies?**

Type I often has antibodies to islet cells, insulin, and GABA-synthesizing enzyme glutamic acid decarboxylase.

❑❑  **In general terms, what are some of the factors involved in the etiology of type I DM?**

It appears to be an autoimmune-mediated process in genetically predisposed patients with association of various environmental factors.  The precise interplay of these factors remains incompletely understood.

❑❑  **Regardless of type of diabetes, what are some of the typical symptoms of diabetes mellitus?**

Polyuria, polydipsia, and polyphagia.  That is, these patients urinate excessively, drink excessively, and often eat excessively.  Paradoxically, in type I DM, the polyphagia is typically associated with weight loss.

❏❏   **What would you expect to see histologically in a patient with insulin-dependent diabetes mellitus (type I DM)?**

Acutely, there is a lymphocytic inflammatory infiltrate seen associated with the islets. The lymphocytes are predominantly T-cells and this infiltrate can be rather patchy. In the long term, there is marked atrophy of the pancreas with profound loss of beta cells thereby making the islets very small, irregular and sometimes difficult to identify.

❏❏   **Although there is beta cell dysfunction in type II diabetes mellitus, what is the primary defect resulting in development of diabetes mellitus in these patients?**

Insulin resistance. These patients have a relative insulin deficiency secondary to some beta cell dysfunction in the face of peripheral insulin resistance.

❏❏   **What is the mode of inheritance in maturity-onset diabetes of youth (MODY)?**

Autosomal dominant.

❏❏   **What is amylin?**

It is also known as islet amyloid polypeptide (IAPP). It is found in beta cells in all patients (diabetic or non-diabetic) and is co-secreted with insulin. It has an unknown function and has been found to be deposited between beta cells in capillaries in the form of amyloid fibrils in type II diabetes mellitus.

❏❏   **How common is diabetes mellitus in end stage chronic pancreatitis?**

Ultimately some 70% of patients develop diabetes mellitus in chronic pancreatitis.

❏❏   **Describe the histologic appearance of the islets in patients with type II diabetes mellitus.**

They are most often normal. Sometimes there is stromal amyloidosis; however, there is no reduction of beta cells or degranulation of beta cells as can be seen in type I diabetes mellitus.

❏❏   **How common is diabetes mellitus in association with cystic fibrosis?**

It occurs in about 10% of patients.

❏❏   **What type of diabetes mellitus develops in hemochromatosis?**

At first, a non-insulin dependent diabetes mellitus develops. However, as the disease progresses insulin dependency occurs.

❏❏   **How does hemochromatosis cause diabetes mellitus?**

Interestingly, iron is preferentially deposited within the beta cells of the islets. The beta cells are then markedly degranulated indicating that somehow iron interferes with the synthesis, storage, and release of insulin.

❏❏   **How are the long term complications of uncontrolled diabetes different in type I and type II diabetes mellitus?**

They aren't. The long term complications ranging from diabetic retinopathy, neuropathy, and small and large vessel disease occur in poorly controlled diabetes regardless of the etiology.

❏❏   **Classically, what is the difference between the comas seen in marked hyperglycemia of type I diabetes mellitus and type II diabetes mellitus?**

Patients with type I diabetes mellitus typically develop diabetic ketoacidosis while the coma seen in type II diabetes mellitus is classically a nonketotic, hyperosmolar coma.

❑❑ **What is the classic renal lesion seen in the kidneys of diabetics?**

Nodular glomerulosclerosis.

❑❑ **What effect does glucose have on insulin in the cells?**

Glucose serves to promote production and release of insulin.

❑❑ **What are the two major causes of death in diabetics?**

Myocardial infarction is the most common cause followed by complications related to diabetic nephropathy.

❑❑ **What substance accumulates in the lens of diabetics resulting in cataracts?**

Sorbitol.

❑❑ **What substance is cleaved from proinsulin in the Golgi apparatus and is stored and secreted in the beta cells?**

C-peptide.

❑❑ **What are some of the reasons for insulin resistance which occurs in type II diabetes mellitus?**

There is a decrease in the number of insulin receptors and there is abnormal cellular transmembrane signaling.

❑❑ **What is the effect on low density lipoprotein (LDL) and high density lipoprotein (HDL) in diabetics?**

Glycosylation of HDL causes it to be broken down more easily. LDL becomes more readily recognized by the LDL receptor when it is glycosylated. In concert, these two factors cause increased development of atherosclerosis in medium and large vessels in diabetic patients.

❑❑ **What are some of the lesions that characterize diabetic retinopathy?**

This is characterized by retinal hemorrhages, exudates, edema, microaneurysms, and microangiopathy.

❑❑ **What would you expect to see histologically in the islets in infants of diabetic mothers?**

There is typically islet hyperplasia secondary to the hyperglycemia that the infant "sees" in utero because of the mother's hyperglycemia.

❑❑ **What is the term given to describe a neuroendocrine tumor of the pancreas which is less than 0.5 cm in diameter?**

Microadenoma, most "functioning" neuroendocrine tumors of the pancreas are greater than 0.5 cm in diameter.

❑❑ **What are the histologic features of a neuroendocrine tumor of the pancreas which help delineate whether it is benign or malignant and what type of hormone it produces?**

There really are no reliable microscopic features to identify any of those characteristics; however, if there is amyloid present this tends to indicate insulin production by the tumor (insulinoma) and somatostatinomas of the ampullary and periampullary region sometimes contain gland formations with psammoma bodies.

❏❏ In general, are insulinomas benign or malignant?

Over 90% of them are benign.

❏❏ In general, are most non-insulin producing neuroendocrine tumors of the pancreas benign or malignant?

Most are malignant.

❏❏ What is the most frequent functioning neuroendocrine tumor of the pancreas?

Insulinoma.

❏❏ What are the criteria necessary for the diagnosis of a malignant islet cell tumor?

The presence of regional lymph node or hepatic metastases are necessary for the diagnosis of malignancy. Supportive findings would include infiltrative borders, increased mitotic activity, and vascular invasion; however, these are very unreliable "predictors" and the only true determining factor is behavior.

❏❏ What is a typical clinical presentation for a patient with insulinoma?

They present with symptoms related to hypoglycemia which is relieved by eating.

❏❏ What is the typical treatment for an insulinoma?

Surgical resection.

❏❏ What is the second most common functioning neuroendocrine tumor of the pancreas?

Gastrinoma.

❏❏ Compared to insulinoma, what is the likelihood of malignancy in a gastrinoma?

In contrast to insulinoma, the vast majority of gastrinomas are malignant. Remember, insulinomas are overwhelmingly benign.

❏❏ What is the triad that characterizes Zollinger-Ellison syndrome?

Severe peptic ulcer disease, gastric hypersecretion, and a gastrinoma.

❏❏ How common is gastrinoma in the duodenum?

Although the vast majority arise in the pancreas, up to 15% occur in the duodenum.

❏❏ What is the incidence of malignancy in "VIPomas"?

Like gastrinomas, the vast majority are malignant (80%).

❏❏ What is the typical clinical presentation of a patient with a glucagonoma?

These are more common in women and occur between the ages of 40 and 70. Patients develop a rash called necrolytic migratory erythema, anemia, glucose intolerance, deep venous thrombosis, weight loss, and depression.

❏❏ What is the favored location of somatostatinomas of the pancreas?

The head of the pancreas followed by the second portion of the duodenum.

❏❏ **What other conditions are somatostatinomas associated with?**

Neurofibromatosis type I and pheochromocytomas.

❏❏ **What substance can be measured in the serum of diabetics to get a "picture" of what their blood glucose control has been like in the preceding several weeks?**

Glycated hemoglobin.

# KIDNEY AND URINARY TRACT

☐☐ **What is the name of the fascia which surrounds the kidneys?**

Gerota's fascia.

☐☐ **What are the main components of the nephron?**

The glomerulus which extends into Bowman's capsule, the renal tubules, and the interstitium.

☐☐ **Which receives more of the renal blood supply, the renal cortex or medulla?**

The renal cortex by far receives more blood, 90% of the total renal circulation.

☐☐ **What is the name of the epithelium which lines the urinary tract?**

Transitional epithelium or urothelium.

☐☐ **What is the term for the gap between adjacent foot processes in the glomerulus?**

It is called the filtration slit and the membrane which drains the adjacent foot processes is called the slit-pore diaphragm.

☐☐ **What type of collagen makes up the glomerular basement membrane (GBM)?**

The predominant collagen is type IV with small amounts of type V.

☐☐ **In addition to collagen, what are the other components of the glomerular basement membrane?**

Laminin, proteoglycans (predominantly heparan sulfate), fibronectin, intactin, and other glycoproteins.

☐☐ **Ultrastructurally, what are the three general layers of the glomerular basement membrane?**

1. Lamina rara externa (electron lucent)
2. Lamina densa (central electron dense)
3. Lamina rara interna (electron lucent)

☐☐ **What is the net charge of the GBM as well as the epithelial and endothelial surfaces of the glomerulus?**

Negative.

☐☐ **What are the two main factors which determine a molecule's permeability in the GBM?**

Size and charge.

☐☐ **Given the nature of the GBM permeability characteristics, what would you expect the permeability of albumin to be?**

Albumin is impermeable secondary to its size (70,000 molecular weight) and negative charge. Small and cationic molecules are typically permeable.

❏❏  **Where is the majority of filtered sodium and water resorbed?**

The proximal tubules.

❏❏  **What are the typical antibodies employed when performing immunofluo rescent studies on kidney biopsies?**

IgG, IgA, IgM, C1q, C3, albumin, fibrinogen, kappa and lambda.

❏❏  **In general, what are the etiologies for glomerular-based diseases compared to tubular-based diseases?**

Glomerular diseases tend to be immunologic while tubular diseases are often toxic or infectious in nature.

❏❏  **What is azotemia?**

This is a rise in blood urea nitrogen (BUN) and creatinine typically secondary to a decreased glomerular filtration rate (GFR).

❏❏  **What is the term used to describe an accumulation of cells or debris within the urinary space (Bowman's space)?**

Crescent.

❏❏  **What are the four terms used to describe the distribution of lesions within a glomerulus?**

The terms focal and diffuse describe whether the lesion effects some or all of the glomeruli within a kidney, respectively. The terms segmental and global describe whether a lesion effects a portion of a particular glomerulus or the entire glomerulus, respectively.

❏❏  **What are the two embryologic origins, both mesodermal, from which the kidney originates?**

The mesonephros and metanephros.

❏❏  **What structures are derived from the urogenital sinus?**

The bladder, female urethra, and parts of the male urethra.

❏❏  **What is the basic etiologic mechanism which results in the development of a crescent?**

Damage to capillary walls resulting in leakage of cells and extracellular material into Bowman's space.

❏❏  **What are the components of acute nephritic syndrome?**

Uremia, oliguria, hematuria, proteinuria, hypertension, and red cell casts. It is a glomerular syndrome and is classically seen in acute poststreptococcal glomerulonephritis.

❏❏  **What are the components of nephrotic syndrome?**

Marked proteinuria (greater than 3.5 g/day), hypoalbuminemia, marked edema, hyperlipidemia, and lipiduria.

❏❏  **What are the basic components of disorders associated with renal tubular defects?**

Polyuria, nocturia, and electrolyte disturbances.

❏❏  **What are the basic electrolyte disturbances one sees in chronic renal failure?**

Hyperkalemia, hyperphosphatemia, hypocalcemia, and resultant metabolic acidosis.

❑❑  **What types of symptoms would one expect to see in a patient who has a glomerular filtration rate (GFR) of 60% of normal?**

None.

❑❑  **How much reduction in GFR is typically necessary for symptoms to become manifest?**

Less than 50% of normal GFR.

❑❑  **What are the requirements for the diagnosis of true renal hypoplasia?**

There must be no other reason such as scars to account for the hypoplasia, and there should be six or fewer renal pyramids.

❑❑  **What is the term used to describe a congenital fusion of the two kidneys?**

Horseshoe kidney and 90% are fused at the lower pole as opposed to the upper pole.

❑❑  **What are tubular casts composed of?**

A mucoprotein produced by the cells found in the thick ascending limb of the loop of Henle called Tamm-Horsfall protein.

❑❑  **How common are other congenital anomalies in patients with bilateral renal agenesis?**

It is quite common to have other abnormalities, occurring in up to half of patients.  Bilateral renal agenesis is incompatible with life and the patient is stillborn or dies shortly after birth.

❑❑  **What is the most common site of an ectopic kidney?**

The pelvis.

❑❑  **List some glomerular causes of the nephrotic syndrome in adults.**

Membranous glomerulonephropathy, focal segmental glomerulosclerosis, diabetes mellitus, minimal change disease, lupus, and membranoproliferative glomerulonephritis type I.

❑❑  **What are some of the glomerular causes of acute nephritic syndrome in adults?**

IgA nephropathy (Berger's disease), lupus, acute postinfectious glomerulonephritis (GN), ANCA-associated GN, membranoproliferative GN, and antiglomerular basement membrane disease (Goodpasture's syndrome).

❑❑  **What are some causes of the nephrotic syndrome in children?**

Focal segmental glomerulosclerosis, membranous nephropathy, minimal change disease, membranoproliferative glomerulonephritis type I and II, and lupus.

❑❑  **What are some causes of acute nephritic syndrome in children?**

IgA nephropathy or Berger's disease, acute postinfectious GN, membranoproliferative GN, and lupus.

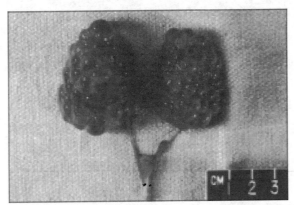

AUTOSOMAL RECESSIVE POLYCYSTIC KIDNEY DISEASE WITH RENAL DYSPLASIA

☐☐  **In this example of cystic renal dysplasia, would you expect other congenital abnormalities of the genitourinary tract?**

Yes, about 90% of the time there are other congenital abnormalities. Histologically, these kidneys feature immature ductules and undifferentiated or immature mesenchyme, often cartilage.

☐☐  **What are some of the components of Meckel's syndrome?**

Meckel's syndrome or Meckel-Gruber is inherited in an autosomal recessive fashion.  There is renal dysplasia with associated hypoplasia of the ureters and bladder in association with an occipital encephalocele, polydactyly, ambiguous genitalia, cleft lip/palate, microphthalmia, and pancreatic dysplasia.

☐☐  **In addition to Meckel's syndrome, what are some other syndromes that feature a component of renal dysplasia?**

Zellweger's syndrome (deficiency of dihydroxyacetone phosphate acyltransferase, hypotonia, seizures, and biliary dysgenesis), Caroli's syndrome, Jeune's syndrome (asphyxiating thoracic dystrophy with a small thorax, pulmonary hypoplasia, polydactyly, biliary dysgenesis, and other features).  There are many other syndromes which may have a component of renal dysplasia.

☐☐  **How is the adult, heritable form of polycystic kidney disease inherited?**

It is autosomal dominant with high penetrance.

☐☐  **Where is the gene located which is responsible for the adult form of polycystic kidney disease?**

The gene is called PKD1 and is found on chromosome 16p13.3.  This gene causes about 90% of the cases.  The PKD2 gene found on chromosome 4q13-23 is causative in around 10% of the cases.  The PKD3 gene is a rare cause of the adult, autosomal dominant polycystic kidney disease and is not yet mapped.

☐☐  **What are some important clinical associations seen in adult, autosomal dominant polycystic kidney disease?**

Mitral valve prolapse is found in about a quarter of the patients and intracranial berry aneurysms are quite common, occurring in up to 40% of patients.  In addition, cysts in other organs like the spleen, pancreas, and lungs also occur.

☐☐  **What is the most common cause of death in patients with adult polycystic kidney disease?**

Almost half die of hypertensive heart disease or coronary artery disease.

❏❏ **What is the difference in presentation of patients with polycystic kidney disease of the PKD2 genotype?**

They tend to be older patients and develop renal failure later in the course of the disease. Black males with hypertension demonstrate a more rapid clinical course.

❏❏ **What are the clinical characteristics of children with familial juvenile nephronophthisis?**

They exhibit polydipsia, polyuria, sodium wasting, and tubular acidosis.

❏❏ **Is there any association with renal cell carcinoma and adult, autosomal dominant polycystic kidney disease?**

Yes, there is an increased incidence of renal cell carcinoma.

❏❏ **What are the various forms of medullary cystic disease?**

1. Sporadic, nonfamilial (about 20% of cases)
2. Familial juvenile nephronophthisis
3. Renal-retinal dysplasia (autosomal recessive, 15% of cases)
4. Adult-onset medullary cystic disease (autosomal dominant, 15%)

❏❏ **What is the typical size of the kidneys in autosomal dominant polycystic kidney disease, autosomal recessive polycystic kidney disease, and medullary cystic disease?**

The kidneys are enlarged in the autosomal dominant and recessive polycystic kidney diseases while they are small in medullary cystic disease.

❏❏ **Is there a risk of development of renal cell carcinoma in acquired or dialysis-associated cystic disease?**

Yes, over the course of 10 years, almost 10% of patients on chronic dialysis will develop renal cell carcinoma in association with acquired cystic disease.

❏❏ **What syndrome is characterized by a defect in type IV collagen in the glomerular basement membrane, hearing loss, and occasional ocular abnormalities?**

Alport's syndrome or hereditary nephritis.

❏❏ **What is the most common inheritance pattern of Alport's syndrome?**

X-linked dominant.

❏❏ **What is the appearance of the glomerular basement membrane by electron microscopy in Alport's syndrome?**

Electron microscopy is critical for the diagnosis as the light microscopy and immunofluorescence are both nonspecific. The GBM is variable along its course from thinned to markedly thickened ranging from 60 nanometers to1200 nanometers. The thickened basement membrane demonstrates alternating electron dense and electron lucent areas creating a lamellated appearance of the basement membrane. The visceral epithelial cell foot processes are effaced.

❏❏ **What is the typical clinical presentation of Alport's syndrome?**

In males, the disease is more severe and occurs earlier. It is characterized by microscopic hematuria with occasional periods of gross hematuria and the characteristic hearing loss.

❏❏ **What is the pathologic finding in thin basement membrane nephropathy?**

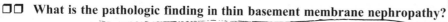

As the name suggests, the only abnormality is thinning of the glomerular basement membrane. By definition, to qualify for this entity the adult GBM must be less than 250 nanometers while in children it is less than 200 nanometers.

❑❑ **Which layer of the GBM is thinned in thin basement membrane nephropathy?**

The lamina densa.

❑❑ **What is the relative prognosis for patients with thin basement membrane disease?**

It is excellent with no significant loss of renal function.

❑❑ **What is the enzyme deficiency in Fabry's disease?**

Alpha-galactosidase A.

❑❑ **Where is the gene for Fabry's disease located?**

Xq22-24.

❑❑ **What is the pathologic effect of Fabry's disease on the kidney?**

There is accumulation of ceramide trihexoside within the epithelial cells of the glomerulus and, to a lesser degree, the distal collecting tubules.

❑❑ **What are the classic ultrastructural structures seen in Fabry's disease?**

"Zebra bodies".

❑❑ **In general terms, what is the most common type of basement membrane thickening?**

Subepithelial deposits as seen in membranous glomerulonephritis.

❑❑ **What is the cause of nephrosclerosis?**

Nephrosclerosis is an ischemic injury of tubules, glomeruli, and interstitium secondary to arteriosclerosis and arteriolosclerosis.

❑❑ **What is the most common etiology of nephrosclerosis?**

Hypertension.

❑❑ **What is the pattern of immunofluorescence in the thrombotic microangiopathies?**

There is a linear pattern of fibrin in the walls of capillaries, arterioles, and arteries.

❑❑ **What is the most common cause of nephrotic syndrome in children?**

Minimal change disease.

❑❑ **What are some of the disease associations with minimal change disease?**

It often occurs in association with both Hodgkin's and non-Hodgkin's lymphoma as well as renal cell carcinoma. Interestingly, it has been found to wax and wane with the status of the lymphoma. In addition, numerous medications are associated with minimal change disease including nonsteroidals and lithium carbonate.

❑❑  **What is the typical immunofluorescence finding in minimal change disease?**
It is usually negative.

❑❑  **What is the characteristic histologic finding in the tubular epithelial cells in minimal change disease?**

The tubular epithelium classically contains lipid vacuoles sometimes termed "lipid degeneration" hence the alternative term of lipoid nephrosis.

❑❑  **What is the predominant ultrastructural finding in minimal change disease?**

Near total effacement of the podocytes or foot-processes with associated microvillus transformation.

❑❑  **What is the typical clinical presentation, therapy, and response in patients with minimal change disease?**

Again, they present with nephrotic syndrome. It typically responds to steroids. Although it can relapse, it typically responds again to steroids. Those that are resistant to this therapy are worthy of a biopsy to rule out another etiology for the clinical picture.

❑❑  **Describe the typical immunofluorescence findings in patients with mesangial proliferative glumerulonephritis.**

They have widespread deposition of IgM in a granular pattern in the mesangium.

❑❑  **What is the typical presentation of patients with focal segmental glomerulosclerosis?**

They typically present with heavy proteinuria and the other features of nephrotic syndrome. It is more common in African-Americans.

❑❑  **What is the prognosis in patients with focal segmental glomerulosclerosis?**

It varies, some pursue an aggressive course with resultant end stage disease while others respond to extended courses of steroids. The disease has a poor prognosis and much poorer steroid response rate than minimal change disease. In addition, it can recur in transplanted kidneys.

❑❑  **What is the most common cause of nephrotic syndrome in adults?**

Membranous glomerulonephritis.

❑❑  **What is the typical clinical presentation in membranous glomerulonephritis?**

The nephrotic syndrome is the most common presentation. In a small number of cases, it may present with asymptomatic proteinuria or microscopic hematuria.

❑❑  **What are some of the underlying etiologies in the secondary form of membranous glomerulonephritis?**

Systemic lupus erythematosus, hepatitis, and malignancy.

❑❑  **Describe the typical or classic ultrastructural finding in membranous glomerulonephritis.**

Classically, there is effacement of the foot-processes and deposition of irregular dense deposits which are positive for IgG and complement in the subepithelial region. Between these deposits, there are irregular protrusions of basement membrane material producing "spikes" of glomerular basement membrane. Eventually, this basement membrane material continues to be laid down and covers the subepithelial deposits resulting in "domes" Thus, the precise appearance ultrastructurally depends on the stage of the disease.

❑❑  **What is the general prognosis of patients with membranous glomerulonephritis?**

50% will experience spontaneous remission of varying degrees, 25% maintain persistent nephrotic syndrome, and 25% progress to end stage renal disease and renal failure. In the secondary form, the underlying disease and treatment of it is clearly the critical factor in progression or remission of the renal disease.

❑❑  **What is the etiology of the majority of cases of membranous glomerulonephritis?**

Some 85% of cases are idiopathic or primary, while the secondary form (SLE, hepatitis, diabetes, syphilis, malignancy, and drugs such as penicillamine and gold) makes up the remaining cases.

❑❑  **What are the three types of membranoproliferative glomerulonephritis (MPGN)?**

Type I -  hypercellular mesangium, lobular glomeruli, and "tram track" or "double contour" basement membrane

Type II  (aka dense deposit disease) - lobular glomerulonephritis, markedly thickened capillary walls with intramembranous electron dense material

Type III - like type I plus subepithelial deposits similar to membranous GN

❑❑  **In the secondary forms of MPGN type I, what is the most common disease association?**

Hepatitis C.

❑❑  **Describe the pattern of immunofluorescence in type I MPGN.**

Immunofluorescence reveals deposition of IgG and C3 in a granular pattern in both the capillaries and mesangium.

❑❑  **What is different about type II MPGN compared to type I in immunofluorescent studies?**

Both exhibit granular immunofluorescence; however, type II is positive for C3 while negative for IgG.

❑❑  **Which of the MPGN diseases is associated with mesangium-cellular interposition?**

Type I.

❑❑  **What are the typical electron microscopy findings in type I MPGN?**

There are deposits in the subendothelium, mesangial migration and interposition, and mesangial deposits.

❑❑  **What are the typical electron microscopy findings in type II MPGN?**

They have so-called "intramembranous deposits" in which the lamina densa is replaced by granular electron dense material. Immune complex deposits can be found in the subepithelium and mesangium and there is foot process effacement.

❑❑  **Does MPGN recur in renal allografts?**

Yes, particularly type II where the recurrence rate is well over 90%.

❑❑  **What is the difference in the activation of complement in type I and type II MPGN?**

Type I activates complement via the classic pathway secondary to the presence of immune complexes in the circulation. Type II activates complement via the alternate pathway owing to an antibody to C3 convertase which is called the C3 nephritic factor. This factor stabilizes the C3 convertase and it allows for unopposed complement activation.

❐❒ **A patient presents with recurrent gross hematuria and mild proteinuria. The kidney biopsy demonstrates mesangial proliferation and IgA deposits in the mesangium. What is the diagnosis?**

IgA nephropathy or Berger's disease.

❐❒ **Worldwide, what is the most common primary glomerulopathy?**

Berger's disease.

❐❒ **What will be increased in the serum in many, but not all, patients with Berger's disease?**

IgA and IgA-fibronectin complexes.

❐❒ **What would one find on immunofluorescence in patients with Berger's disease?**

Mesangial deposits of IgA and often C3. IgG and IgM can be found, but with lesser intensity. The IgA can be seen as granular deposits in some of the capillary walls within a few glomeruli as well.

❐❒ **What is the treatment and prognosis for patients with Berger's disease or IgA nephropathy?**

One can treat the effects of IgA nephropathy but not the underlying etiology. Thus, it progresses to end stage renal disease in a third of the patients within 20 years. If transplanted, IgA deposits will recur in the allograft, but this rarely results in renal failure.

❐❒ **What are some of the components of Henoch-Schonlein purpura?**

This is a small vessel vasculitis with deposits of IgA in the vessels in association with renal, skin, joint, and gastrointestinal symptoms. The kidney lesion is characterized by a mesangial IgA deposition and a proliferative glomerulonephritis.

❐❒ **Describe the typical patient and presentation of Henoch-Schonlein purpura.**

This disease primarily occurs in adolescents and children. The patients present with lower abdominal pain, joint pain, and palpable purpura in the lower extremities. Manifestation of the renal disease occurs in a minority of patients and includes gross or microscopic hematuria and proteinuria.

❐❒ **What is the organism which is classically associated with postinfectious glomerulonephritis?**

Streptococcus. However, numerous other organisms including other bacteria, viruses, and even parasites can cause the same picture.

❐❒ **What is the typical clinical presentation of postinfectious glomerulonephritis?**

Patients have a sudden onset of gross hematuria, proteinuria, hypertension, and edema. They develop decreased levels of serum complement (C3).

❐❒ **What is the classic electron microscopy finding in postinfectious glomerulonephritis?**

They have very large, "hump-shaped" subepithelial deposits which are irregularly distributed.

❐❒ **Where do the autoantibodies present in patients with Goodpasture's disease bind on the glomerular basement membrane?**

They bind to an epitope in the globular noncollagenous domain of the type IV collagen found in the basement membrane. The Goodpasture antigen is a peptide on the alpha3 chain of type IV collagen molecules.

❏❏ **What is the pattern of staining in the immunofluorescence studies of patients with antiglomerular basement membrane disease?**

There is a diffuse, linear staining with IgG.

❏❏ **When does a patient have Goodpasture's disease compared to one that only has antiglomerular basement membrane nephritis?**

Goodpasture's disease or syndrome is when the antibasement membrane autoantibodies affect other organs, particularly the lungs, in addition to the kidney.

❏❏ **Is there crescent formation in antiglomerular basement membrane disease?**

Yes, at least in many of the glomeruli.

❏❏ **What is lacking in the basement membrane of patients with Alport's syndrome?**

These patients lack the Goodpasture antigen.  Thus, if they receive a renal allograft they will develop circulating antiglomerular basement membrane antibodies.

❏❏ **What are the two types of ANCA?**

c-ANCA and p-ANCA.

❏❏ **Which ANCA is associated with Wegener's granulomatosis and corresponds with anti-proteinase3 antibody?**

c-ANCA.

❏❏ **Which ANCA is associated with pauci-immune glomerulonephritis?**

p-ANCA.

❏❏ **What specific disease is indicated by the presence of crescents?**

There is no specific "crescentic" renal disease.

❏❏ **According to the World Health Organization (WHO) classification of lupus nephritis, what class is a renal lesion exhibiting focal and segmental proliferative glomerulonephritis in a patient with SLE?**

Class III.

❏❏ **What are the five categories of the WHO classification of lupus nephritis?**

Class I -   no abnormalities
Class II -  mesangial glomerulonephritis
Class III - focal and segmental proliferative glomerulonephritis
Class IV - diffuse proliferative glomerulonephritis
Class V -  membranous glomerulonephritis
            A - "pure" membranous glomerulonephritis
            B - with mesangial glomerulonephritis
            C - with focal proliferative glomerulonephritis
            D - with diffuse proliferative glomerulonephritis

❏❏ **What renal disease is classically associated with a "full house" immunofluorescence?**

SLE.

⬜⬜ **What is the ultrastructural correlate of the "wire loops" seen histologically in some renal lesions of SLE?**

These are subendothelial immune complex deposits.

⬜⬜ **What are the two basic forms of diabetic nephropathy?**

Diffuse glomerulosclerosis and nodular glomerulosclerosis (Kimmelsteil-Wilson lesions).

⬜⬜ **What would you expect to find on electron microscopy in SLE?**

Immune deposits can be found in the mesangium, subendothelially and in subepithelial locations. In addition, there are characteristic tubuloreticular or tubulovesicular structures.

⬜⬜ **What are the drugs most commonly associated with acute interstitial nephritis?**

Diuretics, various antibiotics (particularly synthetic penicillins) and nonsteroidal anti-inflammatory drugs.

⬜⬜ **What are some poor prognostic indicators for acute interstitial nephritis?**

Older age of patient, longer lasting renal failure (greater than three weeks), and severe cortical inflammation.

⬜⬜ **What is the first histologic lesion seen in analgesic abuse nephropathy?**

Papillary necrosis.

⬜⬜ **What is the most common etiologic agent of acute infectious interstitial nephritis?**

E. coli.

⬜⬜ **What is the difference in the renal involvement in acute infectious interstitial nephritis or acute pyelonephritis depending on if the etiology is an ascending infection or hematogenous spread?**

In ascending infection, the inflammatory response including abundant neutrophils is seen in the medulla and papillae with tubular microabscesses. In contrast, hematogenous spread demonstrates marked cortical inflammation with associated abscesses and the papillae are uninvolved.

⬜⬜ **What is the most common cause of chronic pyelonephritis?**

It is usually related to vesicoureteral abnormalities with subsequent reflux.

⬜⬜ **What is the most common location for the cortical scars seen in patients with chronic pyelonephritis?**

The poles.

⬜⬜ **What organism is classically associated with the development of "staghorn" calculi with subsequent development of obstruction?**

Proteus vulgaris.

⬜⬜ **What cells in the kidney are most susceptible to ischemia?**

The cells of the thick ascending limb of the loop of Henle.

❐❐ **What toxic injury to the kidneys can result in acute tubular necrosis and occasionally abundant intratubular oxalate crystal formation?**

Ethylene glycol (antifreeze).

❐❐ **In particular, what renal tubular cells are susceptible to mercury poisoning and exhibit total necrosis?**

The proximal tubular cells.

❐❐ **What is the most common cause of acute renal failure?**

Acute tubular necrosis of varying etiologies.

❐❐ **What type of antibiotic would a patient most likely have received if they developed renal failure and acute tubular necrosis with myeloid bodies in the proximal tubular cells?**

An aminoglycoside.

❐❐ **What type of immune deposits are present in diabetic nephropathy?**

There are no immune deposits in diabetic nephropathy.  Trick question.

❐❐ **What happens to the mesangium in diabetic nephropathy?**

It is expanded and mildly hypercellular.

❐❐ **How common is renal disease in diabetics?**

It is very common.  More than 1/3 of patients with type I diabetes mellitus will develop end stage renal disease after 20 years.  The rate is lower in patients with type II diabetes mellitus.

❐❐ **What might you see in the capillary loops in nodular glomerulosclerosis (Kimmelsteil-Wilson lesions)?**

There can be microaneurysmal dilatation of the peripheral capillary loops in association with the Kimmelsteil-Wilson lesions.

❐❐ **What are the two general categories or etiologies of acute tubular necrosis?**

1.  Toxic
2.  Ischemic

❐❐ **What are the three types of rapidly progressive (crescentic) glomerulonephritis?**

Type I - Idiopathic and Goodpasture's syndrome
Type II (immune complex) - Idiopathic, postinfectious, SLE, Henoch-Schonlein purpura
Type III - (pauci-immune) - Idiopathic, Wegener's granulomatosis, microscopic polyarteritis nodosa

❐❐ **What alpha chain in the structure of type IV collagen is the Goodpasture antigen?**

The alpha3 chain.

❐❐ **What is the definition of microalbuminuria?**

This is urinary excretion of albumin at the rate of 30-300 mg/day.

❐❐ **Discuss how light chains cause renal dysfunction in patients with multiple myeloma.**

The free light chains (Bence-Jones proteins) are directly nephrotoxic to the proximal tubular cells. They precipitate out in the tubular lumen and combine with Tamm-Horsfall proteins to form casts which then elicit an inflammatory response including multinucleated giant cells (cast nephropathy).

❏❏  **What are the three types of cryoglobulins?**

Type I - monoclonal immunoglobulin (plasma cell dyscrasias)
Type II - polyclonal IgG, monoclonal IgM (infection, autoimmune, lymphoma, and idiopathic)
Type III - polyclonal IgG, polyclonal anti-IgG (autoimmune and chronic infections)

❏❏  **What is the most common type of cryoglobulin which affects the kidney?**

Type II is by far the most common. About a third of the cases are idiopathic, while the remainder are found in association with other conditions such as lymphoma.

❏❏  **What is the typical clinical presentation in patients with mixed cryoglobulinemia?**

These patients develop purpura, arthralgia, and hypertension. The renal involvement varies from proteinuria to renal failure. Complement is low and rheumatoid factor is elevated.

❏❏  **List some of the causes of papillary necrosis.**

Analgesics, acute pyelonephritis, sickle cell disease, NSAIDS, diabetes mellitus, and urinary obstruction.

❏❏  **What systemic disease gives arterioles a similar appearance as that seen in malignant hypertension?**

Progressive systemic sclerosis (scleroderma).

❏❏  **Is there an increased risk for renal cell carcinoma in patients with acquired renal cystic disease?**

Yes.

❏❏  **In renal transplant pathology, what is the name of the process of activation of T-lymphocytes by several cytokines including interferon-gamma and interleukin-2 resulting in infiltration and injury to the allograft?**

Acute (cellular) rejection.

❏❏  **When, following transplantation, would you be most likely to find acute (cellular) rejection?**

Within the first three to six months.

❏❏  **What is the most common renal disease (non-recurrent) that occurs in a transplanted kidney?**

Membranous nephropathy.

❏❏  **In a patient who is status post renal transplantation eight years ago, a biopsy shows tubular atrophy and "striped" interstitial fibrosis with essentially no associated inflammation. The glomeruli appear ischemic and the arterioles are hyalinized with expansion of the juxtaglomerular apparatus. What is the most likely diagnosis?**

Chronic cyclosporine toxicity.

❏❏  **Name two diseases which recur frequently in renal allografts and do so at an early stage.**

Focal and segmental glomerulosclerosis and membranoproliferative glomerulonephritis type II.

❑❑  **What disease recurs frequently in the renal allograft; however, is not typically clinically significant?**

IgA nephropathy.

❑❑  **What condition can result in renal artery stenosis and hypertension and tends to occur in younger females?**

Fibromuscular dysplasia.

❑❑  **You receive a renal tumor that has a mahogany color grossly and is composed of cells with abundant granular, eosinophilic cytoplasm histologically. What is the origin of this benign tumor?**

This is a renal oncocytoma and they arise from the distal tubules.

❑❑  **Describe the typical patient who develops an angiomyolipoma.**

These tumors are twice as common in women, occur typically in the fourth and fifth decades, and present most commonly with flank pain.  Half of the cases occur in association with tuberous sclerosis.

❑❑  **What is the most common renal tumor in the 0-3 month age group?**

Mesoblastic nephroma (benign nephroblastoma).

❑❑  **What syndrome is characterized by acute renal failure and hematemesis and/or melena following an episode of diarrhea or an influenza-like prodrome?**

Hemolytic uremic syndrome which is most commonly associated with infection with E. coli type O157:H7.

❑❑  **What are some conditions that are most commonly associated with development of diffuse renal cortical necrosis?**

Obstetric emergencies, septic shock, and significant surgery.

❑❑  **What is the most common type of renal stone?**

Calcium oxalate accounts for about 75% of the cases while struvite, uric acid, and cystine are the next most common in descending order of frequency.

❑❑  **How frequently do patients with tubulous sclerosis develop angiomyolipoma?**

Up to half of the patients with tubulous sclerosis develop angiomyolipoma.

❑❑  **Name the three basic types of renal cell carcinoma.**

Clear cell, chromophil, and chromophobe.

❑❑  **Where is the von Hippel-Lindau syndrome gene located?**

Chromosome 3p25.3.

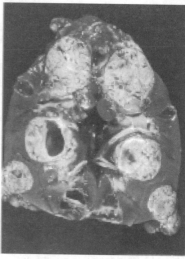

RENAL CELL CARCINOMA IN VON HIPPEL-LINDAU SYNDROME
*(Photo courtesy of Julie Breiner, MD - University of Nebraska Medical Center)*

❏❏  **What are the components of the von Hippel-Lindau syndrome?**

Hemangioblastomas of the cerebellum and retina in association with bilateral renal cysts and often multiple renal cell carcinomas.

❏❏  **What are the most common sites of metastases of renal cell carcinoma?**

Lungs, bones, regional lymph nodes, liver, adrenal glands, and brain.

❏❏  **What is the classic presentation of renal cell carcinoma and how common is it?**

The classic triad includes costovertebral angle pain, palpable mass, and hematuria.  Unfortunately, this "classic" triad occurs in no more than 10% of cases.

❏❏  **What is the number one risk factor for development of renal cell carcinoma?**

Tobacco use.

❏❏  **Where is the Wilms' tumor associated gene located?**

Chromosome 11p13.

❏❏  **What are the two types of Wilms' tumor histology?**

The two categories are favorable and unfavorable histologic features which are based on the presence or absence of anaplasia as indicated by high nuclear grade and abnormal mitotic figures.

❏❏  **What are some important prognostic features in Wilms' tumor?**

A better prognosis is associated with young age (less than 2 years old), lack of capsular penetration by tumor, absence of venous invasion and/or distant metastases, and presence of tubular/glomerular differentiation in a setting of favorable histology.

❏❏  **What is the WAGR syndrome and what is its association with Wilms' tumor?**

The WAGR syndrome is comprised of Wilms' tumor, aniridia, genital abnormalities, and mental retardation.  The Wilms' tumor develops in a third of the cases.

🔲🔲 **In general terms, what is the prognosis for patients with Wilms' tumor?**

It is excellent, with some 90% of patients cured with varying combinations of surgical resection, chemotherapy, and radiation.

🔲🔲 **Where in the kidney is the most common location of congenital calyceal diverticulum?**

Upper pole.

🔲🔲 **What is the most common location for fibroepithelial polyps in the urinary tract?**

Ureter, left greater than right.

🔲🔲 **What is urothelial hyperplasia?**

This is hyperplastic urothelium (greater than 5 cell layers) which is devoid of papillary architecture and significant dysplasia.

🔲🔲 **What is the term given to describe an invagination of the normal urothelium into the underlying lamina propria in the bladder?**

Von Brunn's nests.

🔲🔲 **What is the most common site for the development of cystitis cystica in the urinary bladder?**

Trigone.

🔲🔲 **What is the term given to describe the absence of the anterior musculature of the bladder resulting in protrusion of the opened bladder on the anterior abdominal wall?**

Exstrophy.

🔲🔲 **What are the most common symptoms found in cystitis?**

Frequency, suprapubic pain, and dysuria.

🔲🔲 **What is the most likely diagnosis in a female with significant frequency, urgency, and pain beyond that which is normally seen in a routine urinary tract infection?**

Interstitial cystitis.

🔲🔲 **What are the major risk factors for the development of bladder carcinoma?**

Cigarette smoking, exposure to arylamines, Schistosoma haematobium, chronic analgesic use, and history of extensive cyclophosphamide exposure.

🔲🔲 **What is the lesion in the bladder which can develop following transurethral resection or spontaneously and can be mistaken for malignancy?**

Pseudosarcoma or post operative spindle cell nodule.

🔲🔲 **What is the most common malignant tumor of the bladder?**

Transitional cell carcinoma (urothelial carcinoma).

🔲🔲 **What is the benign lesion of the external urethral meatus found in females which appears as a red, painful mass?**

Urethral caruncle.

**□□  What is an inverted papilloma?**

This is a benign lesion found in the urinary tract, most commonly the bladder, composed of urothelial cells which extends into the lamina propria but which is not truly invasive.  They are five times more common in men and are most frequently associated with painless hematuria.

**□□  What is the most common cytogenetic abnormality seen in high grade invasive transitional cell carcinomas?**

Abnormalities of chromosome 17p (p53 gene).

**□□  In addition to transitional cell carcinoma of the bladder, what are some other malignant tumors of the bladder?**

Squamous cell carcinoma, adenocarcinoma, carcinosarcoma, leiomyosarcoma, and rhabdomyosarcoma.

**□□  What is the cell of origin of the most common renal cell carcinoma (clear cell)?**

The proximal tubular epithelium.

**□□  In the WHO classification of lupus nephritis, what is the most common form of renal disease seen?**

Class IV (mesangial proliferation).

**□□  What is the name of the syndrome characterized by an autosomal dominant inheritance with fingernail dysplasia, hypoplasia or agenesis of the patella, and other skeletal and ocular abnormalities?**

Hereditary onycho-osteodysplasia.  The gene has been mapped to chromosome 9q.  Renal disease occurs in up to half of the patients with asymptomatic proteinuria being the most common abnormality.

**□□  What is the most common age of development of clear cell sarcoma of the kidney?**

This is a tumor of childhood with the greatest incidence occurring from 12-24 months of age.

**□□  What common benign renal tumor shows positive immunoreactivity for the marker HMB-45?**

Angiomyolipoma.

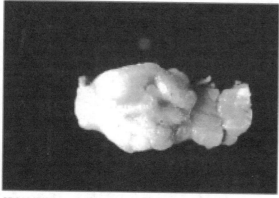

GROSS PHOTO OF URETER WITH PAPILLARY TUMOR

**□□  What is the most likely diagnosis of this tumor seen in the ureter?**

Transitional cell (urothelial) carcinoma.

❏❏  **What is the term given to the condition of the bladder which is characterized by the presence of gas-filled vesicles in the bladder wall?**

Emphysematous cystitis.

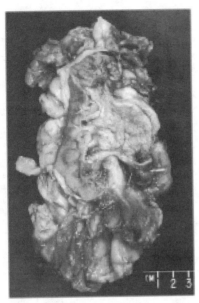

CARCINOMA OF RENAL PELVIS

❏❏  **What is the most common malignant tumor arising in the renal pelvis as shown above?**

Transitional cell carcinoma.

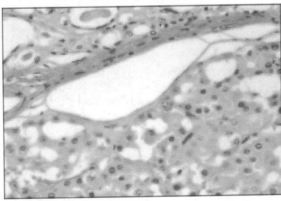

BENIGN RENAL TUMOR

❏❏  **This tumor in the kidney was mahogany in color and had a central, stellate scar. Ultrastructurally, the tumor cells were filled with numerous mitochondria. What is your diagnosis?**

Renal oncocytoma.

# MALE REPRODUCTIVE SYSTEM

❏❏ **What are the terms given to describe the congenital abnormality of abnormal openings of the penile urethra on either the ventral or dorsal surface?**

Hypospadias and epispadias, respectively.

❏❏ **Of the two conditions listed above, which is more common?**

Hypospadias occurs in 1 in 300 male births.

❏❏ **What is phimosis and what causes it?**

This is an abnormally small orifice of the prepuce which makes it difficult to retract the prepuce appropriately. This can be either a congenital abnormality or, more commonly, it can occur as a result of previous bouts of infection leading to scarring. In either case, secondary infection is common and even carcinoma of the penis can develop.

❏❏ **What is the term used to describe the inability to retract the prepuce over the glans secondary to scarring or a congenitally narrow orifice?**

Paraphimosis.

❏❏ **What is the term used to describe inflammation of the penis which usually involves the glans, prepuce, and/or the urethra?**

Balanoposthitis.

❏❏ **What is the major risk factor for development of balanoposthitis?**

This occurs typically as a result of poor hygiene in patients who are uncircumcised. Buildup of various cells and debris termed smegma occurs and serves to continually irritate the area.

❏❏ **What is the name of the lesion which occurs on the penile shaft, prepuce, or glans as the result of infection with Haemophilus ducreyi?**

Chancroid.

❏❏ **Where on the penis is the chancre of syphilis located?**

The glans.

❏❏ **What is the causative agent of lymphogranuloma venereum?**

Chlamydia trachomatis.

❏❏ **What is Peyronie's disease?**

This is a type of fibromatosis which appears to arise from Buck's fascia of the shaft of the penis and causes deformity of the penis.

❐❐  **What virus is strongly associated with condyloma acuminatum?**

Human papillomavirus (HPV) type 6 and, less commonly, type 11.

❐❐  **What are three lesions of the penis which may represent three separate entities or variants of squamous cell carcinoma in situ?**

Bowen's disease, erythroplasia of Queyrat, and bowenoid papulosis.

❐❐  **What type of human papillomavirus (HPV) is associated with development of squamous cell carcinoma in situ of the penis?**

HPV type 16 is the most common type found.  Overall, HPV DNA is found in 8 out of 10 cases.

❐❐  **What is the difference between erythroplasia of Queyrat and Bowen's disease?**

Erythroplasia of Queyrat is carcinoma in situ that occurs on the glans penis, while Bowen's disease occurs on the shaft of the penis.

❐❐  **How commonly does Bowen's disease evolve into invasive squamous cell carcinoma?**

About 10% of the time.

❐❐  **What types of human papillomavirus are associated with bowenoid papulosis?**

Types 16 and 18 are most commonly isolated, which are the types most commonly associated with malignancy in the cervix and elsewhere.  However types 6, 11, 31, and 33 have also been isolated.

❐❐  **What effect does circumcision have on the risk for developing squamous cell carcinoma of the penis?**

It may be protective.  Squamous cell carcinoma of the penis is a rare tumor, but it is even more rare in circumcised individuals.

❐❐  **What is the most important factor in determining survival in patients with penile squamous cell carcinoma?**

Stage, as in all tumors.  When the tumor is limited to the glans penis or prepuce, the patients have a greater than 90% survival.

❐❐  **What are the different clinical characteristics of patients with bowenoid papulosis compared to Bowen's disease?**

Bowenoid papulosis occurs in young males (less than 30) and is characterized by multiple plaques on the shaft or glans of the penis.  Also, it essentially never proceeds to an invasive squamous cell carcinoma, unlike Bowen's disease which does.

❐❐  **What is the name of the crystalline structures seen in a small number of Leydig cells?**

Reinke crystals.

❐❐  **What is cryptorchidism?**

This refers to the congenital condition of undescended testes.  It is usually unilateral but may be bilateral in a fourth of patients.

❐❐  **What are the two phases of testicular descent?**

1 Transabdominal phase - This is where the testis comes to reside within the lower abdomen or upper pelvis. Mullerian-inhibiting substance is thought to control this phase.

2. Inguinoscrotal phase - This is where the testes descend through the inguinal canal into the scrotum. This phase is under androgen control.

The most common abnormality in the pathway of normal testicular descent occurs in the second (inguinoscrotal) phase .

☐☐ **Is there an increased risk for testicular cancer in patients with cryptorchidism?**

Yes, or I would not have asked. It is 5 to 10 times more common for cryptorchid patients to develop testicular cancer than patients without cryptorchidism. Most believe that early surgical correction of the cryptorchidism reduces the risk.

☐☐ **What substance is produced by Sertoli cells and serves as a negative-feedback on the pituitary secretion of FSH and LH?**

Inhibin.

☐☐ **What are some causes of testicular atrophy within the scrotum?**

Atherosclerotic disease, previous orchitis, hypopituitarism, alcoholism, malnutrition, radiation therapy, cryptorchidism, exogenous female sex hormones, and semen outflow obstruction.

☐☐ **Is infection more common in the epididymis or the testis?**

Epididymis. Gonorrhea and tuberculosis almost always arise in the epididymis and may secondarily involve the testis. In contrast, syphilis tends to arise in the testis more that the epididymis.

☐☐ **What testicular tumor should be carefully ruled out in a testis with granulomatous inflammation?**

Seminoma.

☐☐ **What is Sertoli cell only syndrome?**

This is also known as del Castillo syndrome and is a form of germ cell aplasia in which the seminiferous tubules are devoid of spermatogonia and contain only Sertoli cells. Obviously, this results in infertility and is seen not infrequently in biopsy specimens from infertile males.

☐☐ **What is a hydrocele?**

This is fluid from the abdominal cavity which accumulates in the tunica vaginalis.

☐☐ **What is a spermatocele?**

This is a dilated cyst which originates from the rete testis or epididymis and contains spermatozoa.

☐☐ **What is Fournier's gangrene?**

This is a necrotizing fasciitis which involves the scrotum and penis and carries a fairly high morbidity and even mortality rate.

☐☐ **How common is testicular involvement in adult patients with mumps?**

Quite common, about 25% of adults have involvement of the testicle (mumps orchitis) while fewer than 1% of children do.

❑❑  **Other than mumps virus, what is the most common viral cause of orchitis?**

Coxsackie B virus.

❑❑  **Briefly, what are the stages of spermatogenesis?**

There are two types of stem cell spermatogonia, light and dark. They become primary spermatocytes and pass through various stages called preleptotene, leptotene, zygotene, pachytene, and diplotene. Following that, at the end of the first meiotic division, they are termed secondary spermatocytes. They then undergo a second meiotic division to become round spermatids. Gradually, the cells become elongated, develop a tail, and lose cytoplasm which results in a mature spermatozoa or sperm.

❑❑  **What is the most common location of sperm granuloma following a vasectomy?**

The vast majority are found in the vas deferens with less than 10% occurring in the epididymis. Sperm granulomas can occur in other instances; however, almost half occur following vasectomy.

❑❑  **What venous plexus is involved in patients with a varicocele?**

The pampiniform plexus. Varicoceles are found on the left side in almost 90% of cases.

❑❑  **What is priapism?**

This is a condition in which the patient develops intractable, very painful erections.

❑❑  **Which specific types of germ cell tumors occur at an increased frequency in patients with cryptorchidism?**

Seminoma and embryonal carcinoma.

❑❑  **What painful condition of the testicle results in decreased blood supply and subsequent potential for necrosis and gangrene?**

Torsion of the spermatic cord.

❑❑  **In a patient with Klinefelter's syndrome, what would you expect the gross appearance of the testes to be?**

Atrophic.

❑❑  **What are the most common etiologic agents of epididymitis?**

Neisseria gonorrhoeae, Chlamydia trachomatis, Escherichia coli, and Mycobacterium tuberculosis.

❑❑  **Which male reproductive structures are derived from the Wolffian ducts?**

The seminiferous tubules, rete testis, epididymis, vas deferens, ejaculatory duct, and seminal vesicles.

❑❑  **What are the terms used to describe a decrease or complete absence of spermatozoa in the ejaculate?**

Oligospermia and azospermia, respectively.

❑❑  **What are the most common etiologic agents of acute orchitis?**

Escherichia coli, staphylococci, and streptococci.

❑❑  **What are the two major causes of granulomatous orchitis?**

Trauma and an autoimmune reaction.

❏❏ **In elderly males, what is the usual etiology of epididymitis and orchitis?**

These conditions usually occur secondary to recurrent urinary tract infections in elderly males with benign prostatic hyperplasia. Thus, the coliform bacteria are the most common etiologic agents.

❏❏ **What is thought to be the most common cause of male infertility?**

Varicocele.

❏❏ **Which cells in the testes are not significantly altered by radiation?**

The Leydig cells.

❏❏ **What is the most common tumor in males between the ages of 15 and 34?**

Germ cell tumors.

❏❏ **How frequently is there a single histologic pattern in germ cell tumors in males?**

Less than half the time.

❏❏ **What are the two broad categories of germ cell tumors which form the basis for treatment and prognosis?**

Seminomas and non-seminomas.

❏❏ **What is the incidence of germ cell tumors of the testes in African-Americans compared to Caucasians?**

It is much more common in Caucasians (5:1) than African-Americans.

❏❏ **What congenital testicular development disorder has the highest incidence of subsequent development of germ cell tumors?**

Testicular feminization.

❏❏ **What is the most common type of germ cell tumor?**

Seminoma accounts for about 50% of cases.

❏❏ **What is the female tumor counterpart to the male seminoma?**

Dysgerminoma.

❏❏ **What is the peak incidence age of seminoma?**

The mid 30s.

❏❏ **What is the effect of trauma on the development of germ cell tumors?**

Trauma seems to be associated with an increased risk of development of germ cell tumors.

❏❏ **Discuss the treatment and prognosis of seminoma.**

Seminomas are radiosensitive and are treated with orchiectomy and radiation therapy with or without associated chemotherapy. The prognosis is excellent with a five year survival of greater than 90%.

🗆🗆  **What immunoperoxidase stains are positive in seminoma cells?**

PLAP and, when syncytial giant cells are present, they are positive for human chorionic gonadotropin (HCG).

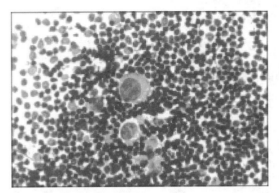 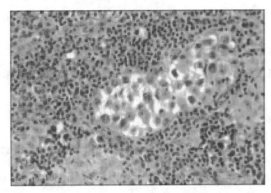

GRANULOMATOUS SEMINOMA
*(Photos courtesy of Cary J. Buresh, M.D. - University of Nebraska Medical Center)*

🗆🗆  **In general terms, describe the basic histologic appearance of seminoma.**

Classic seminomas are composed of large, polyhedral cells with prominent, central nucleoli and abundant glycogenated cytoplasm.  Fibrous septa extend into the tumor with associated lymphocytes.  As shown above, a prominent granulomatous reaction can exist which is sometimes mistaken for granulomatous orchitis.

🗆🗆  **Describe a simple immunoperoxidase method by which one can distinguish between seminoma and embryonal carcinoma.**

Seminomas are PLAP+ while embryonal carcinomas are negative.  In contrast, seminoma is keratin negative while embryonal carcinomas are positive.

🗆🗆  **Which germ cell tumor is most commonly bilateral?**

Spermatocytic seminoma is bilateral in up to 5% of cases.

🗆🗆  **What is the most common combination of cell types in a mixed germ cell tumor?**

Embryonal carcinoma and teratoma (teratocarcinoma).

🗆🗆  **What is the second most common type of pure germ cell tumor (one cell type)?**

Embryonal carcinoma.

🗆🗆  **Compare the prognosis in spermatic seminoma with that of classic seminoma.**

While classic seminoma has a good prognosis with excellent response to radiation and chemotherapy, spermatocytic seminoma is essentially benign, slow-growing and may, in fact, never metastasize.

🗆🗆  **What is the typical age of a patient with spermatocytic seminoma?**

They are older than the classic seminoma; most patients are over 65.  In a 60 year old male, the top two tumors in the differential of a testicular tumor are lymphoma and spermatocytic seminoma.

🗆🗆  **What is the peak age of incidence of embryonal carcinoma?**

Between ages 25 and 35.

❑❑  **Which has a better prognosis, seminoma or embryonal carcinoma?**

Seminoma.  Embryonal carcinoma has lymph node metastases in 2/3 of the patients upon initial presentation.

❑❑  **What is the most common testicular tumor in children younger than 3?**

Yolk sac tumor (endodermal sinus tumor).

❑❑  **What is the classic immunoperoxidase stain which is found in the tumor cells of yolk sac tumor?**

Alpha-fetoprotein (AFP).

❑❑  **Histologically, you see a germ cell tumor which contains numerous papillary projections with fibrovascular cores extending into the tumor cell lined spaces (Schiller-Duval bodies).  What is your diagnosis and what immunoperoxidase stain would you use to confirm it?**

Yolk sac tumor which, of course, is AFP positive.

❑❑  **How common are pure yolk sac tumors in adults?**

They are very rare, and are usually found in association with other types of germ cell tumors in adults.

❑❑  **Which is more likely to exhibit distant metastases, a pure yolk sac tumor or embryonal carcinoma?**

Embryonal carcinoma.

❑❑  **What are the cell types that are found in choriocarcinomas?**

Cytotrophoblasts and syncytial trophoblasts.

❑❑  **What is the typical gross appearance of a choriocarcinoma?**

They are classically very hemorrhagic and can be quite small.

❑❑  **How common is pure choriocarcinoma?**

It is very rare, less than 1% of all germ cell tumors.  In contrast, it is a fairly common component in mixed germ cell tumors.

❑❑  **What is the typical immunohistochemical staining pattern of choriocarcinoma?**

They are positive for HCG as well as human placental lactogen.

❑❑  **What germ cell tumor is occasionally characterized by a small scar in the testis only, without other evidence of solid tumor or hemorrhage and necrosis?**

Occasionally choriocarcinoma leaves only a scar of fibrous tissue behind, and the normal appearance of extensive hemorrhage and necrosis is not evident.

❑❑  **After yolk sac tumor, what is the next most common testicular tumor in male infants?**

Teratoma.

❑❑  **In adults, are teratomas more commonly found in association with other germ cell tumors or as a pure tumor?**

They are uncommon as a pure tumor (less than 3%) but are quite commonly found in association with other germ cell tumors.

❑❑  **What are the two forms or types of teratomas?**

Mature and immature.

❑❑  **Compare the incidence of malignant transformation in testicular teratomas and ovarian teratomas.**

Both can undergo malignant transformation; however, it is much less common in testicular teratomas.

❑❑  **What is the behavior of mature teratomas in prepubertal boys?**

They behave in a benign fashion.  Those that occur in postpubertal boys may metastasize even in the absence of immature elements.  The metastases are often in the form of a nonseminomatous germ cell tumor.

❑❑  **What is the five year survival for yolk sac tumor?**

About 50%.

❑❑  **A patient presents to you at age 7 with precocious puberty and a testicular tumor.  When you examine the testicular tumor histologically, you note lipid vacuoles, abundant cytoplasm, brown cytoplasmic pigment, a vaguely nodular growth pattern focally and the presence of Reinke's crystals within the tumor cells.  What is your diagnosis?**

Leydig cell tumor.

❑❑  **What is the treatment of choice for Leydig cell tumor?**

Orchiectomy.

❑❑  **What is the typical behavior of Leydig cell tumor?**

They are typically benign, but malignancy can develop in less than 10% of cases.

❑❑  **Which lymph nodes are most commonly involved when lymphatic spread of germ cell tumors occurs?**

The retroperitoneal para-aortic lymph nodes.

❑❑  **Which is the most aggressive type of germ cell tumor?**

Choriocarcinoma.

❑❑  **In a patient with a testicular mass and a markedly elevated serum AFP, what is your best diagnosis?**

A yolk sac tumor.

❑❑  **In a patient with a testicular mass and a markedly elevated serum HCG, what is your best diagnosis?**

Choriocarcinoma.

❑❑  **What is the most common age of presentation for a patient with a Leydig cell tumor?**

Most occur between the ages of 20 and 60, although they can occur in children.

❏❏  **What is another term for a Sertoli cell tumor?**

Androblastoma.

❏❏  **In general, what is the clinical behavior of both Leydig cell tumors and Sertoli cell tumors?**

In each case, most are benign; however, about 10% of each will pursue a malignant or aggressive course.

❏❏  **What is the most common malignant tumor of the testicles in men over the age of 60?**

Lymphoma.

❏❏  **What type of lymphoma is typically found in testicular lymphoma?**

Non-Hodgkin's lymphoma of diffuse large cell type.

EPIDIDYMAL TUMOR

❏❏  **The tumor shown above is the most common benign epididymal tumor and is derived from mesothelial origin.  What is your diagnosis?**

Adenomatoid tumor.

❏❏  **What substance is secreted by Sertoli cells and is responsible for regression of the mullerian duct in male gonadal development?**

Mullerian-inhibiting factor (MIF).

❏❏  **What structures are derived from the Wolffian duct?**

The epididymis, vas deferens, and seminal vesicles.

❏❏  **What are some proteins or substances which are produced by the Sertoli cells?**

Androgen-binding protein, transferrin, ceruloplasmin, and testibumin.

❏❏  **What substance is produced by the action of 5 alpha-reductase on testosterone?**

Dihydrotestosterone.

❏❏  **What is the action of dihydrotestosterone (DHT) late in male gestational  development?**

DHT results in the final development of male external genitalia including elongation of the phallus. In the absence of DHT, female external genitalia will develop.

❏❏  **What is the term used to describe the presence of XY chromosomes, testicular gonads, and a female or ambiguous phenotype?**

Male pseudohermaphroditism.

❏❏  **What are some adrenal cortical enzymatic defects which can result in male pseudohermaphroditism?**

20, 22 desmolase; 3-beta-hydroxysteroid dehydrogenase; 17-alpha-hydroxylase; 17, 20 desmolase; and 17-beta-hydroxysteroid dehydrogenase.

❏❏  **What is the most frequent cause of male pseudohermaphroditism?**

Testicular feminization or androgen insensitivity syndrome which results from a lack of androgen receptors.

❏❏  **What is the most common tumor that develops at an increased rate in patients with mixed gonadal dysgenesis?**

Gonadoblastoma.

❏❏  **In patients with one of the gonadal dysgenesis syndromes, what is the most common genotype?**

45 XO/46XY mosaic with 46 XY being the next most common.

❏❏  **What is the typical genotype, phenotype, and type of gonads present in patients with androgen insensitivity syndrome or testicular feminization?**

These patients are females with a 46XY genotype, and they have testes which may be found anywhere from the abdomen to the labia.

❏❏  **What is the most common type of sex cord-stromal tumor that occurs in patients with testicular feminization?**

Sertoli cell tumor.

❏❏  **What is the most common malignant germ cell tumor occurring in patients with testicular feminization?**

Seminoma.

❏❏  **What type of germ cell tumor is known for its propensity to exhibit calcification?**

Gonadoblastoma.

❏❏  **What are the most common benign and malignant tumors of the spermatic cord?**

Lipoma and rhabdomyosarcoma, respectively.

❏❏  **What is the most common cyst of the testicles?**

Epidermoid cysts.

❏❏  **What testicular tumor is associated with Carney's syndrome?**

Large cell calcifying Sertoli cell tumor.

❑❑  **How frequently are gonadoblastomas bilateral?**

1/3 of the cases.

❑❑  **Which zone of the prostate usually harbors carcinoma as opposed to hyperplasia?**

Most carcinomas arise in the peripheral zone while hyperplasias occur in the transitional and periurethral zones.

❑❑  **What are the three cell types of the prostatic epithelium?**

1.  Secretory luminal cells
2.  Basal cells
3.  Neuroendocrine cells

❑❑  **Which of the prostatic epithelial cells produces prostate-specific antigen (PSA), prostatic acid phosphatase (PAP), and scant mucin?**

The secretory luminal cells.

❑❑  **Is acute inflammation ever normal within the prostate?**

Yes, a small amount of patchy, acute, and/or chronic inflammation is a normal finding and does not merit a diagnosis of prostatitis.

❑❑  **What are the most common bacterial etiologic agents of acute prostatitis?**

E. coli, enterococci, staphylococci, and other gram-negative rods.  Acute prostatitis is typically a progression from a urethral or bladder infection.

❑❑  **What is the most common etiologic agent of chronic prostatitis?**

E. coli.  Chronic bacterial prostatitis is a common cause of recurrent urinary tract infections.  There is also a nonbacterial form of chronic prostatitis which, in contrast, rarely follows or causes recurrent urinary tract infections.

❑❑  **Of the various causes or categories of granulomatous prostatitis, what is the most common?**

Idiopathic or unknown cause.

❑❑  **What does a needle biopsy of prostate containing granulomatous inflammation and Michaelis-Gutmann bodies indicate for a diagnosis?**

Malakoplakia.

❑❑  **What bacterial organism is most commonly isolated in cultures from patients with malakoplakia of the prostate?**

E. coli.

❑❑  **How common is benign prostatic hyperplasia in men older than 70?**

Extremely.  It is found in over 95% of patients.

❑❑  **What are some of the common clinical symptoms of benign prostatic hyperplasia?**

PATHOLOGY MEDICAL STUDENT PEARLS OF WISDOM

These patients get symptoms which are due to urinary outflow obstruction such as urgency, weakened urine stream, difficulty in starting and stopping the flow of urine, and nocturia.

⬚⬚ **What is the risk for the development of carcinoma in benign prostatic hyperplasia?**

BPH is not a pre-malignant condition and does not seem to predispose to carcinoma.

⬚⬚ **What is the most common form of cancer in men?**

Prostate, of course. It is second only to lung as the leading cause of cancer-related death.

⬚⬚ **How common is prostate cancer in patients age 80?**

At age 80, 80% have cancer.

⬚⬚ **Is prostate cancer more common in blacks or whites?**

Blacks.

⬚⬚ **What hormones are essential for development of both benign prostatic hyperplasia and growth of prostate cancer?**

Testosterone and dihydrotestosterone.

⬚⬚ **Is heredity an important component in the development of prostate cancer?**

Yes, a man has twice the incidence of prostate cancer if he has a father or brother who has prostate cancer.

⬚⬚ **What are two histologic lesions within the prostate which are premalignant in nature?**

Prostatic intraepithelial neoplasia (PIN) and atypical adenomatous hyperplasia.

⬚⬚ **What are the four architectural patterns found in high grade PIN?**

1. Tufting
2. Micropapillary
3. Cribriform
4. Flat

⬚⬚ **What part of the prostate is most likely to contain PIN?**

Like prostatic carcinoma, the periphery of the prostate is the most likely location for PIN.

⬚⬚ **In the Gleason system of grading prostatic adenocarcinoma, what forms the basis of assigning a grade - the cytologic appearance of the tumor cells or the architectural appearance of the tumor?**

The architecture.

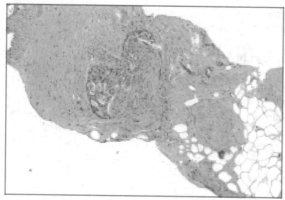

PERINEURAL INVASION BY PROSTATIC ADENOCARCINOMA

❑❑  **What are some of the histologic features of adenocarcinoma of the prostate?**

1. An infiltrative pattern
2. Loss of the basal cell layer
3. Prominent nucleoli
4. Perineural invasion (see photo above)
5. Acidic mucin
6. Crystalloids
7. Vascular invasion
8. Extraprostatic extension by tumor

❑❑  **What do the two numbers that make up a total score mean in the Gleason grading system?**

The first number represents the primary pattern of tumor and the second number represents the secondary pattern of tumor. These numbers may be the same if there is only one pattern exhibited. The two numbers are combined to create a score which has significant prognostic implications. The higher the score or total of the two patterns, the worse the prognosis.

❑❑  **In comparing the Gleason score on a needle biopsy to the subsequent prostatectomy specimen, what normally happens to the score?**

The Gleason score is often upgraded once the entire gland has been received. It is uncommon for the score given on the needle biopsy to be lower on the prostatectomy specimen.

❑❑  **What effect does prostatitis have on the serum prostate-specific antigen (PSA)?**

PSA can be elevated in prostatitis, benign prostatic hyperplasia, and for a short time following biopsy.

❑❑  **What are the most common sites of spread of prostatic carcinoma?**

Regional lymph nodes, bones, lungs, liver, and brain.

❑❑  **What is the nature of the bony metastases that are typically found in prostate cancer?**

They are typically osteoblastic rather than osteolytic.

❑❑  **How does prostate-specific antigen exist in the serum?**

Most is bound to alpha-1-antichymotrypsin and the remaining portion is unbound or free.

❑❑  **What happens to the ratio of free or unbound and bound PSA in patients with prostate cancer?**

Generally there is less free or unbound PSA and more bound PSA in patients with prostate cancer.

❑❑ **What are three melanotic lesions which can occur in the prostate?**

Two of the lesions are benign and one is malignant. Prostatic melanosis occurs when there is melanin pigment within the stroma of the prostate. Blue nevus is similar histologically to the lesion of the same name which occurs in the skin. Finally, melanoma can also be found in the prostate and represents a metastatic lesion.

❑❑ **What are the most common sarcomas that occur in the prostate of children and adults?**

In children, rhabdomyosarcoma is most common while leiomyosarcoma is most frequent in adults.

❑❑ **What type of leukemia most frequently involves the prostate?**

Chronic lymphocytic leukemia.

❑❑ **What congenital abnormalities of the seminal vesicles can be seen in association with ipsilateral renal agenesis?**

Unilateral agenesis of the seminal vesicles and congenital cysts.

❑❑ **In schistosomiasis (secondary to S. haematobium), which is more likely to be involved - the seminal vesicles or the prostate?**

The seminal vesicles.

❑❑ **What is the usual source of acute vesiculitis?**

Bacterial infection of the seminal vesicles is usually secondary to infection of adjacent or nearby organs including the bladder and prostate.

❑❑ **What is the typical histologic appearance of a granuloma secondary to previous transurethral resection?**

These granulomas features central fibrinoid necrosis with a ring of palisaded epithelioid histiocytes.

❑❑ **Are most adenocarcinomas of the prostate derived from the acini or the ducts?**

Acini, less than 1% are derived from prostatic ducts.

# FEMALE REPRODUCTIVE SYSTEM

❑❑ **What is the sex-determining region Y gene?**

The SRY gene is found in the 1A1 region at the distal end of chromosome Yp. Its presence dictates development of testicles while its absence results in ovarian differentiation.

❑❑ **What two substances are responsible for development of the wolffian duct system and regression of the mullerian ducts?**

Testosterone and mullerian-inhibiting substance (MIS) which are produced by the testes.

❑❑ **What is a hermaphrodite?**

The presence of both ovarian and testicular tissue in a single individual.

❑❑ **What is the most common karyotype in Turner's syndrome?**

XO.

❑❑ **What is the most common cause of male pseudohermaphroditism?**

Androgen insensitivity syndrome (testicular feminization).

❑❑ **What is the most common cause of ambiguous genitalia?**

Congenital adrenal hyperplasia.

❑❑ **What are the causative agents of granuloma inguinale and lymphogranuloma venereum?**

Calymmatobacterium granulomatis and Chlamydia, respectively.

❑❑ **What is the name of the cytology preparation whereby one scrapes the base of a fresh vesicle, spreads the material on a slide, and stains it in an attempt to diagnose herpes?**

Tzank prep.

❑❑ **What is the most common cause of a Bartholin's cyst abscess?**

Gonorrhea.

❑❑ **What happens to a large number of cases of lichen sclerosus et atrophicus of the vulva in children when they reach puberty?**

A large percentage of these cases involute or regress spontaneously.

❑❑ **What is the most common age of development of lichen sclerosus et atróphicus?**

Postmenopausal women, but it can occur at any age and sex.

❏❏  **What are some ectopic tissues that can occur in the labia?**

Breast (along the milk line), salivary gland tissue, and mesothelial cysts. In addition, various rests of embryonic tissues can occur.

❏❏  **What benign lesion can occur in the vulva and is thought to arise from sweat glands?**

Papillary hidradenoma (hidradenoma papilliferum).

❏❏  **Describe the typical patient who develops papillary hidradenoma.**

This tumor is rare overall; however, it tends to occur in white females after puberty. This correlates with the development of the apocrine sweat glands which is the origin of this tumor.

❏❏  **What types of human papillomavirus are typically recovered from condylomatous lesions of the vulva?**

As in other locations with HPV lesions, the benign appearing condyloma acuminata tend to have HPV types 6 and 11. While squamous cell carcinoma in situ and invasive squamous cell carcinoma of the vulva tends to be associated with types 16, 18, and 31.

❏❏  **What tumor that most commonly occurs in the soft tissue of the vulva of young to middle-aged women, is characteristically well-circumscribed, shows positive immunoreactivity for vimentin and desmin, and has been reported to occur in males?**

Angiomyofibroblastoma.

❏❏  **What tumor typically occurs in women less than 40 and involves the genitalia, is poorly circumscribed, and has distinct myxoid and vascular areas histologically?**

Aggressive angiomyxoma.

❏❏  **What is the most common type of HPV found in vulvar intraepithelial neoplasia (VIN) and invasive squamous cell carcinoma of the vulva?**

HPV type 16.

❏❏  **What is the most common malignant tumor of the vulva?**

Squamous cell carcinoma.

❏❏  **What are some of the features in staging a vulvar carcinoma which are important in determining prognosis?**

Diameter of the tumor, depth of invasion, and status of regional lymph nodes.

❏❏  **What is the classic presentation of bowenoid papulosis of the vulva?**

A pigmented papule in a young pregnant female.

❏❏  **What is the name of the tumor that is an intraepidermal adenocarcinoma which can occur in the vulva?**

Extramammary Paget's disease.

❏❏  **What is the characteristic immunoperoxidase staining pattern of Paget's disease cells in the vulva?**

The cells are positive for low molecular weight keratin, epithelial membrane antigen, carcinoembryonic antigen, B72.3, and fibrocystic disease fluid protein (GCBFP-15). These cells fail to react with S-100 and HMB-45.

☐☐ **How common is the presence of an underlying, invasive adenocarcinoma in a patient with vulvar Paget's disease?**

One third to half the time.

☐☐ **What are some risk factors involved in development of squamous cell carcinoma of the vulva?**

Cigarette smoking, diabetes mellitus, presence of HPV (particularly younger patients), and immunosuppression.

☐☐ **How common is lymph node metastases in verrucous carcinoma of the vulva?**

While this tumor is locally recurrent, it does not metastasize in the absence of altered, aggressive behavior secondary to radiation therapy.

☐☐ **What tumor, more characteristically found in the salivary glands, can occur in the vulva and is characterized by late hematogenous spread and perineural invasion?**

Adenoid cystic carcinoma.

☐☐ **Does melanoma occur in the vulva?**

Yes, or I would not have asked, although it represents less than 5% of the vulvar malignancies.

☐☐ **What is Sampson's theory regarding endometriosis?**

This hypothesis states that endometriosis (endometrial glands and stroma) occurs outside of the uterine mucosa via "reflux menstruation" through the fallopian tubes and into the abdominal cavity.

☐☐ **What is Novak's theory regarding endometriosis?**

This theory, favored by many, states that tissue derived from the mullerian system may undergo metaplasia to become endometrial tissue.

☐☐ **What are the two most common causes of vaginitis?**

Candida albicans and Trichomonas vaginalis.

☐☐ **What is the most common cause of bacterial vaginosis?**

Gardnerella vaginalis.

☐☐ **What organism is occasionally seen in Pap smears classically in association with use of an intrauterine device (IUD)?**

Actinomyces israelii.

☐☐ **What is the organism which, in association with the use of tampons, is associated with toxic shock syndrome?**

Staphylococcus aureus. Specifically, the enterotoxin F and exotoxin C produced by the organism and absorbed by the patient are the cause of this syndrome.

❏❏   **What is the name of the rare simple vaginal cyst which is typically found in the lateral or anterolateral wall of the vagina and is lined by a single layer of cuboidal-type cells?**

Gartner's duct cyst (mesonephric cyst).

❏❏   **What is the most common benign tumor of mesenchyme in the vagina?**

Leiomyoma.

❏❏   **What is vaginal adenosis and what is it associated with?**

This is a collection of benign mucinous endocervical glands in the vagina and is associated with exposure to diethylstilbesterol (DES) in utero by the patient's mother.  Specifically, the critical time of exposure is prior to the 18th week of gestation.

❏❏   **What is the more serious complication associated with in utero exposure to DES?**

Development of clear cell adenocarcinoma of the vagina and cervix.

❏❏   **What is the most common site in the vagina of adenosis and clear cell adenocarcinoma?**

The upper 1/3 of the vagina on the anterior wall.

❏❏   **What benign polypoid lesion occurs in the vagina and tends to protrude from the introitus and can be confused with sarcoma botryoides?**

Fibroepithelial polyp.

❏❏   **What is the most common malignant vaginal tumor found in children?**

Embryonal rhabdomyosarcoma, also known as sarcoma botryoides.

❏❏   **What is the most common age of presentation of sarcoma botryoides?**

A diagnosis is made at age 5 or less in almost every case.  The mean age is about 3 years old.  Tumors arising in the cervix occur at a somewhat older age.

❏❏   **What is the natural history of vaginal intraepithelial neoplasia or squamous dysplasia of the vagina?**

The vast majority of lesions will regress following biopsy only.  Slightly more than 10% will persist and less than 10% will progress to an invasive squamous cell carcinoma.

❏❏   **What is the most common primary germ cell tumor of the vagina?**

These are quite rare; however, yolk sac tumor is the most common and, in reported cases, always occurs in children age 3 or less.

❏❏   **What is the most common malignant mesenchymal tumor of the vagina?**

Leiomyosarcoma.

❏❏   **What are some of the melanocytic lesions that occur not infrequently in the vagina?**

Lentigo, blue nevus, cellular blue nevus, and melanoma.

❏❏   **What type of herpes simplex virus is typically associated with genital infection?**

Type 2 (HSV-2).

❑❑ **What are the typical signs and symptoms of pelvic inflammatory disease (PID)?**

Pelvic pain, vaginal discharge, fever, and adnexal tenderness on bimanual examination.

❑❑ **What are some of the potential complications of PID?**

Infertility, bacteremia, abdominal adhesions with resultant bowel obstruction, peritonitis, and chronic pain.

❑❑ **What is the term given to describe the junction of the ectocervix and endocervix?**

The squamocolumnar junction, and the transformation zone is the area between the original squamocolumnar junction and the new squamocolumnar junction that changes depending on the patient's age and hormonal status.

❑❑ **What is the name of the process whereby columnar epithelium of the cervix is replaced by squamous epithelium?**

Squamous metaplasia.

❑❑ **What benign glandular proliferative lesion of the cervix is associated with the use of oral contraceptives in young females?**

Microglandular hyperplasia.

❑❑ **What is the risk of subsequently developing an adenocarcinoma in an endocervical polyp?**

Essentially no increased risk.

❑❑ **What is the most common type of HPV associated with flat condylomas of the cervix?**

Types 6 and 11.

❑❑ **What is the most common type of HPV found in high grade squamous intraepithelial lesions and invasive carcinomas of the cervix?**

Type 16.

❑❑ **What are some risk factors for development of cervical carcinoma?**

Smoking, oral contraceptives, multiple sexual partners, early age at initial sexual activity, and the presence of HSV and/or HPV.

❑❑ **What is the classic colposcopic appearance of a high grade squamous intraepithelial lesion of the cervix?**

A mosaic pattern.

❑❑ **What is the classic colposcopic appearance of an invasive carcinoma of the cervix?**

Irregular, tortuous blood vessels extending across the cervix.

❑❑ **What is the natural course or potential for progression to an invasive carcinoma in low grade squamous intraepithelial lesions of the cervix?**

Up to 20% in 5 years, 30% in 10 years, 33% in 15 years, and just under 40% in 20 years.

❑❑  **Is HPV found in association with adenocarcinoma in situ of the cervix?**

Yes, HPV types 16 and 18 have been found in adenocarcinoma in situ of the cervix indicating a possible causal factor in development of adenocarcinoma of the cervix.

❑❑  **Briefly, what is the staging system for carcinoma of the cervix?**

Stage I - Confined to cervix
Stage II - Beyond the cervix but limited to the upper 2/3 of the vagina
Stage III - Beyond the cervix extending to either the lateral pelvic wall or the lower 1/3 of the vagina
Stage IV - Beyond the cervix extending to the bladder, rectum, or beyond the pelvis

❑❑  **What is the most common cause of death in patients with cervical carcinoma?**

Cervical carcinoma tends to spread locally and via lymphatics, not hematogenously.  Thus, the ureters are frequently obstructed resulting in hydronephrosis, pyelonephritis, and renal failure which is the most common cause of death.

❑❑  **Which has a higher prevalence of HPV, vulvar/vaginal invasive squamous cell carcinoma or cervical invasive squamous cell carcinomas?**

Cervical, 90% of the lesions have detectable HPV while only around 20% of vulvar/vaginal tumors do.

❑❑  **While only a small minority of low grade squamous intraepithelial lesions (mild dysplasia) progress to severe dysplasia/carcinoma in situ, what is the mean time interval to the higher grade lesion?**

It has varied in many studies; however, it is approximately 18-24 months.

❑❑  **What types of human papillomavirus (HPV) have been isolated in verrucous carcinoma of the vagina/vulva?**

Types 6 and 16.

❑❑  **Does one find HPV in adenocarcinomas of the cervix?**

Yes, at about the same rate (90%) as in squamous cell carcinoma.

❑❑  **What is the pattern of spread and prognosis in papillary villoglandular adenocarcinoma of the cervix?**

This unusual tumor is found in younger women and, although it can be deeply invasive, it does not appear to metastasize.

❑❑  **What is the name of the benign lesion of the cervix which is composed of a nodular, circumscribed aggregate of dilated endocervical glands which are superficially located beneath the epithelial surface?**

Tunnel clusters.

❑❑  **What part of the cervix is the commonest site of development of dysplasia and invasive carcinoma?**

The transformation zone.

❑❑  **How common is an associated squamous dysplastic lesion of the cervix in association with adenocarcinoma in situ of the cervix?**

Very common, ranging from 50% to nearly 100% in a variety of studies.

❏❏  **What is a Nabothian cyst?**

This is a large, benign cystic dilatation of an endocervical gland or glands.

❏❏  **In an endometrial biopsy, you see pronounced stromal edema, moderate glandular secretions, an absence of stromal/glandular mitoses, markedly tortuous glands and no significant decidual change.  Approximately what day of the 28-day cycle is the biopsy obtained from?**

Approximately day 22.  Day 22 is when stromal edema is maximal and glandular secretions are just beyond their peak (day 20 or 21) and predecidual change has not become evident yet.

❏❏  **What is the most common site of endometriosis?**

The ovary.

❏❏  **What substances are produced by the corpus luteum and are important in regulating the secretory phase of the endometrium?**

Estradiol and progesterone.

❏❏  **What is the name of the phenomenon which tends to occur in pregnancy and is characterized by a focus of tightly clustered endometrial glands which appear hypertrophic and demonstrate nuclear pleomorphism and cytoplasmic vacuolization?**

Arias-Stella reaction.

❏❏  **What is the basic mechanism by which clomiphene citrate is useful as a fertility drug?**

Clomiphene citrate decreases endogenous estrogen thus resulting in secretion of gonadotropin-releasing hormone and then FSH and LH.  This, hopefully, results in ovulation.

❏❏  **What is the most common cause of dysfunctional uterine bleeding in reproductive age women?**

Anovulatory cycles.

❏❏  **What is the term given to describe the presence of an inadequate corpus luteum resulting in dysfunctional uterine bleeding?**

Inadequate luteal phase.

❏❏  **What is the most common cause of postmenopausal endometrial bleeding?**

Endometrial atrophy.  Remember, endometrial carcinoma has to be ruled out.

❏❏  **What is the most common etiology of chronic endometritis?**

It is most commonly an ascending infection by way of the cervix following such things as abortion or instrumentation.

❏❏  **What is the hallmark inflammatory cell of chronic endometritis?**

Plasma cells.  Some believe that the presence of a single plasma cell in the endometrium is indicative of chronic endometritis.  Eosinophils are also harbingers of chronic endometritis.

❏❏  **What are the most common etiologic agents of chronic endometritis?**

Chlamydia trachomatis and Neisseria gonorrhoeae.

❏❏ **What is the name of the endometrial polypoid lesion which has abundant smooth muscle, tends to occur in the lower uterine segment, and occurs in women of reproductive age?**

Atypical polypoid adenomyoma.

❏❏ **What is the most common type of metaplasia seen in the endometrium?**

Tubal (ciliated) metaplasia.

❏❏ **What are the four types of endometrial hyperplasia according to the World Health Organization?**

Simple hyperplasia without atypia, simple hyperplasia with atypia, complex hyperplasia without atypia, and complex hyperplasia with atypia.

❏❏ **What is the relative risk of development of malignancy within the various types of endometrial hyperplasia?**

Simple hyperplasia without atypia - approximately 1%
Simple hyperplasia with atypia - less than 10%
Complex hyperplasia without atypia - less than 5 %
Complex hyperplasia with atypia - approximately 30%

❏❏ **What is the mechanism of development of endometrial hyperplasia in obese women?**

Androstenedione is converted to estrone in the adipose tissue which serves as the stimulation for development of hyperplasia.

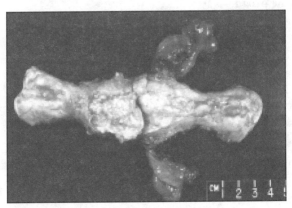

GROSS PHOTO OF ENDOMETRIAL CARCINOMA

❏❏ **What is the nature of the endometrial carcinomas that develop in obese women secondary to peripheral conversion to estrogens?**

The tumors tend to be well-differentiated, superficially invasive, and have a very good prognosis.

❏❏ **What are some associations with development of adenocarcinoma of the endometrium?**

Obesity, diabetes mellitus, infertility, late menopause, any source of continuous unopposed estrogen, and hypertension.

❏❏ **What is the prognosis of clear cell carcinoma of the endometrium compared to typical endometrioid carcinoma?**

Clear cell carcinoma tends to occur in older women and carries a poor prognosis.

**❏❏  What is the embryologic origin of the tumor cells in clear cell carcinoma?**

They are of mullerian origin.  Histologically, they are characterized by clear cells, frequently showing a "hobnail" pattern and focal papillary configuration.

**❏❏  In general terms, what is the five year survival for endometrial carcinoma?**

If the tumor is limited to the endometrium, 90% five year survival.  If the tumor invades less than 1/2 of the myometrium, the five year survival is approximately 70%.  If the tumor has spread beyond the uterine corpus, the five year survival is poor at approximately 15%.

**❏❏  What is the name of the tumor which occurs both in the uterus and the ovary, is characterized by a papillary pattern, high nuclear grade, and psammoma bodies?**

Serous papillary adenocarcinoma.

**❏❏  Which is more important in prognosis of endometrial carcinoma, the progesterone receptor status or estrogen receptor status?**

The progesterone receptor status.

**❏❏  What is the term given to describe the presence of endometrial glands and stroma deep within the myometrium?**

Adenomyosis.

**❏❏  How does the presence of carcinoma in a focus of adenomyosis in addition to typical endometroid adenocarcinoma of the uterus effect the prognosis?**

It doesn't.

**❏❏  Is there a history of estrogen replacement in most patients with clear cell carcinoma of the endometrium?**

No, most patients are older and do not have that history.

**❏❏  What tumor of the endometrium is characterized by a population of cells which are histologically similar to the stromal cells of a normal proliferative endometrium but exhibit an infiltrative pattern and extensive intravascular involvement by tumor?**

Low-grade endometrial stromal sarcoma.

**❏❏  What is the prognosis in low-grade endometrial stromal sarcoma?**

It is excellent, although it can recur quite late (decades later).  The most important factor is stage at presentation.

**❏❏  What is an alternative term  for mixed mullerian tumors?**

Carcinosarcoma which depicts the nature of the neoplasm - a mixture of carcinoma and sarcoma.

**❏❏  What is the classic  clinical  presentation  for patients with mixed mullerian tumor?**

They most commonly present with bleeding and on exam have a protuberant polypoid mass protruding through the cervical os.

❑❑  **What do the designations homologous and heterologous elements mean in mixed mullerian tumors?**

Homologous refers to the state of an undifferentiated sarcoma, while heterologous refers to the presence of differentiated sarcomatous elements which are not derived from the normal uterus such as chondrosarcoma, osteosarcoma, or skeletal muscle differentiation (rhabdomyosarcoma).

❑❑  **What is the prognosis of patients with mixed mullerian tumor?**

It is very poor, and these tend to occur in older patients.  It does not appear that the presence of homologous or heterologous elements markedly effects survival.

❑❑  **What are some of the complications of acute salpingitis?**

Infertility, small bowel obstruction (secondary to adhesions), pyosalpinx, and tubo-ovarian abscess.

❑❑  **What is Gardnerella and what is its importance in the female genital tract?**

It is a small gram-negative rod which can cause vaginitis and is associated with "clue cells" which are epithelial cells covered by bacteria.

❑❑  **What is the best preparation by which one can demonstrate Trichomonas vaginalis at the time of pelvic examination?**

The use of a wet mount is ideal because one can see the flagellated and motile organism swimming in the saline after direct application to the slide from a sampling of the cervix.

❑❑  **What is uterus didelphys?**

This is a congenital abnormality whereby the patient has a double uterus accompanied by a septate or double vagina as a result of lack of complete fusion of the mullerian ducts.

❑❑  **In a setting of chronic cervicitis, you note a prominent plasma cell infiltrate and distinct germinal center formation.  What organism should you suspect most strongly as the etiologic agent?**

Chlamydia trachomatis.

❑❑  **What organism should you suspect in a case of chronic cervicitis where there is significant epithelial spongiosis (intraepithelial edema)?**

T. vaginalis.

❑❑  **Is there a uniform progression in cervical squamous cell carcinoma from mild dysplasia to severe dysplasia and subsequent invasive squamous cell carcinoma?**

No, some lesions clearly do not arise from mild dysplasia.  As stated before, the majority of lesions never progress at all.

❑❑  **How commonly do patients with severe dysplasia/squamous cell carcinoma in situ that have been treated progress to invasive squamous cell carcinoma?**

About 1 in 500.

❑❑  **At what age are you most likely to find a patient with anovulatory cycles?**

They occur most commonly at menarche and in perimenopausal women.

❑❑  **After the ovaries, what are the most common sites of endometriosis?**

1. Ovaries
2. Uterine ligaments
3. Rectovaginal septum
4. Pelvis
5. Previous laparotomy scars
6. Umbilicus, vagina, vulva, appendix

❏❏  **What are some of the typical clinical signs and symptoms of endometriosis?**

Dysmenorrhea, dyspareunia, pelvic pain, gastrointestinal abnormalities, and infertility.  The disorder is most common in women in their 20s and 30s.

❏❏  **What is the most common tumor in women?**

Leiomyoma (fibroids).

❏❏  **What is the most reliable indicator of a leiomyosarcoma as opposed to a cellular leiomyoma?**

Mitotic rate.

❏❏  **What are the three general locations of leiomyomas within the uterus?**

Submucosal, subserosal, and intramural.

❏❏  **Do most leiomyosarcomas arise from a pre-existing leiomyoma?**

No, most believe that leiomyosarcomas arise de novo and that if they do arise within a pre-existing leiomyoma, that it is extremely rare.

❏❏  **How common is recurrence of leiomyosarcoma following resection?**

Quite common, greater than 50% of cases will metastasize hematogenously most commonly to the lungs.

❏❏  **What is the typical histologic appearance of a benign endometrial polyp?**

These are polypoid portions of endometrial mucosa containing both glands and stroma with thick-walled vessels.

❏❏  **What is the most common bacteria associated with acute salpingitis?**

Chlamydia trachomatis followed by Neisseria gonorrhoeae.

❏❏  **How frequently are the fallopian tubes involved when there is tuberculosis involving the female genital tract?**

Essentially always.

❏❏  **What are the histologic features of salpingitis isthmica nodosa?**

This represents bilateral nodules typically in the tubal isthmus which are composed of tubal epithelial lined channels with admixed, prominent, smooth muscle bundles.

❏❏  **What are some  risk  factors for a tubal ectopic pregnancy?**

A history of salpingitis isthmica nodosa, chronic salpingitis, and previous tubal pregnancy.

❐❐  **What is the term given to describe small, simple cysts filled with clear serous fluid which occur commonly next to the fallopian tubes?**

Paratubal cysts or, when larger and near the fimbria, they are called hydatids of Morgagni.

❐❐  **What benign mesothelial-derived tumor can occur in the fallopian tubes?**

Adenomatoid tumor, remember from the previous chapter this is the most common tumor of the epididymis.

❐❐  **How commonly is primary adenocarcinoma of the tube bilateral?**

1 in 5 cases.

❐❐  **What is the prognosis in tubal adenocarcinoma?**

It is quite poor with about 30% survival at five years.

❐❐  **A patient has an ulcerative lesion on the vulva and you are told that microscopically there are Donovan bodies. What are those and what is the disease and organism?**

The disease is granuloma inguinale which is caused by Calymmatobacterium granulomatis. The Donovan bodies are vacuolated macrophages which are filled with the organism and are seen with the aid of a Giemsa stain.

❐❐  **On the cervical smear from a patient with vaginal discharge and dysuria, you note the presence of gram-negative diplococci. What would you expect the culture to grow?**

Neisseria gonorrhea.

❐❐  **By dark-field exam, you are able to detect spirochete organisms taken from a painless ulcer from the genitalia of a female. What is your diagnosis?**

Syphilis (Treponema pallidum).

❐❐  **Where in the process of cell division are the oocytes of the ovary at the time of birth?**

They are in a resting stage of the first meiotic division. They will not complete that process until ovulation and fertilization occurs.

❐❐  **In a primary follicle of an infant, what are the cells which lie around the oocyte?**

Granulosa cells.

❐❐  **What is a Call-Exner body?**

This is a small, round collection of eosinophilic material which is surrounded by a ring of granulosa cells. These are normal but can be neoplastic.

❐❐  **What is the primary source of estrogen in the preovulatory stage of menses?**

The theca cells.

❐❐  **What is the primary source of progesterone in the ovary which is responsible for regulation of the secretory phase of menses?**

The corpus luteum.

☐☐  **If fertilization occurs, when does primary production of progesterone no longer occur in the corpus luteum?**

After about eight weeks the placenta begins taking over primary production of progesterone from the corpus luteum.

☐☐  **How common is the resistant ovary syndrome?**

It accounts for about 20% of the cases of premature ovarian failure.

☐☐  **At what age do solitary follicle cysts and corpus luteum cysts occur?**

The solitary follicle cysts occur in perimenopausal women and after menarche while corpus luteum cysts occur in women of childbearing age.

☐☐  **How common is polycystic ovary disease?**

It occurs in about 5% of females.

☐☐  **What is the typical patient presentation in polycystic ovary disease?**

The patients are classically in their 20s and present with oligomenorrhea, infertility, and hirsutism.

☐☐  **Where are the cysts typically located in polycystic ovary disease?**

They are found in the periphery of the ovary and contain a densely fibrotic/sclerotic stroma.

☐☐  **What is the most common etiologic agent of vaginitis?**

Candida albicans.

☐☐  **Why do leiomyomas often increase in size during pregnancy and decrease in size in postmenopausal women?**

They are estrogen sensitive, thus during the times of high estrogen (pregnancy) they get larger and in times of low estrogen they decrease in size.

☐☐  **What is the most common benign tumor in the fallopian tubes?**

Adenomatoid tumor.

☐☐  **What is the name of the condition whereby the patient has numerous follicle cysts in association with oligomenorrhea?**

Polycystic ovarian disease (Stein-Leventhal syndrome).

☐☐  **In patients with polycystic ovarian disease, how common is true virilism?**

It is rare.  They typically have persistent anovulation, hirsutism, and almost half are obese.

☐☐  **What is the histologic picture of an ovary in polycystic ovarian disease?**

The cortex is hypocellular and fibrotic.  The cystic follicles are lined by nonluteinized granulosa cells with an outer layer of luteinized theca interna cells.  The primordial follicles are normal, but corpora lutea and albicantia are typically absent.

☐☐  **In polycystic ovarian syndrome, what are the levels of follicle-stimulating hormone (FSH)?**

FSH is normal as is 17-ketosteroid production. Androgens, on the other hand, are elevated in the cyst fluid and urine.

□□ **Describe the typical clinical presentation in massive ovarian edema.**

The condition is usually unilateral and the patients are young with an average age of 20 years. They present with abdominal or pelvic pain and an associated palpable abdominal mass.

□□ **How can you differentiate between fibromatosis and an ovarian fibroma?**

Fibromatosis occurs in younger patients (mean of 25 years) who sometimes have menstrual abnormalities and contains entrapped follicles and their derivatives. In contrast, fibromas are found in older patients, do not contain entrapped normal structures, and are not associated with menstrual abnormalities.

□□ **What lesion of the ovary is related to hCG stimulation, and typically occurs in black multiparous females who are in their 20s or 30s?**

The pregnancy luteoma.

□□ **How common is extraovarian spread by ovarian malignancies at the time of initial presentation?**

It is very common (70% of patients) thus the high mortality rate.

□□ **What are some of the risk factors for development of ovarian carcinoma?**

Nulliparity, family history, and history of fertility drug use in the absence of pregnancy.

□□ **What are three syndromes that have been described related to ovarian cancer?**

Lynch II syndrome (cancer of the ovary, endometrium, and colon), breast-ovary syndrome, and ovary-specific syndrome.

□□ **What serum marker is useful in determining the presence or recurrence of ovarian carcinoma?**

CA-125.

□□ **What is the most common cell of origin resulting in ovarian neoplasms (example germ cells, stromal cells, surface epithelium, etc.)?**

By far, the surface epithelium gives rise to the most ovarian neoplasms (more than 60% overall and more than 90% of malignant tumors).

□□ **What is the most common malignant tumor of the ovary?**

Serous cystadenocarcinoma, and it is frequently bilateral (more than half the time).

□□ **What are the three general categories which surface epithelial tumors of the ovary are divided into?**

Benign, borderline (low malignant potential), and malignant.

□□ **What are some of the histologic features that determine classification into the borderline category?**

These are tumors that are composed of the same cell type but generally lack "high grade" nuclear features, complex architecture, and destructive stromal invasion.

❏❏ **What is the benign version of the serous tumors of the ovary?**

Benign serous cystadenoma, remember the malignant version is the serous cystadenocarcinoma.

❏❏ **Do borderline tumors (low malignant potential) spread beyond the ovary?**

Yes. The majority (60-70%) present confined to the ovary while up to 40% will spread beyond the ovary, particularly as peritoneal implants. Overall, the prognosis is markedly better than the malignant counterpart with 100% five year survival when confined to the ovary and 90% when spread to the peritoneum.

❏❏ **What is the name of the benign epithelial tumor of the ovary which is characterized by mucin production?**

Benign mucinous cystadenoma, of course the malignant counterpart would be mucinous cystadenocarcinoma.

❏❏ **What is the overall five year survival of the mucinous cystadenocarcinoma compared to the serous cystadenocarcinoma?**

The serous cystadenocarcinoma has a much worse prognosis with an overall five year survival of 20-30%, while the mucinous cystadenocarcinoma has an overall five year survival of 50-60%.

❏❏ **What is the name of the lamellated calcific concretions which are commonly found in papillary serous cystadenocarcinomas?**

Psammoma bodies.

❏❏ **What are the two histologic types of mucinous tumors of the ovary based on histologic appearance?**

In addition to be divided into benign, borderline and malignant varieties, the mucinous tumors may resemble endocervical mucosa or intestinal epithelium. Thus, the tumors are divided into endocervical-type and intestinal-type.

❏❏ **What is pseudomyxoma peritonei?**

This is so-called mucinous or gelatinous ascites as a result of implantation of cells in the peritoneal cavity which produce abundant mucous. This can be a result of a mucinous borderline tumor of the ovary or a mucinous tumor of the appendix. Although benign, death can occur as a result of extensive spreading and compression of abdominal viscera.

❏❏ **Which has a better prognosis, borderline mucinous tumors of the endocervical or intestinal type?**

Endocervical-type.

❏❏ **What tumor is fairly commonly found concomitantly with an endometrioid carcinoma of the ovary?**

Approximately 1/3 of patients with an endometrioid carcinoma of the ovary have a co-existent adenocarcinoma of the endometrium. These are thought to be separate primaries.

❏❏ **What ovarian epithelial tumor is characterized by large epithelial cells with abundant intracytoplasmic glycogen and form a so-called "hobnail" appearance as they protrude into the lumen of small tubules/cysts?**

Clear cell carcinoma.

❑❑  **Is a Brenner tumor more commonly benign or malignant?**

Nearly 99% of them are benign; however, there are proliferative or borderline as well as malignant versions reported.

❑❑  **How are most Brenner tumors discovered?**

Incidentally, as about half are microscopic in nature.  The vast majority are less than 2 cm.

❑❑  **How common is bilaterality in endometrioid carcinoma of the ovary?**

It is quite common, up to 50% of patients have bilateral tumors at the time of surgery.

OVARIAN TUMOR

❑❑  **The tumor shown above occurred in the ovary of a 20-year-old female with hypercalcemia which resolved following resection of her ovary.  What is the diagnosis?**

Small cell carcinoma of the ovary.

❑❑  **What is the most common benign tumor of the ovary?**

Dermoid cyst or mature cystic teratoma.

❑❑  **An 18-year-old female has a large (20 cm) ovarian mass for which she undergoes oopherectomy.  Histologically, the mass contains tissue derived from ectoderm, endoderm, and mesoderm and abundant areas of small blue cells thought to be neuroblasts.  What is your diagnosis?**

Immature teratoma.

❑❑  **What is the term given to a benign ovarian teratoma where almost all of the tissue is composed of benign thyroid elements?**

Struma ovarii.

❑❑  **Do mature teratomas undergo malignant change?**

The vast majority (99%) do not; however, it can occur and has been well described and is most commonly a squamous cell carcinoma.

❑❑  **What is the ovarian counterpart of the testicular seminoma?**

Dysgerminoma.

❐❐  **Are dysgerminomas benign or malignant?**

They are malignant but have a very good prognosis particularly if limited to the ovary.  In addition, they are extremely radiosensitive and thus the overall survival rate is greater than 80%.

❐❐  **What is Meigs' syndrome?**

This is the presence of a large ovarian fibroma with associated ascites and pleural effusion both of which resolve upon resection of the fibroma.

❐❐  **What is produced by the majority of granulosa cell tumors which result in "feminizing" signs and symptoms?**

Estrogenic hormones.

❐❐  **What is the characteristic shape of the nuclei of granulosa cells?**

They are round to oval, haphazardly arranged, and frequently contain a longitudinal groove imparting a "coffee bean" appearance.

❐❐  **What ovarian tumor is associated with the basal cell nevus syndrome?**

Fibromas, which are almost universally bilateral, multinodular, and at least focally calcified in these patients.

❐❐  **What is the typical age of presentation in patients with a thecoma?**

They are almost always postmenopausal with a mean age of about 60.

❐❐  **Although this can be true in several ovarian tumors, which sex cord-stromal tumor is associated with the classic yellow gross tumor appearance?**

Thecoma.

❐❐  **In contrast to thecomas, what is the typical age of patients with Sertoli-Leydig cell tumors?**

They occur during reproductive years with a mean of 25 years old.

❐❐  **What syndrome is found in about a third of patients with the sex cord tumor called "sex cord tumor with annular tubules"?**

Peutz-Jeghers syndrome.

❐❐  **What is a so-called Krukenberg's tumor?**

This is a gastric carcinoma which is metastatic to the ovary.

❐❐  **In general, what is the prognosis for dysgerminoma?**

It is excellent as the tumor is quite radiosensitive and responsive to chemotherapy.  Thus, for a stage I tumor, the five year survival is almost 95%.  Overall, the five year survival is between 70 and 90% for all tumors.

❐❐  **A 17-year-old female has an ovarian tumor which has resulted in an elevated serum alpha-fetoprotein.  What is your diagnosis?**

Yolk sac tumor.

❏❏ **In an ovarian yolk sac tumor, what are some of the characteristic histologic features you would expect to see?**

Schiller-Duval bodies and eosinophilic globules which are PAS positive and diastase resistant.

❏❏ **What is the typical genotype and phenotype in patients with gonadoblastoma?**

They are usually phenotypic females and genotypic males (have a Y chromosome).

❏❏ **What is placental abruption?**

This is when the placenta partially separates from the uterine wall and results in retroplacental hemorrhage.

❏❏ **What placental abnormality is classically associated with painless vaginal bleeding?**

Placenta previa in which the placenta covers, partially or totally, the internal os of the cervix.

❏❏ **What is placenta accreta?**

This is an unusual condition whereby the placenta implants in the myometrium to varying degrees. Placenta increta indicates deeper penetration into the myometrium while placenta percreta indicates penetration through the entire thickness of the myometrium.

❏❏ **What is the most common site of an ectopic pregnancy?**

Ectopic pregnancy simply means pregnancy outside of the uterus and it occurs in the fallopian tubes over 90% of the time.

❏❏ **What is pre-eclampsia?**

This is a syndrome that occurs in some pregnant females whereby they develop hypertension, edema, and albuminuria with associated retention of salt. If seizure activity occurs in this setting, it is termed eclampsia.

❏❏ **What are some conditions which are associated with an increased incidence of hydatidiform mole?**

Poverty, poor nutrition, extremely old or young maternal age, and consanguinity.

❏❏ **What is the most common karyotype in complete hydatidiform mole (CHM) compared to partial hydatidiform mole (PHM)?**

In CHM they are almost always 46XX while in PHM, the majority are 69XXY with 69XXX representing up to 40% of cases.

❏❏ **Which is at a greater risk for development of choriocarcinoma - CHM or PHM?**

CHM results in choriocarcinoma in approximately 5% of cases.

❏❏ **Which type of mole is associated with a higher level of beta-hCG?**

The beta-hCG in CHM is usually twice that of PHM.

# BREAST

❏❏  **How common is breast cancer?**

1 in 9 women will develop it.

❏❏  **What is the name of the cells which are found immediately subjacent to the ductular and lobular epithelium?**

Myoepithelial cells.

❏❏  **What is the most common congenital abnormality of the breast?**

Supernumerary breasts which are accessory glands which can arise at any point along the embryonal milk line.

❏❏  **At what point do the male and female breasts begin to differ histologically?**

Prior to puberty, they are identical; however, after that the female breasts undergo significant development including lengthening and branching of ducts, proliferation of stroma and fat, and development of lobules.

❏❏  **What is microscopically typically lacking in the male breast that distinguishes it from the female breast?**

Lobules.

❏❏  **What liver condition is associated with gynecomastia?**

Cirrhosis.  This is due to the fact that the diseased liver is less able to metabolize estrogens thus the level of estrogen is higher than normal with resultant gynecomastia.

❏❏  **When is juvenile hypertrophy of the breast most likely to develop?**

This is a rare, bilateral condition which comprises massive enlargement of the breast and occurs immediately after menarche.  Actually, this condition is a hyperplasia although it has been incorrectly termed a hypertrophy.

❏❏  **What is another name for the lesion termed periductal mastitis which is characterized by duct dilatation with associated fibrosis and lymphoplasmacytic inflammation and is typically found in perimenopausal women?**

It is also called duct ectasia and can clinically mimic carcinoma by causing nipple alterations.

❏❏  **What are some "risk factors" for development of fibrocystic change?**

Early menarche, nulliparity, and older age at the time of first pregnancy and birth.

❏❏  **What is the most common age of development of fibrocystic change?**

It typically occurs in women ages 20-40 and is a very common cause of biopsy of the breast.

❏❏  **What is the most common cause of a palpable breast mass in women between the ages of 25 and 50?**

Fibrocystic change.

**❑❑  Is there an increased risk for subsequent development of cancer in fibrocystic change?**

The risk of development of carcinoma is related to the degree and type of epithelial hyperplasia present. Thus, assigning a risk of development of breast carcinoma to fibrocystic change must be done with the caveat that this assignment is based on the degree and type of epithelial hyperplasia not the cystic and fibrotic change itself.

**❑❑  What effect does oral contraceptive use have on the development of fibrocystic change?**

It appears to decrease the risk of fibrocystic change development.

**❑❑  What is the most common benign tumor of the breast?**

Fibroadenoma.

**❑❑  What are the two distinct patterns of fibroadenomas which tend to occur even within the same lesion?**

Intracanalicular and pericanalicular.

**❑❑  Besides young age, what are the patient characteristics which are most likely to be found in a patient with fibroadenoma?**

They are more commonly found during pregnancy and are more likely to be multiple in African-American females.

**❑❑  What is the prognostic significance between the intracanalicular and pericanalicular variants of fibroadenoma?**

None.

**❑❑  Is there an increased risk of developing breast carcinoma in a patient with fibroadenoma?**

Yes, but the increased incidence is slight.

**❑❑  What is a juvenile fibroadenoma?**

This is a very large, fast-growing variant of fibroadenoma which occurs in adolescents.  The stroma tends to be more cellular and mitotically active than the typical fibroadenoma.  They are usually solitary, unilateral and do not recur following excision.

**❑❑  Compare the typical age at presentation of fibroadenoma and phyllodes tumor.**

Phyllodes tumor is most commonly seen in women in their 50s while fibroadenoma most commonly occurs in women age 30 or younger.

**❑❑  What is the clinical behavior of the majority of cystosarcoma phyllodes lesions?**

The majority behave in a benign fashion, do not recur or metastasize.

**❑❑  Are phyllodes tumors more common in blacks or whites?**

There is a striking preponderance of this tumor in whites, approximately 90%.

**❑❑  How frequently do phyllodes tumors recur?**

30% recur and most of those occur within the first two years following initial resection.

❑❑ **Describe the typical route of spread in a "malignant" phyllodes tumor.**

Phyllodes tumor spreads hematogenously rather than via lymphatics. The lung is the most common site of metastasis.

❑❑ **What is the recommended treatment of phyllodes tumor?**

If possible, wide local excision should be performed in lieu of mastectomy. Certainly, lymph node dissection is unnecessary.

❑❑ **What is the name of the benign tumor of the breast characterized by a proliferation of small, round tubular structures in a tightly packed, well-circumscribed architecture with a distinct myoepithelial layer?**

Tubular adenoma.

❑❑ **What is the most common presentation of a patient with a duct papilloma?**

Nipple discharge which may be bloody.

❑❑ **What is the typical age at presentation of a patient with an intraductal papilloma?**

Perimenopausal.

❑❑ **Is there an increased risk of carcinoma in patients with a single, central intraductal papilloma?**

There does not appear to be any significant increased risk.

❑❑ **Is there an increased risk for development of carcinoma in a patient with multiple intraductal papillomas?**

There does appear to be some increased risk as multiple papillomas may be associated with concurrent atypical ductal hyperplasia and/or ductal carcinoma in situ.

❑❑ **What are some risk factors for development of carcinoma of the breast?**

Family history, Li-Fraumeni syndrome, Cowden disease (multiple hamartoma syndrome), ataxia-telangiectasia, lower socioeconomic status, increasing age, proliferative epithelial lesions of the breast, contralateral breast carcinoma, endometrial carcinoma, radiation exposure, early menarche and late menopause, nulliparity, older age at birth of first child, and obesity.

❑❑ **Does papillary carcinoma have a generally good or bad prognosis?**

Good, it is an indolent tumor found in older women which is largely intraductal.

❑❑ **What type of hyperplasia poses the greatest risk for development of carcinoma?**

Atypical hyperplasia. In addition, florid intraductal hyperplasia also carries an increased risk of development of carcinoma.

❑❑ **What is the relative risk of development of invasive carcinoma of the breast in a patient with atypical ductal hyperplasia (ADH)?**

4-5 times.

❑❑ **What is the relative risk of development of invasive carcinoma of the breast in a patient with epithelial hyperplasia (mild)?**

1.5-2 times.

❐❐ **What is the relative risk of development of invasive carcinoma of the breast in a patient with atypical lobular hyperplasia (ALH)?**

4-5 times. Interestingly, the tumors that develop in these patients are most commonly ductal carcinomas thus indicative of ALH as a marker for cancer risk rather than a precursor lesion.

❐❐ **Is there a myoepithelial layer in sclerosing adenosis?**

Yes, at least focally.

❐❐ **Is there an increased relative risk of development of invasive breast carcinoma in patients with sclerosing adenosis?**

Yes, a mild one (1.5-2 times).

❐❐ **What two genes account for the vast majority of inherited breast cancers?**

BRCA1 and BRCA2.

❐❐ **Is there a risk of development of other types of malignancies in patients with mutations involving BRCA1 and BRCA2?**

Yes, or I would not have asked. BRCA1 mutations are associated with a pronounced increased risk of development of ovarian cancer (up to 60% by age 70) and it also has risks associated with prostate and colon cancer. BRCA2 is associated with development of male breast cancer, ovarian cancer and cancer of the bladder, prostate, and pancreas.

❐❐ **What is the risk of development of breast cancer in a patient who has two first degree relatives with breast cancer?**

4-6 times.

❐❐ **Do the majority of women with a family history of breast cancer have the BRCA1 and 2 genes?**

No, less than 20% do.

❐❐ **How significant is the risk of development of breast cancer in a patient with Cowden disease?**

This is a mutation found on the long arm of chromosome 10 and these patients have up to 50% risk of development of breast carcinoma by the time they reach age 50.

❐❐ **What is the most common location in the breast in which carcinoma develops?**

The upper outer quadrant. However, this contains the most breast tissue and it stands to reason why it would contain more tumors. Interestingly, the cancer is more frequently found in the left breast than the right.

❐❐ **How common is the presence of estrogen receptors in carcinoma cells?**

About half of the cases contain estrogen receptors.

❐❐ **What is the relative risk of developing invasive breast carcinoma in a patient with atypical ductal hyperplasia and a strong family history of breast cancer?**

Greater than 10 times.

❐❐  **What is the risk of developing breast cancer in association with caffeine consumption and cigarette smoking?**

There is no substantial data to prove a causative effect of either substance.

❐❐  **What structure within the breast gives rise to all carcinomas?**

The terminal duct lobular unit.

❐❐  **What is the most common type of in situ carcinoma and invasive carcinoma?**

Ductal carcinoma accounts for 80% of the in situ lesions and 80% of the invasive lesions.

❐❐  **What is the incidence of ductal carcinoma in situ (DCIS) in a patient with invasive carcinoma of the breast?**

DCIS is present in the contralateral breast in about half of the patients with an invasive carcinoma. In addition, about a third of the cases develop invasive carcinoma of the breast in the ipsilateral breast where DCIS was previously excised.

❐❐  **What is the relative risk of developing an invasive carcinoma in a patient with lobular carcinoma in situ?**

The risk increases approximately 1% per year. The risk is bilateral and the majority of the invasive tumors that develop are actually ductal and not lobular.

❐❐  **What are the various treatment options for a patient with breast carcinoma?**

Surgical resection varies from lumpectomy to variations of mastectomy. Axillary lymph node dissections may or may not be done depending on the surgical excision. Following that, radiation and chemotherapy (including antiestrogens, etc.) may or may not be used depending on patient preference, receptor status of the tumor, surgical resection margins, tumor size, and lymph node status.

❐❐  **What is the rate of bilaterality in infiltrating lobular carcinoma?**

There is a concurrent contralateral tumor in 10-15% of cases and about 1/3 of the cases will develop a contralateral invasive tumor.

❐❐  **What is the characteristic histologic invasion pattern of infiltrating lobular carcinoma?**

They classically invade in a single file fashion and exhibit a "targetoid" or concentric ring formation around normal ducts.

❐❐  **What is the prognosis of medullary carcinoma?**

It has an excellent prognosis, even better than intraductal carcinoma with 10 year survivals of up to 90%.

❐❐  **What is the prognosis for tubular carcinoma?**

It is the best of all invasive carcinomas with a five year survival rate approaching 100%. It, however, is bilateral (concurrent or subsequent) in up to 20% of patients.

❐❐  **What is the prognosis for mucinous (colloid) carcinoma of the breast?**

It too is excellent. It is more common in older females and has a 10 year survival of up to 90% for the typical mucinous carcinoma.

❐❐  **How common are axillary lymph node metastases in tubular carcinoma?**

Uncommon, occurring in less than 10% of cases.

❑❑ **What is the incidence of bilaterality and multifocality in tubular carcinoma?**

Tubular carcinoma occurs in younger women (40s) and is multifocal in up to half of the cases and bilateral in up to 40% of the cases.

❑❑ **What is the maximal tumor measurement to keep a breast carcinoma at stage I?**

2 cm or less.

❑❑ **What is the maximal tumor measurement to keep a breast carcinoma at stage II?**

5 cm or less.

❑❑ **How does the presence or absence of hormone receptors in a tumor effect prognosis?**

Tumors with high numbers of hormone receptors have a slightly better prognosis than those without. Most breast cancers do express estrogen receptors, particularly in postmenopausal women.

❑❑ **How does mammary Paget's disease differ from extramammary Paget's?**

While it is uncommon to have underlying adenocarcinoma in extramammary Paget's, Paget's disease of the nipple is the presence of intraepidermal malignant cells from an underlying invasive ductal carcinoma or comedo DCIS.

❑❑ **How does the status of HER-2/neu (c-erbB-2) effect the prognosis in breast cancer?**

It is associated with decreased survival when overexpressed in tumor cells.

❑❑ **Which is more common, intraductal or infiltrating ductal carcinoma?**

Infiltrating ductal, by far. It accounts for about 70% of breast cancers while intraductal accounts for less than 10%.

❑❑ **What is the characteristic histologic feature of mucinous (colloid) carcinoma?**

It is characterized by pools of mucin within which groups of tumor cells "float".

❑❑ **What does the term "metaplastic carcinoma" describe in breast cancer?**

These are tumors with "sarcomatoid" features or a mixture of malignant epithelial and mesenchymal elements.

❑❑ **What is the most common pure sarcoma to occur in the breast?**

Angiosarcoma.

❑❑ **What is the mean age of development of angiosarcoma of the breast?**

Approximately 40 years.

❑❑ **In general terms, what is the prognosis of angiosarcoma of the breast?**

It varies greatly depending on the grade of the tumor. Low grade tumors have a good prognosis with over 80% 10 year survival; however, that number drops to less than 15% 10 year survival in grade 3 tumors.

□□  **Does non-Hodgkin's lymphoma occur in the breast?**

Of course, many believe them to be a part of the lymphomas related to mucosa-associated lymphoid tissue (MALT).

□□  **What is the typical age at presentation for male breast cancer?**

Around 60, which is some 10 years later than in females.

□□  **In general terms, what is the prognosis of male breast cancer?**

It is poor with a five year survival of around 40%, dropping to less than 20% at 10 years.

□□  **What is the definition of microinvasive carcinoma of the breast?**

This refers to a carcinoma which is almost exclusively in situ; however, there are one or more separate foci of early invasion by tumor. None of the foci can measure greater than 1 mm in diameter to qualify as microinvasive.

# ENDOCRINE

*Please refer to chapter on pancreas for questions regarding the endocrine pancreas.*

□□ **What is the embryonic origin of the adenohypophysis (anterior lobe of the pituitary)?**

It is derived from Rathke's pouch which is an ectodermal upgrowth from the oral cavity.

□□ **What is the embryonic origin of the neurohypophysis (posterior lobe of the pituitary)?**

Diencephalon.

□□ **What are the hormones contained in the posterior pituitary?**

Vasopressin and oxytocin.

□□ **What is the "empty sella syndrome"?**

This is when the dura mater that forms the roof of the sella turcica (sellar diaphragm) is absent resulting in increased pressure from cerebrospinal fluid which compresses the pituitary gland and widens the sella. It is usually not associated with hypopituitarism.

□□ **What is the basic functional difference between the anterior and posterior pituitary?**

The anterior pituitary, owing to its embryonic origin in the ectoderm from the oral cavity, produces its own hormones which then act on target organs after stimulation from the hypothalamic releasing hormones. In contrast, the posterior pituitary, again owing to its embryonic origin in the diencephalon, simply stores its hormones (oxytocin and vasopressin/antidiuretic hormone) which are originally produced in the hypothalamus, specifically the paraventricular and supraoptic nuclei.

□□ **What are the three basic cell types seen in the anterior pituitary?**

Acidophils, basophils, and chromophobes.

□□ **How can you tell the various hormone-producing cells apart in the anterior pituitary?**

Via immunohistochemistry. For instance, although they are broken down into the three cell types described above, one cannot tell apart prolactin-producing cells from growth hormone-producing cells as they are both acidophils.

□□ **What are the hormones produced in the anterior pituitary and their corresponding hypothalamic regulating protein?**

| ANTERIOR PITUITARY HORMONE | HYPOTHALAMIC REGULATOR |
|---|---|
| ACTH | Corticotropin-releasing hormone (CRH) |
| Follicle-stimulating hormone (FSH) | Gonadotropin-releasing hormone (GRH) |
| Luteinizing hormone (LH) | GRH |
| Thyroid-stimulating hormone (TSH) | Thyrotropin-releasing hormone (TRH) |
| Prolactin | TRH |
| Growth hormone | Inhibited by somatostatin |
| Prolactin | Inhibited by dopamine |

□□ **What is the most numerous cell type in the anterior pituitary?**

Almost half the cells are growth hormone-producing, which are acidophilic-type cells.

□□ **What is the most common inflammatory condition affecting the hypothalamus and subsequently the pituitary gland?**

Sarcoidosis.

□□ **What is Sheehan's syndrome?**

This is infarction of the pituitary secondary to hypotension from massive blood loss during childbirth or from postpartum hemorrhage. Remember, during pregnancy the pituitary increases in size greatly making it more susceptible to infarction.

□□ **What would you expect to see in the pituitary gland of a patient with Addison's disease?**

They typically get diffuse and nodular hyperplasia of the ACTH-producing cells. Occasionally, true ACTH-producing adenomas may occur.

□□ **What is the effect of bromocriptine on the pituitary?**

It is a dopamine agonist and thus inhibits prolactin secretion.

□□ **What is Kallmann's syndrome?**

This is isolated gonadotropin deficiency owing to an abnormality in the formation and subsequent transport of gonadotropin releasing hormone and is associated with olfactory bulb agenesis. It is most commonly inherited in an X-linked pattern.

□□ **In anencephaly, what cell type is most commonly reduced in the anterior pituitary?**

ACTH producing cells are reduced in number and the adrenal glands are subsequently usually hypoplastic.

□□ **Approximately how much of the pituitary must be destroyed before patients become symptomatic?**

More than 50%.

□□ **What are some of the general conditions which can result in panhypopituitarism?**

A primary or metastatic pituitary tumor, a tumor of a nearby structure, infarction (Sheehan's syndrome), irradiation, granulomatous disease like sarcoidosis, and empty sella syndrome.

□□ **What pituitary tumor is most commonly associated with deposition of amyloid?**

Prolactin producing pituitary adenomas.

□□ **What is the nature of lymphocytic hypophysitis?**

This is most likely an autoimmune disorder involving the pituitary gland. It classically affects women who are pregnant or postpartum, although older patients have been diagnosed at autopsy. Steroids are the treatment.

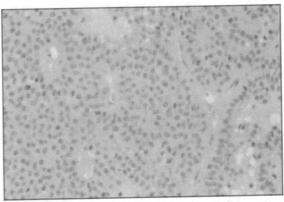

PITUITARY TUMOR

❏❐  **What is the most common cause of hypersecretion of an anterior pituitary hormone?**

Pituitary adenoma.

❏❐  **What is the most common type of pituitary adenoma?**

Prolactin adenoma.

❏❐  **Where do most pituitary adenomas arise, the anterior or posterior pituitary?**

By far, the anterior pituitary is most common with less than 1% of all tumors in the pituitary arising in the posterior pituitary.

❏❐  **What is the definition of a microadenoma in the pituitary?**

They are adenomas which measure less than 1 cm in diameter.

❏❐  **What is the result of excessive growth hormone production in children compared to adults?**

In children, when the growth plates are not closed, excessive GH results in gigantism while in adults it results in acromegaly.

❏❐  **What is the typical age and presentation of patients with prolactin adenomas?**

The patients are typically women of childbearing age who present with amenorrhea, galactorrhea, and infertility.

❏❐  **What is Nelson's syndrome?**

This is a large pituitary corticotroph adenoma which occurs following removal of the adrenal glands in a patient with Cushing's syndrome as treatment of hypercortisolism.

❏❐  **How common is so-called null cell adenoma and oncocytoma in the pituitary?**

Quite common, as they represent about a quarter of the surgically removed pituitary tumors.

❏❐  **How does one diagnose pituitary carcinoma compared to adenoma?**

Although they can show some pleomorphism and other histologic evidence of aggressive behavior, the diagnosis of carcinoma rests on the demonstration of distant metastases as histologic criteria are not reliable. Fortunately, these tumors are exceedingly rare.

**❑❑  What is the second most common neoplasm of the sellar region?**

The most common is pituitary adenoma and second most common is craniopharyngioma.

**❑❑  What is the typical behavior of craniopharyngioma?**

They are almost always benign and do not secrete active hormones.  Their symptoms relate to their anatomic location and compression on surrounding structures to result in such things as headache, visual changes, increased intracranial pressure, and seizures.  Treatment is surgical with radiation for recurrences.

**❑❑  Is there a gender preference in occurrence of ACTH cell adenomas (Cushing's disease) and LH/FSH adenomas?**

Yes, the former occurs more frequently in females and the latter more commonly in males.

**❑❑  What suprasellar tumor is more common in children, usually has a cystic component whose contents are referred to as "machine oil", and contains a squamous epithelial growth pattern?**

Craniopharyngioma.  Remember, there is also a papillary variant which occurs in adults, involves the third ventricle, has clear fluid, and lacks calcification.

**❑❑  What does goiter mean in regard to the thyroid?**

It simply means enlargement of the thyroid gland.  Thus, thyroid adenoma, carcinoma, colloid goiter, iodine deficiency, and many others all are causes of thyroid enlargement or "goiter".

**❑❑  How does the biologic activity compare to circulating levels of T4 and T3?**

T4 is found in much greater amounts in the circulation than T3; however, T3 is four times more active.

**❑❑  What congenital midline cyst occurs predominantly in children as a result of failure of complete regression of a normal embryologic structure?**

Thyroglossal duct cyst.

**❑❑  What are the most common etiologic agents of acute thyroiditis?**

This rare condition is most commonly a result of infection with Staphylococcus aureus, Streptococcus pyogenes, and Streptococcus pneumoniae.

**❑❑  In general terms, what is the most likely cause of subacute thyroiditis?**

It is most likely viral in nature.

**❑❑  Describe the typical patient and signs/symptoms seen in subacute thyroiditis.**

There is an association with HLA-Bw35, and it most commonly occurs in middle-aged females.  Presentation is marked by an abrupt painful enlargement of the thyroid in association with fever, malaise, and other non-specific symptoms.

**❑❑  What is the most common type of autoimmune thyroiditis?**

Hashimoto's thyroiditis.

**❑❑  Describe the typical patient with Hashimoto's thyroiditis.**

As with all autoimmune phenomena, it is much more common in females (10:1), occurs in middle age (30-50 years), and is associated with painless enlargement of the thyroid with hypothyroidism.

❒❒ **What is the typical time course of disease in a patient with subacute thyroiditis?**

It typically resolves of its own accord within about three months.

❒❒ **What are the autoantibodies found in patients with Hashimoto's thyroiditis?**

They develop antibodies to thyroglobulin and thyroid peroxidase (antimicrosomal antibodies). These are not found in all patients.

❒❒ **What is Schmidt's syndrome?**

This is a lymphocytic adrenalitis in the presence of Hashimoto's thyroiditis.

❒❒ **What are some of the histologic features of Hashimoto's thyroiditis?**

There is a massive lymphoplasmacytic infiltrate including germinal center formation with associated small thyroid follicles and Hurthle cell change.

❒❒ **Is there an increased risk for lymphoma in patients with Hashimoto's thyroiditis?**

Of course.

❒❒ **What is juvenile thyroiditis?**

This is a variant of Hashimoto's which tends to occur in children and younger women who are euthyroid. They have lower titers of antibodies and Hurthle cell change is absent or inconspicuous.

❒❒ **What is the typical clinical presentation of patients with Riedel's thyroiditis?**

The average age is 50, and it is more common in women. The thyroid is hard upon palpation and appears fixed to adjacent structures in the neck.

❒❒ **What are the two most common causes of hyperthyroidism?**

Graves' disease and toxic nodular goiter.

❒❒ **Do patients with Graves' disease have circulating autoantibodies?**

Yes, they have antibodies against the thyroid stimulating hormone (TSH) receptor.

❒❒ **Describe the typical clinical presentation of patients with Graves' disease.**

It has a wide age range but occurs most commonly in patients in their 20s and 30s and, of course, has an increased incidence in women. The classic feature in addition to typical hyperthyroidism and thyroid enlargement is a marked exophthalmos.

❒❒ **What is the typical inheritance pattern of patients with enzyme defects resulting in abnormal or deficient thyroid hormone production?**

Autosomal recessive.

❒❒ **What is cretinism?**

This is congenital hypothyroidism with associated consequences including marked mental and growth retardation. This is screened for in all newborns and is certainly preventable by using replacement hormones.

⬜⬜ **What is Plummer's disease?**

This is also referred to as a toxic nodular goiter and refers to the presence of a nodular goiter with associated hyperthyroidism.

⬜⬜ **What is the significance of a "hot" or "cold" nodule on scintogram evaluation of thyroid nodules?**

The terms "hot" and "cold" refer to whether the nodule in question is functional (takes up radioactive iodine) or non-functional (does not take up radioactive iodine), respectively. Most thyroid tumors in general, benign or malignant, are "cold" and most thyroid malignancies are "cold"; however, the majority of "cold" nodules are benign.

⬜⬜ **Compare the prognoses for the various carcinomas of the thyroid which arise from the follicular cells.**

Papillary carcinoma is the most common and has the best prognosis with a greater than 90% ten year survival rate. This is followed by follicular carcinoma, Hurthle cell carcinoma, poorly differentiated carcinoma, and undifferentiated carcinoma (anaplastic) in worsening prognosis.

⬜⬜ **How does one make the distinction between a follicular adenoma and a follicular carcinoma based on histology?**

Multiple histologic sections are necessary to adequately evaluate any thyroid tumor, particularly if a follicular neoplasm is suspected. A follicular carcinoma differs from an adenoma by virtue of increased mitoses, a thicker capsule, capsular penetration by tumor, and vascular space invasion. The latter two criteria are the most important in this distinction. Remember, there is a follicular variant of papillary carcinoma which, although architecturally follicular, cytologically the tumor cells maintain the characteristic features of papillary carcinoma.

⬜⬜ **Are thyroid carcinomas more common in males or females?**

Females by about 2:1.

⬜⬜ **What are the cytologic features of the tumor cells in papillary carcinoma of the thyroid?**

1. Optically clear nuclei
2. Nuclear pseudoinclusions
3. Longitudinal nuclear grooves

⬜⬜ **What are the most common sites of metastases in papillary carcinoma of the thyroid?**

The cervical lymph nodes are the most common site. Distant metastases, as with many tumors, favor the lung. Remember, thyroid cancer is one of the tumors in humans that also metastasizes to bone.

⬜⬜ **What is the definition of papillary microcarcinoma?**

This was previously referred to as "occult sclerosing carcinoma" and refers to a papillary carcinoma which measures less than 1 cm in greatest dimension.

⬜⬜ **What is the prognosis of patients with papillary microcarcinoma involving lymph nodes?**

Even with metastatic spread to lymph nodes, the prognosis for this tumor remains excellent.

⬜⬜ **How does the prognosis for the tall cell variant of papillary carcinoma differ from routine papillary carcinoma?**

It has a worse prognosis; however, it also tends to occur in older patients which calls into question the real reason for the worse prognosis - the histology or simply the older age of the patient.

☐☐  **How does follicular carcinoma tend to spread, in contrast to papillary carcinoma?**

Follicular carcinoma spreads via the hematogenous route rather than via lymphatics as in papillary carcinoma.

☐☐  **What is the prominent ultrastructural feature in the tumor cells of a Hurthle cell tumor of the thyroid?**

They are filled with abnormal mitochondria which vary greatly in size and shape.

☐☐  **How do you make the diagnosis of malignancy in a Hurthle cell tumor?**

It should be treated similar to a follicular lesion of the thyroid in that capsular penetration and vascular invasion should be sought for a diagnosis of malignancy.

☐☐  **What is the treatment of choice for a Hurthle cell carcinoma?**

Total thyroidectomy.

☐☐  **What is the most common cause of hyperthryoidism?**

Diffuse hyperplasia in a setting of Graves' disease.

☐☐  **What is the typical clinical presentation of anaplastic carcinoma of the thyroid?**

These tend to occur in older patients with a slight female preponderance, less striking than in the other thyroid carcinomas.  These patients develop a rapidly progressing neck mass that may cause symptoms of compression of local structures including the airway.

☐☐  **What is the prognosis in anaplastic carcinoma of the thyroid?**

It is dismal with fewer than 10% of patients alive after five years and a mean survival of six months.

☐☐  **What is the cell of origin of medullary carcinoma of the thyroid?**

The C-cells (calcitonin producing cells).

☐☐  **What syndrome are some medullary carcinomas of the thyroid a part of?**

Multiple endocrine neoplasia type 2A (MEN 2A).  The other components of the syndrome are parathyroid hyperplasia or adenoma and adrenal medullary hyperplasia or pheochromocytoma.

☐☐  **How is MEN type 2A inherited?**

Autosomal dominant.

☐☐  **How do the sporadic and familial medullary carcinomas of the thyroid differ?**

The sporadic tumors are typically unilateral while the familial tumors tend to be multicentric and bilateral.

☐☐  **What substance is found in the stroma of up to 80% of cases of medullary carcinoma of the thyroid?**

Amyloid.

❏❏ **What is the treatment for medullary carcinoma of the thyroid?**

Total thyroidectomy.

❏❏ **What is the general survival of medullary carcinoma of the thyroid?**

The five year survival is approximately 60-70%. It improves for patients younger than 40 and is better in women.

❏❏ **Is there a difference in prognosis in medullary carcinomas occurring in association with MEN type 2A, 2B, or sporadically?**

In general, tumors in association with MEN type 2B are more aggressive than either sporadic tumors or those in association with MEN type 2A.

❏❏ **What is the treatment of choice for patients with C-cell hyperplasia?**

Total thyroidectomy.

❏❏ **What are some of the typical clinical manifestations of hyperthyroidism?**

They all relate to an increase in the basal metabolic rate and include tachycardia, palpitations, occasionally arrhythmias, lid lag with a staring gaze, proximal muscle weakness, warm and moist skin, increased gut motility, and osteoporosis among many other symptoms.

❏❏ **What is myxedema?**

This is hypothyroidism in older children and adults and is characterized by numerous symptoms including generalized fatigue, slow mentation, slow speech, cold intolerance, occasional obesity, decreased cardiac output with dyspnea, deposition of glycosaminoglycans and hyaluronic acid in the skin and other sites, coarse facial features, macroglossia, and many other symptoms.

❏❏ **What HLA haplotypes are strongly associated with Graves' disease?**

HLA-B8 and HLA-DR3.

❏❏ **What is the typical age and gender of patients with sporadic goiter?**

This is more common in females, particularly at puberty or in young adulthood.

❏❏ **What is the inheritance pattern of the enzymatic defects resulting in ineffective thyroid hormone synthesis and subsequent goiter formation?**

Autosomal recessive.

❏❏ **What is the major risk factor which predisposes individuals to development of thyroid cancer?**

Previous exposure to ionizing radiation, particularly at a young age.

❏❏ **What are the three morphologic patterns in anaplastic carcinoma of the thyroid?**

1. pleomorphic giant cells
2. spindle cells (sarcomatous)
3. small cell-like

❏❏ **What is the most common cause of hyperthyroidism in children?**

Interestingly, it is Graves' disease.

## ❑❑ What is the embryologic origin of the parathyroid glands?

The inferior parathyroids develop from the third branchial pouch (along with the thymus) and the superior parathyroids develop from the fourth branchial pouch.

## ❑❑ What happens to the cellularity of the parathyroid gland as one ages?

The cellularity decreases making the relative fat content increase.

## ❑❑ What are the two cell types (not including the adipocytes or fat cells) in the parathyroid gland?

Chief cells are the first and only cells in the glands until puberty. After puberty, they are joined by the oxyphil cells.

## ❑❑ Where is the majority of parathyroid hormone (PTH) stored in the parathyroid glands?

Chief cells.

## ❑❑ What are some of the actions of PTH?

PTH increases serum calcium by activating osteoclasts, increasing renal tubular resorption of calcium, increasing the level of active (dihydroxy) vitamin D, and increasing calcium absorption in the gut.

## ❑❑ Where is PTH synthesized in the parathyroid glands?

In the chief cells.

## ❑❑ Where is the biologically active portion of the PTH molecule located?

The N-terminal 34 amino acids are responsible for the majority of its activity.

## ❑❑ How is the majority of PTH found or represented in the circulation?

About 95% of the circulating PTH is represented by a C-terminal fragment.

## ❑❑ What does the mnemonic MISHAP stand for regarding causes of hypercalcemia?

Malignancy (myeloma)
Intoxication (vitamin D)
Sarcoidosis
Hyperpararthyroidism
Alkali (milk-alkali syndrome)
Paget's disease of bone

## ❑❑ What are some of the symptoms of hypercalcemia?

They are vague and include "stones, moans, and groans". That is, urolithiasis, gastrointestinal complaints including constipation, and musculoskeletal pain.

## ❑❑ What are some causes of hypoparathyroidism?

Inadvertent surgical resection of the parathyroid glands, congenital absence (example DiGeorge syndrome), idiopathic atrophy of the glands (autoimmune in nature), familial hypoparathyroidism (mucocutaneous candidiasis and primary adrenal insufficiency), and pseudohypoparathyroidism (end organ resistance to PTH).

❏❏  **What is the most common clinical presentation of primary hyperparathyroidism?**

Now, with the advent of chemical screening, more than half the patients are asymptomatic. Renal disease is the next most common presentation.

❏❏  **What is the most common parathyroid pathology in patients with primary hyperparathyroidism?**

Adenomas account for about 80% of the cases, followed in frequency by hyperplasia and carcinoma (less than 1%).

❏❏  **An x-ray performed on a patient is diagnosed as having "osteitis fibrosa cystica", what is your diagnosis?**

Primary hyperparathyroidism.

❏❏  **What is the major cell type of parathyroid adenomas?**

Chief cells.

❏❏  **What are the features necessary to make the diagnosis of parathyroid adenoma?**

Size/weight is critical.  An adenoma is enlarged by weight and the three remaining parathyroid glands should be identified and shown to be normal in size.  Histologically, they are composed of solid nests of tumor cells. There is a conspicuous absence of the normal adipose tissue within the adenoma.  Ideally, one would see a thin rim of compressed normal parathyroid immediately outside the fibrous capsule of the parathyroid adenoma.

❏❏  **What is the name of the parathyroid tumor composed of a mixture of fat and chief cells in an enlarged pararthyroid?**

Lipoadenoma.

❏❏  **What is the distinguishing histologic feature between a given histologic section of pararthyroid hyperplasia and parathyroid adenoma?**

There is none, that is why it is important to know what the other glands look like in order to render the correct diagnosis.

❏❏  **What are some of the microscopic features that aid in the diagnosis of parathyroid carcinoma versus adenoma?**

In carcinoma, the cells tend to be larger with capsular and angioinvasion. Interestingly, the malignant tumors tend to be more monotonous with the more pleomorphic lesions likely representing adenomas.  As with all endocrine malignancies, behavior not histology is the only reliable indicator of malignancy or benignity.

❏❏  **What is the most common cause of secondary hyperparathyroidism?**

Renal disease.

❏❏  **What is the most common cause of hypoparathyroidism?**

It is typically iatrogenic following thyroid surgery, tracheal surgery, neck dissection, or other head and neck surgeries.

❏❏  **What is Chvostick's sign?**

This is the elicitation of tetany in hypocalcemic patients by tapping on the facial nerve.

**□□  How is DiGeorge's syndrome inherited?**

It is found on chromosome 22q11 and is inherited in an autosomal dominant fashion.

**□□  What are the three cell layers of the adrenal cortex and their associated products?**

1. zona glumerulosa (outermost) - mineralocorticoids (aldosterone)
2. zona fasciculata - glucocorticoids (cortisol)
3. zona reticularis - androgens/gonadotropins

**□□  What effect does Beckwith-Wiedemann's syndrome have on the adrenal glands?**

The adrenal glands are typically enlarged and feature cytomegaly.

**□□  What effect does anencephaly have on the adrenal glands?**

They are typically quite small.

**□□  What is adrenoleukodystrophy?**

This is a congenital abnormality by which patients are unable to oxidize very long chain fatty acids resulting in an accumulation of lipid within the tissues.  It is a degenerative, demyelinating process with associated adrenocortical atrophy with enlarged cortical cells imparting a "striated" appearance to the cells.

**□□  What is the inheritance pattern of congenital adrenal hyperplasia (CAH)?**

Autosomal recessive.

**□□  What is the most common cause of ambiguous genitalia in the newborn?**

Congenital adrenal hyperplasia.

**□□  Where is the gene locus for 21-hydroxylase?**

It is associated with the HLA major histocompatibility complex on chromosome 6p.

**□□  What is the most common form of Addison's disease?**

Addison's disease is primary adrenal insufficiency and the most common type is idiopathic which is thought to be autoimmune in nature.

**□□  What is Schmidt's syndrome?**

It is Addison's disease with associated lymphocytic thyroiditis.

**□□  What are some of the clinical features of Addison's disease?**

Generalized weakness, wasting, and cutaneous pigmentation.

**□□  What is Waterhouse-Friderichsen syndrome?**

This is hemorrhagic necrosis of the adrenal glands in the setting of sepsis (classically meningococcal) with associated circulatory collapse and shock.

**□□  What is the most common cause of noniatrogenic Cushing's syndrome?**

Pituitary-dependent overproduction of ACTH resulting in hypercortisolism (so-called Cushing's disease) is the most common cause.

☐☐ **What is the most common cause of Cushing's syndrome in children less than 8?**

Adrenocortical tumors, either adenoma or carcinoma.

☐☐ **What are the most frequent symptoms and signs of Cushing's syndrome regardless of etiology?**

Truncal obesity is seen in about 90% of cases. This is followed closely by "moon facies", generalized malaise, hirsutism, hypertension, plethora, glucose intolerance or even frank diabetes, osteoporosis, menstrual changes, and abdominal stria.

☐☐ **What is primary pigmented nodular adrenocortical disease (PPNAD)?**

This is a descriptive term for a rare kind of Cushing's syndrome which is pituitary independent hypercortisolism, that is, the ACTH level may be normal to undetectable. These patients have hypercortisolism and do not exhibit suppression of serum cortisol with dexamethasone administration nor do they respond to metyrapone or ACTH administration.

☐☐ **What is the treatment for PPNAD?**

Bilateral adrenalectomy.

☐☐ **Do adrenal adenomas have a gender preference?**

Yes, 80% of cases occur in females.

☐☐ **What is the only method by which one can determine if an adrenal tumor is a carcinoma or adenoma?**

Adrenal carcinoma can only definitively be diagnosed in a setting of metastatic disease.

☐☐ **What is Conn's syndrome?**

This is hyperaldosteronism as a result of an adrenocortical adenoma.

☐☐ **What are some of the electrolyte abnormalities seen in Conn's syndrome?**

The excess aldosterone produced in this condition results in increased total plasma volume, sodium retention, increased renal artery pressure and subsequent inhibition of renin secretion. This occurs most commonly in females, and they typically have hypertension and hypokalemic alkalosis.

☐☐ **What cell type in the adrenal cortex comprises an adrenal adenoma resulting in Cushing's syndrome?**

Remember, the zona fasciculata is the source of cortisol production thus this is the cell in adrenal adenomas which would result in hypercortisolism.

☐☐ **What is the cell type that comprises an adrenocortical adenoma which results in Conn's syndrome?**

Zona glomerulosa.

☐☐ **What is the prognosis, in general terms, for adrenocortical carcinoma?**

Extremely poor, most patients die within a year and present with metastatic disease (liver and lung most commonly).

❑❑ **How commonly are pheochromocytomas malignant?**

10% of cases.

❑❑ **How commonly are pheochromocytomas bilateral?**

10% of the cases.

❑❑ **How commonly are pheochromocytomas found in association with MEN type 2A and 2B?**

10% of cases.

❑❑ **How commonly do pheochromocytomas occur outside of the adrenal medulla?**

10% of the cases. Notice a pattern? Remember the "rule of 10s" in pheochromocytomas.

❑❑ **What are the most common signs and symptoms of patients with pheochromocytomas?**

Severe headaches, palpitations, diaphoresis, nervousness, anxiety, angina, and carbohydrate intolerance.

❑❑ **What is the predominant substance found in the secretory granules in pheochromocytomas?**

Norepinephrine, in contrast to the normal chromaffin cells which contain predominantly epinephrine.

❑❑ **What is the Verner-Morrison syndrome, also known as WDHA syndrome (watery diarrhea, hypokalemia and achlorhydria)?**

This is a pheochromocytoma which secretes vasoactive intestinal polypeptide (VIP).

❑❑ **What is the most common malignancy in infants less than one year of age?**

Neuroblastoma.

❑❑ **What are the most frequent sites of neuroblastoma?**

Adrenal medulla, and the cervical, thoracic and abdominal sympathetic ganglia.

❑❑ **What are the two most important factors in determining survival in patients with neuroblastoma?**

1. Age at diagnosis (younger is better)
2. Stage of disease

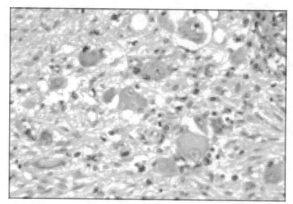

GLANGLIONEUROMA

**☐☐  How commonly does a ganglioneuroma like the one shown arise in the adrenal gland?**

About 10% of the cases.

# CENTRAL NERVOUS SYSTEM

❑❑ **What conditions are associated with the following neuronal inclusions: neurofibrillary tangles, Pick bodies, granulovacuolar degeneration, Hirano bodies, Bunina bodies, Lewy bodies, Lafora bodies?**

Neurofibrillary tangles -    Alzheimer's disease, progressive supranuclear palsy, and postencephalitic Parkinson's disease
Pick bodies -    Pick's disease
Granulovacuole degeneration -  Alzheimer's disease
Hirano bodies -    Alzheimer's disease
Bunina bodies -    Amyotrophic lateral sclerosis (ALS)
Lewy bodies -    Parkinson's disease and diffuse Lewy body disease
Lafora bodies -    Lafora body disease (myoclonus epilepsy)

❑❑ **How common is cerebrovascular disease?**

It is the third leading cause of death in the United States.

❑❑ **What is a transient ischemic attack (TIA)?**

These are brief neurologic deficits that resolve fully and last no more than 24 hours.

❑❑ **What is the characteristic gross finding in the brain of a patient with a fat embolism?**

Classically, there are widespread petechiae found throughout the white matter.

❑❑ **What is Binswanger's disease?**

This is a rare cause of vascular dementia which is notable for diffuse or multifocal white matter degeneration. There is myelin loss/destruction with associated gliosis and scattered macrophages. The small vessel walls in the brain are thickened and hyalinized. This is also called subcortical arteriosclerotic leukoencephalopathy. It is thought to be a result of sustained hypertension.

❑❑ **What is a Charcot-Bouchard aneurysm?**

This is a fusiform segmental dilatation of a small arteriole in the brain as a result of the degenerative changes of the media that occurs in association with hypertension.

❑❑ **What are some common sites of hypertensive hemorrhage in the brain?**

Basal ganglia, subcortical white matter, cerebellum, and the basis pontis.

❑❑ **What is the most frequent cause of a spontaneous subarachnoid hemorrhage?**

Berry or sacular aneurysms.

❑❑ **What is a berry aneurysm?**

This an aneurysm that occurs in the circle of Willis at branch points of vessels.

❑❑ **Within the circle of Willis, are berry aneurysms more common in the anterior portion or the posterior portion of the circle?**

The anterior portion of the circle accounts for 90% of cases.

❏❏ **How commonly are berry aneurysms multiple rather than single lesions?**

Fairly frequently, up to 20% of cases.

❏❏ **Where is the most common location for atherosclerotic (fusiform) aneurysms in the brain?**

They typically effect the vertebrobasilar arteries and rarely rupture.

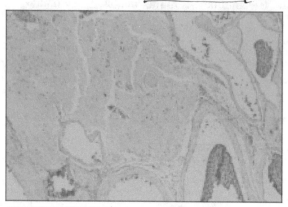

ARTERIOVENOUS MALFORMATION OF THE BRAIN

❏❏ **What is the most common location for an arteriovenous malformation (AVM) in the brain?**

They typically are found supratentorially and most commonly in the Sylvian fissure region supplied by the middle cerebral artery.

❏❏ **Does the presence of cerebral amyloid angiopathy (CAA) mean that the patient has systemic amyloidosis?**

No, CAA occurs independently and the patient may or may not have dementia or Alzheimer's disease.  It most commonly occurs in the frontal, parietal, and occipital lobes and is associated with cerebral hemorrhages.

❏❏ **What are the most common etiologic agents of bacterial meningitis?**

Neonatal (0-1 month)  Escherichia coli, Group B streptococci, Listeria monocytogenes
3 months - 6 years  Haemophilus influenzae, Streptococcus pneumoniae, Neisseria meningitidis
6 years - young adult  Neisseria meningitidis, Streptococcus pneumoniae
Older adults   Streptococcus pneumoniae

❏❏ **What is the most common mycosis that involves the CNS in patients with AIDS?**

Cryptococcus neoformans.

❏❏ **How does the ameba Nigleria fowleri result in meningoencephalitis?**

It is acquired while swimming in poorly sanitized pools or water containing the ameba. It reaches the CNS through the cribiform plate by traversing the olfactory nerves.

❏❏ **In a newborn that demonstrates convulsions, chorioretinitis, hydrocephalus and cerebral calcifications, what parasitic infection should one consider highly?**

Toxoplasma gondii.

❏❏  **What is the cause of cerebral cysticercosis?**

The larvae of the pork tapeworm, Taenia solium.

❏❏  **Which of the major Schistosoma species is known to sometimes involve the brain?**

S. japonicum, while S. mansoni and S. haematobium tend to involve the spinal cord.

❏❏  **Where specifically in the brain do the enteroviruses have an affinity for infecting?**

The large motor neurons of the anterior horns and the brain stem including the reticular formation.  In addition, neurons in the hypothalamus and posterior horns are also often involved.

❏❏  **What is the prognosis in symptomatic CNS involvement by rabies?**

It is nearly 100% fatal.

❏❏  **Sections of a brain demonstrate Negri bodies in Purkinje cells in hippocampal pyramidal neurons, what is your diagnosis?**

Rabies.

❏❏  **What virus tends to cause brain necrosis in an ependymal and subependymal distribution following intrauterine infection?**

Cytomegalovirus (CMV).

❏❏  **In an immunocompromised host, a severe meningoencephalitis develops with extensive cortical necrosis involving the medial temporal lobes.  What is your best diagnosis?**

Herpes simplex virus type I.

❏❏  **In general terms, what are the basic features of human immunodeficiency virus (HIV) meningoencephalitis?**

This is characterized by microglial nodules with multinucleated giant cells and, occasionally, areas of myelin pallor and gliosis.

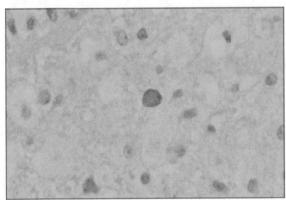

PROGRESSIVE MULTIFOCAL LEUKOENCEPHALOPATHY

❏❏  **What is the causative agent of progressive multifocal leukoencephalopathy (PML)?**

It occurs in immunocompromised patients and is caused by the JC strain of papova virus group B (see viral inclusion above).

**□□  What are the terms used to describe brain contusions at the site of direct impact and the site opposite of the direct impact?**

Coup and contrecoup, respectively.

**□□  What is the source of bleeding (arterial or venous) in epidural and subdural hemorrhages?**

Epidural - arterial usually in association with fracture of the thin squamous portion of the temporal bone
Subdural - arterial or venous, but more commonly the latter (bridging veins)

**□□  What type of injury or trauma results in diffuse axonal injury?**

This is a process which is related to acceleration or deceleration injury particularly during motor vehicle accidents or falls.  Actual impact is not necessary.  The shearing force of the injury results in tearing of small vessels and axons.

**□□  What is the most common cause of organic dementia?**

Alzheimer's disease (AD).

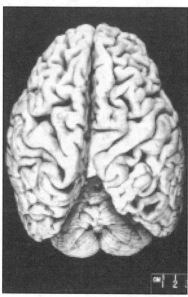

ALZHEIMER'S DISEASE WITH MARKED GYRAL ATROPHY

**□□  What are the characteristic gross findings of the brain in Alzheimer's disease?**

There is atrophy of the gyri and sulcal widening which may be most prominent in the frontal and temporal lobes.

**□□  What two microscopic features are the hallmarks of Alzheimer's disease?**

Neurofibrillary tangles and senile plaques.

**□□  What makes up the core of a mature senile plaque in AD?**

Amyloid.

**□□  What congenital disease is associated with an increased incidence of Alzheimer's disease?**

Down syndrome (trisomy 21).

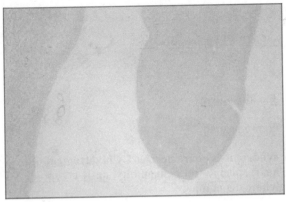

PICK'S DISEASE

❑❑  **What part of the brain is classically most severely affected by atrophy in Pick's disease?**

The frontal and anterior temporal regions imparting a so-called "knife-edge" gyral appearance which is demonstrated above in the low power photomicrograph.

❑❑  **What are Pick cells and Pick bodies?**

Pick cells are "ballooned" neurons with abundant cytoplasm and eccentric nuclei and Pick bodies are so named by virtue of the presence of intracytoplasmic blue globular inclusions.

❑❑  **Where is the gene located and what is the mode of inheritance of Huntington's disease?**

The gene is found on chromosome 4p and the condition is inherited in an autosomal dominant fashion with a high degree of penetrance.

❑❑  **What is the classical clinical triad of Huntington's disease?**

1. Emotional abnormalities
2. Chorea
3. Dementia

❑❑  **What are some of the clinical features of Parkinson's disease?**

Cogwheel rigidity, resting tremor ("pill rolling"), akinesia, and mask-like facies.

❑❑  **Describe the gross appearance of the substantia nigra and locus ceruleus in patients with Parkinson's disease.**

They are both hypopigmented secondary to loss of their pigmented neurons.

❑❑  **What is the name of the slightly enlarged, pale neurons with intracytoplasmic, eosinophilic, spherical inclusions that persist in Parkinson's disease?**

Lewy bodies.

❑❑  **How common is concomitant dementia in patients with Parkinson's disease?**

It is fairly common, occurring in up to 15% of patients, which is greater than one would expect in age matched controls.

❑❑  **What ocular abnormality would one expect to find in a patient with progressive supranuclear palsy?**

They have abnormal or impaired vertical eye motions.

□□  **In general terms, what is the pharmacotherapy for Parkinson's disease?**

Exogenous L-dopa.

□□  **What is the most common cause of secondary Parkinsonism?**

Extended use of antipsychotic medications (example, chlorpromazine).

□□  **What hereditary degenerative spinocerebellar syndrome is characterized by involvement of organ systems outside of the CNS, particularly the heart, peripheral neuropathy, optic atrophy, hearing loss and a fairly rapid progression to wheelchair dependency?**

Friedreich's ataxia.  It is usually inherited in an autosomal recessive fashion and the causative gene is on chromosome 9.

□□  **If a patient had paralysis with a Babinski sign and hyperactive deep tendon reflexes, would you expect the disease process to be involving the upper or lower motor neurons?**

Upper motor neurons.

□□  **What is Lou Gehrig's disease?**

It is the most common degenerative disease of motor neurons which is also called amyotrophic lateral sclerosis (ALS) and is characterized by upper and lower motor neuron signs.  It is slightly more common in males with an average age of 55.  Its course is fairly rapid and always fatal.  Most cases are sporadic although about 1 in 10 are inherited.

□□  **What is the typical appearance of an infant with Werdnig-Hoffmann disease?**

They present very soon after birth as "floppy babies".  They have diffuse muscle wasting and are said to assume a "frog leg" appearance.

□□  **What are some of the clinical features of progressive multifocal leukoencephalopathy?**

Hemiparesis, mental impairment, blindness, and aphasia.

□□  **What is tabes dorsalis?**

This is one of the forms of neurosyphilis which occurs approximately 10 years following infection in a minority of patients.  The posterior columns of the spinal cord are small and there is degeneration of axons and myelin in the dorsal roots.  This all results in a wide gait and ataxia with loss of deep tendon reflexes and vibratory sense.

□□  **What is the central nervous system equivalent of the peripheral nervous system's Schwann cell?**

Oligodendrocytes.

□□  **What are the hemorrhagic lesions found in association with transtentorial herniation which classically occur in the mid brain and pons ?**

Duret hemorrhages.

□□  **What is the most common site of intraparenchymal hemorrhage in the brain resulting from hypertension?**

The putamen accounts for up to 60% of cases.

❑❑ **In viral meningitis, what is the protein and glucose content in the CSF?**

The CSF typically exhibits a moderate elevation of protein and the sugar content is normal.

❑❑ **In bacterial meningitis, what is the protein and glucose content in the CSF?**

The protein level is elevated and there is a markedly diminished glucose content in the CSF.

❑❑ **In general, how does the location of primary pediatric CNS tumors differ from those in adults?**

Pediatric CNS neoplasms are generally infratentorial while in adults they tend to be supratentorial.

❑❑ **What are some of the histologic features which are used to help grade astrocytomas?**

Nuclear atypia, mitotic activity, endothelial proliferation, cellularity, and necrosis.

❑❑ **How common is evolution of gemistocytic astrocytomas into glioblastoma multiforme (GBM)?**

Very common, 8 out of 10 cases will evolve into GBM.

❑❑ **What feature is lacking in anaplastic astrocytoma (grade III) that would otherwise make it qualify for glioblastoma multiforme?**

Necrosis.

GLIOBLASTOMA MULTIFORME

❑❑ **What is the prognosis for glioblastoma multiforme like the one shown above?**

Dismal, the average survival rate is from 6 to 18 months.

❑❑ **List the most common tumors involving the brain in children.**

Astrocytomas, medulloblastoma, ependymoma, and craniopharyngioma - listed in decreasing order of frequency.

❑❑ **List the most common tumors involving the brain in adults.**

Metastatic lesions, astrocytomas, and meningiomas - listed in order of decreasing frequency.

❑❑ **What are some of the common secondary effects of CNS tumors?**

Edema, compression and compromise of vascular structures, compression of vital structures by tumor or resultant edema, herniation, obstruction of CSF, and papilledema.

❑❑ **What is the most common general location of pilocytic astrocytomas?**

They tend to occur in children/young adults and are found in the cerebellum and midline structures particularly the optic chiasm, the third ventricle, brain stem, and spinal cord. They also occasionally occur in the temporal lobes in young adults.

❑❑ **What is the prognosis for juvenile pilocytic astrocytoma?**

The prognosis is excellent with the majority of patients surviving greater than 20 years.

❑❑ **A 40-year-old male presents with a history of seizures and is found to have a tumor in the deep white matter with a "fried egg" appearance and a "chicken wire" vascular pattern. What is the diagnosis?**

Oligodendroglioma.

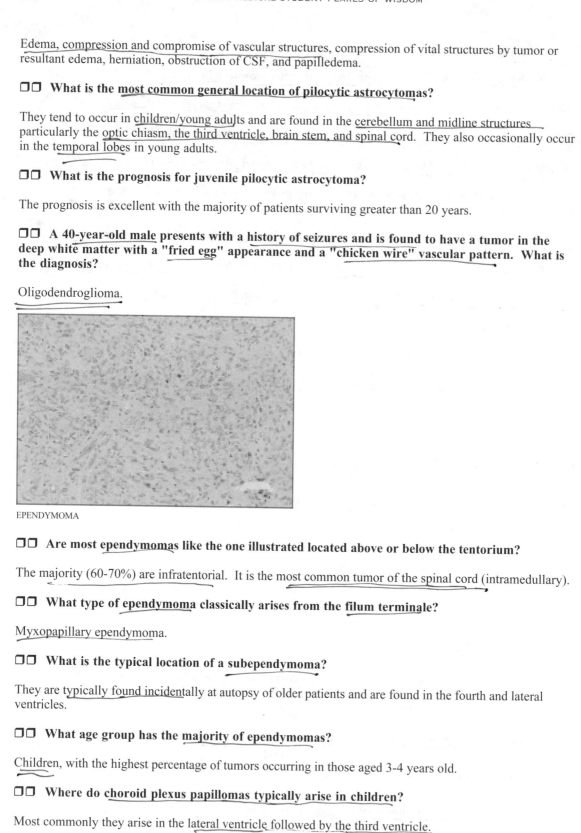

EPENDYMOMA

❑❑ **Are most ependymomas like the one illustrated located above or below the tentorium?**

The majority (60-70%) are infratentorial. It is the most common tumor of the spinal cord (intramedullary).

❑❑ **What type of ependymoma classically arises from the filum terminale?**

Myxopapillary ependymoma.

❑❑ **What is the typical location of a subependymoma?**

They are typically found incidentally at autopsy of older patients and are found in the fourth and lateral ventricles.

❑❑ **What age group has the majority of ependymomas?**

Children, with the highest percentage of tumors occurring in those aged 3-4 years old.

❑❑ **Where do choroid plexus papillomas typically arise in children?**

Most commonly they arise in the lateral ventricle followed by the third ventricle.

❑❑ **Where do choroid plexus papillomas typically arise in adults?**

Fourth ventricle.

❑❑  **What is the most common clinical manifestation of a choroid plexus papilloma?**

Most patients present with hydrocephalus either due to obstruction or overproduction of cerebrospinal fluid by the tumor.

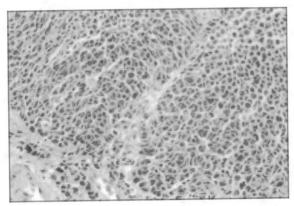

MEDULLOBLASTOMA

❑❑  **What is the typical age of presentation for the medulloblastoma depicted above?**

It has a bimodal peak at around age 10 (most common) and 20.  It is second to cerebellar astrocytomas in frequency for pediatric intracranial primary brain tumors.

❑❑  **What is the classic site of origin of the medulloblastoma?**

Vermis.

❑❑  **What is the typical age of presentation of esthesioneuroblastomas (olfactory neuroblastomas)?**

The age distribution is bimodal with peaks occurring at age 20 and 50.

❑❑  **What is the typical age of occurrence of pineoblastomas?**

They tend to occur in children and young adults.

❑❑  **What is the prognosis for pineoblastomas?**

Although they are extremely sensitive to radiation therapy, they tend to recur and can spread via the subarachnoid space resulting in a poor prognosis overall.

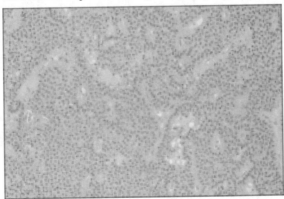

PITUITARY ADENOMA

❑❑ **What are the two most common tumors involving the sellar region in adults?**

Pituitary adenomas (see above) and meningiomas.

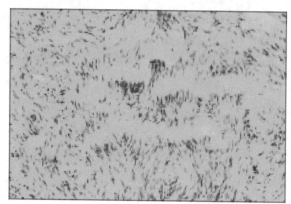

BRAIN TUMOR INVOLVING THE CEREBELLOPONTINE ANGLE

❑❑ **An adult male presents with acute unilateral hearing loss and a mass at the cerebellopontine angle. Based on the histology (above) and history, what is your diagnosis?**

Schwannoma.

❑❑ **What is the most common intramedullary tumor of the spinal cord in children?**

Astrocytoma.

❑❑ **Do spinal meningiomas have a gender preference?**

Yes, or I would not have asked. They are 10 times more common in women.

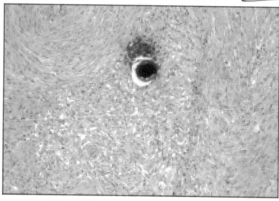

DURAL BASED TUMOR

❑❑ **A patient presents with a dural mass over the frontoparietal lobe on the right. The mass is resected and demonstrates the above histology including cells arranged in whorls and extensive psammoma bodies. What is your diagnosis?**

Meningioma.

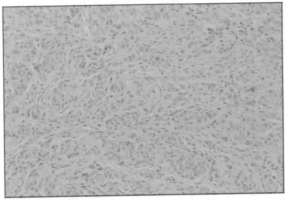

DURAL BASED TUMOR

❏❏  This neoplasm was discovered arising from the dura in a middle-aged male and in other tissue sections demonstrated "pseudopsammoma bodies".  What is your diagnosis?

Meningioma, specifically a secretory meningioma.

❏❏  What disease condition is associated with multiple hemangioblastomas?

von Hippel-Lindau disease.

❏❏  What is the chromosome and inheritance pattern of von Hippel-Lindau disease?

Chromosome 3, autosomal dominant.

❏❏  What are the other components of von Hippel-Lindau disease?

In addition to hemangioblastomas, these patients have renal, hepatic and pancreatic cysts, pheochromocytomas, and renal cell carcinomas.

❏❏  What immunoperoxidase stain is strongly positive in schwannomas and typically completely negative or only focally positive in a minority of meningiomas?

S-100 protein.

❏❏  What is the basic immunophenotype (B or T cell) of most CNS lymphomas?

B-cell type.

❏❏  What is the most common primary CNS neoplasm in immunocompromised patients?

Lymphoma.

❏❏  What tumor of the sella turcica may be solid or cystic, may be a remnant of Rathke's duct, and most commonly occurs in children?

Craniopharyngioma.

❏❏  Compare the cyst fluid found in Rathke cleft cysts and craniopharyngiomas.

Remember, the fluid in craniopharyngiomas is said to have a "motor-oil" look and feel while Rathke cysts contain a pearly-white fluid.

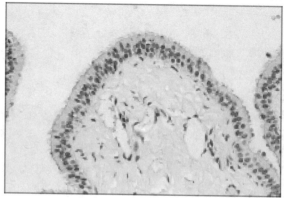

COLLOID CYST

❐❐  **Where was this colloid cyst most likely located in the brain?**

The anterior roof of the third ventricle is the most frequent location as a result of abnormally placed endoderm.

❐❐  **What is the most common location of a chordoma?**

The clivus followed by the lumbosacral spine.

❐❐  **What congenital CNS abnormality is seen in about two thirds of cases of Patau's syndrome (trisomy 13)?**

Holoprosencephaly.

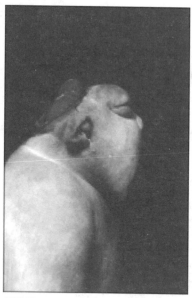

ANENCEPHALY

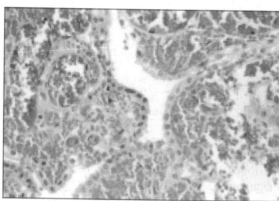

AREA CEREBROVASCULOSA

❑❑ What is the term given to describe this vascular, disorganized tissue which is often found on the base of the skull in patients with anencephaly?

Area cerebrovasculosa.

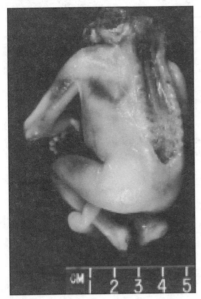

NEURAL TUBE DEFECT

❑❑ What is the name of the condition shown above whereby the neural tube defect extends the entire length of the spinal column?

Craniorachischisis.

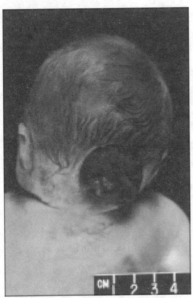

POSTERIOR SKULL DEFECT

❑❑ What is the name of the condition shown above?

Occipital encephalocele.

□□ **What is the difference between communicating and noncommunicating hydrocephalus?**

As the terms imply, noncommunicating refers to a partial or complete obstruction of the flow of CSF with dilatation of the proximal ventricular system. Communicating hydrocephalus, on the other hand, shows no such lack of "communication" and is generally a defect of either overproduction by the choroid plexus or resorption by the arachnoid granulations.

□□ **What is the Arnold-Chiari malformation?**

There are three types but, in general, it refers to the downward displacement of the cerebellum and medulla into the cervical vertebral canal. It is often seen in association with lumbar spina bifida and hydrocephalus owing to the imposed stenosis of the aqueduct.

□□ **Which specific type of Arnold-Chiari malformation is characterized by an occipital bony defect through which the cerebellum herniates (posterior encephalocele)?**

Type III.

□□ **What is the most common neural tube defect overall?**

Spina bifida.

□□ **What is the term used to describe the congenital herniation of the spinal arachnoid and dura through a vertebral defect?**

Meningocele.

□□ **What is the term used to describe the congenital abnormality whereby a portion of the spinal cord or a spinal root is included with the arachnoid and dura herniation through the vertebral defect?**

Meningomyelocele.

□□ **What is the Dandy-Walker malformation?**

This is a congenital abnormality whereby the vermis is hypoplastic, there is cystic dilatation of the fourth ventricle, and upward displacement of the tentorium with enlargement of the posterior fossa.

□□ **What is the term used to describe the congenital abnormality whereby there is incomplete separation of the cerebral hemispheres?**

Holoprosencephaly.

□□ **What is the term used to describe the congenital absence of the surface gyri and sulci?**

Agyria (lissencephaly).

□□ **A patient presents to you with bilateral acoustic neuromas (schwannomas), what is your suspected diagnosis?**

Neurofibromatosis 2.

□□ **Where is the gene locus found for neurofibromatosis 2?**

Chromosome 22q12.

□□ **In addition to neurofibromas and schwannomas, what other CNS tumors are patients with neurofibromatosis 2 prone to develop?**

Pilocytic astrocytomas of the third ventricle, optic gliomas, ependymomas, and glioblastoma multiforme.

❏❏ **A patient presents to you with cortical tubers, subependymal nodules, and retinal hamartomas (phakomas). What is your diagnosis?** *"Candle drippings"*

Tuberous sclerosis.

❏❏ **What are the typical skin lesions found in patients with tuberous sclerosis?**

They get pale macules, angiofibromas of the face, shagreen patches, and subungual fibromas.

❏❏ **What is the most likely diagnosis of a patient who presents with so-called port-wine angiomas which follow the distribution of the sensory trigeminal nerve?**

Sturge-Weber syndrome.

❏❏ **Are there HLA haplotypes that are associated with multiple sclerosis (MS)?**

Yes, these include HLA A3, B7, D2, Dw2, and Drw2.

❏❏ **What are some of the sites of involvement of MS lesions?**

Optic nerves and chiasm, basis pontis, and periventricular white matter.

❏❏ **What is the inheritance pattern of adrenoleukodystrophy?**

X-linked.

❏❏ **What is the most likely pathogenesis of central pontine myelinolysis?**

It is likely the result of rapid correction of serum osmolality.

❏❏ **What is Wernicke's encephalopathy?**

This is found in chronic alcoholics as a result of thiamine (vitamin B1) deficiency and is characterized by confusion, ataxia, and visual changes.

❏❏ **What structure in the brain is typically involved by the hemorrhage and necrosis seen in Wernicke's encephalopathy and is believed to be responsible for the amnesia seen in Wernicke-Korsakoff syndrome?**

The mammillary bodies and the medial dorsal nucleus of the thalamus.

❏❏ **What are some of the clinical and pathologic characteristics of Zellweger syndrome (cerebrohepatorenal syndrome)?**

This is a peroxisomal disorder which is characterized by dysmorphic facies and pronounced hypotonia with seizures which develop as an infant. There is polymicrogyria and pachygyria in association with hepatic fibrosis, renal cysts and adrenocortical striated cells.

❏❏ **What is your diagnosis in a 19-year-old male who presents with extrapyramidal signs, hepatic failure, Kayser-Fleischer rings, spongiosis, and necrosis in the brain?**

Wilson's disease (hepatolenticular degeneration).

❏❏ **What is the name of the X-linked disorder of copper metabolism which occurs as a result of abnormal gastrointestinal tract absorption of copper and abnormal mitochondrial function?**

Menkes' or kinky hair disease.

❑❑  **What protein is used in the screening of maternal serum and is elevated in neural tube defects?**

Alpha-fetoprotein.

❑❑  **What is the risk of rupture of a berry aneurysm measuring 1 cm or more in diameter?**

There is a 50% risk of rupture per year.

❑❑  **What is the characteristic, general feature histologically in Creutzfeldt-Jakob disease (CJD)?**

It is part of a spectrum of diseases called spongiform encephalopathies which, as the term implies, are characterized by a spongiform change as a result of intracellular vacuoles.

❑❑  **What substance accumulates in the neural tissue of patients with CJD and appears to be the cause of the pathology?**

Prion protein which has assumed an abnormal beta pleated sheet isoform (PrPsc).

❑❑  **What is the prognosis for CJD?**

It is typically fatal within about 6 months. It is characterized by a very rapid progression from subtle memory loss to profound dementia and death.

❑❑  **What does one typically find on electrophoresis of the CSF of patients with multiple sclerosis?**

Most MS patients have oligoclonal bands in their CSF and an increased portion of gamma globulin with a mild protein elevation overall.

❑❑  **Describe the typical clinical presentation of progressive supranuclear palsy.**

It most commonly affects males (2:1) in their 40s to 60s. They develop truncal rigidity with dysequilibrium, nuchal dystonia, ocular abnormalities (vertical gaze palsy), mild dementia, abnormal speech, and pseudobulbar palsy. These patients are dead typically within 7 years of onset of symptoms.

❑❑  **What syndrome is characterized by degeneration of neurons in the intermediolateral column of the spinal cord and a combination of extrapyramidal, autonomic system dysfunction, and parkinsonism?**

Shy-Drager syndrome.

❑❑  **What vitamin deficiency is associated with the combined degenerative changes of the ascending and descending tracts of the spinal cord?**

Vitamin B12.

# PERIPHERAL NERVOUS SYSTEM AND MUSCLES

▢▢ **What are some conditions which are characterized by peripheral neuropathy with a predominant motor component?**

Guillain-Barre syndrome, lead neuropathy, and porphyria among others.

▢▢ **What are some causes of a subacute sensorimotor neuropathy?**

When symmetric causes include vitamin deficiency, alcoholism, toxic damage, and paraneoplastic neuropathy. When asymmetric, diabetes, vasculitis, and sarcoid are all considerations.

▢▢ **What is Charcot-Marie-Tooth disease (CMT)?**

This is a slowly progressive hereditary peripheral neuropathy which often presents with symmetric muscular atrophy of the calves. There are both the motor symptoms as described and sensory deficits. There is a type I and type II.

▢▢ **What is the characteristic finding in the peripheral nerves of patients with Charcot-Marie-Tooth type I?**

They get "hypertrophic" peripheral nerves with onion bulb formation indicative of multiple demyelination and remyelination episodes.

▢▢ **How is Charcot-Marie-Tooth type I inherited?**

Autosomal dominant.

▢▢ **How does the conduction velocity differ in patients with Charcot-Marie-Tooth type I and type II?**

In type I, the velocity is decreased while in type II it is usually normal.

▢▢ **What would you expect to see histologically in type II Charcot-Marie-Tooth disease?**

There is loss of both small and large myelinated axons, and onion bulb formation is absent or not frequent.

▢▢ **What hereditary motor and sensory neuropathy is characterized by onset between the ages of 5 and 15, palpably enlarged peripheral nerves, clubfoot, kyphoscoliosis, and muscular atrophy?**

Dejerine-Sottas disease (hereditary motor and sensory neuropathy type III).

▢▢ **How is Dejerine-Sottas disease inherited?**

Autosomal recessive.

▢▢ **What hereditary neuropathy is characterized by the presence of pigmentary retinopathy, cerebellar ataxia, elevated serum phytanic acid, and onion bulb change histologically?**

Refsum disease (HMSN type IV).

❒❒  **What is the natural course of neuroaxonal dystrophy?**

These children are normal at birth and early life; however, they become symptomatic by age 2 and progress to death in childhood.

❒❒  **What hereditary neuropathy (autosomal dominant) has characteristic bulbous fusiform areas of thickened myelin, segmental demyelination and Schwann cell hyperplasia with diffuse slowing on nerve conduction studies?**

Tomaculous neuropathy.

❒❒  **Where is the amyloid deposited in hereditary amyloid neuropathy?**

It is found within the endoneurial space and in the walls of blood vessels in the endoneurium.

❒❒  **What is the typical course of disease in hereditary amyloid neuropathy?**

It exhibits a progressive course with impairment of pain, temperature, touch, and vibratory sensation. In addition, there are gastrointestinal symptoms including nausea, vomiting, and incontinence. Death typically occurs within 10 years although liver transplantation has resulted in clinical improvement.

❒❒  **What are some common characteristics of vasculitic neuropathy?**

Ischemic injury to peripheral nerves, asymmetric neuropathy, acute onset with rapid progression, clinical improvement with steroids or other immunosuppressants and, of course, vasculitis.

❒❒  **In arsenic toxicity, which is more pronounced - motor or sensory impairment?**

Sensory with the potential for distal muscle weakness to occur.

❒❒  **What vitamin deficiency results in neuropathic beri beri?**

Vitamin B1 (thiamine).

❒❒  **Name some vitamin deficiencies which can result in axonal neuropathies.**

Vitamin B1 (thiamine), B6 (pyridoxine), B12 (cobalamin) and E (alpha-tocopherol).

❒❒  **How common is peripheral neuropathy in longstanding diabetes?**

It is present in about half of patients with diabetes of 25 years or greater duration.

❒❒  **What are some of the forms of neuropathy which occur in patients with diabetes mellitus?**

1. Symmetric sensorimotor neuropathy - most common, distal, symmetric, sensory and motor
2. Asymmetric sensorimotor neuropathy - asymmetric, subacute, worse at night, older patients
3. Autonomic neuropathy - symmetric, usually associated with sensory deficits as well
4. Mononeuropathy - third cranial nerve commonly involved

❒❒  **In general terms, what are two processes which may cause diabetic neuropathy secondary to hyperglycemia?**

1. Increased expression of aldose reductase (increased sorbitol)
2. Nonenzymatic glycation of proteins

❒❒  **Can one develop a peripheral neuropathy in the setting of uremia?**

Of course, that was a leading question. Some 60% of patients with chronic renal failure will manifest symptoms of uremic neuropathy when dialysis is initiated.

❑❑ **What ganlion serves as a common site of latency for herpes simplex virus type I?**

Trigeminal ganglion.

❑❑ **Describe the characteristic nerve involvement in the tuberculoid form of leprosy?**

Well-formed granulomas involving nerves are the characteristic lesions.

❑❑ **Of the four neuropathies found in AIDS, which is the most common?**

A distal symmetric axonal neuropathy is most common. A cauda equina syndrome caused by CMV also occurs, as does a vasculitic neuropathy and a demyelinating peripheral neuropathy (similar to Guillain-Barre).

❑❑ **What are the two basic types of paraneoplastic neuropathies and which is more common?**

Sensory and sensorimotor, with the latter being more common. Each is most commonly associated with lung carcinoma and may have something to do with antibodies to the circulating tumor antigen Hu.

❑❑ **What is a common preceding event in patients that develop acute inflammatory demyelinating polyradiculoneuropathy (Guillain-Barre syndrome)?**

Most patients report a typical antecedent viral illness prior to the neuropathic symptoms. Demyelination, most notably in spinal roots, is the characteristic feature.

❑❑ **What is the natural course of Guillain-Barre syndrome?**

Reliance on a ventilator secondary to respiratory paralysis is a not uncommon feature. In spite of that, more than 95% of patients survive typically with a complete recovery. Less than 20% have residual neurologic deficits.

❑❑ **What is the most common tumor of peripheral nerves?**

Schwannoma.

❑❑ **What syndrome is characterized by multiple meningiomas and bilateral acoustic schwannomas?**

Type II neurofibromatosis (NF2), autosomal dominant.

❑❑  What is the term given to describe the cellular, compact areas and the loose myxomatous areas in Schwannomas?

Antoni A and Antoni B, respectively.

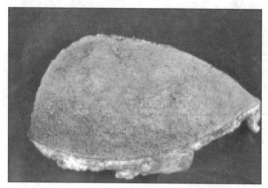

SKIN SURFACE WITH DARK PIGMENTATION

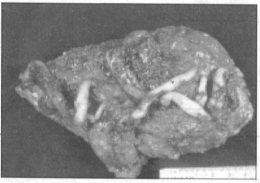

DEEP SURFACE WITH ROPE-LIKE NERVES

❑❑  Based on the resection specimen shown above, what is your diagnosis of this patient?

The photo depicts extensive plexiform neurofibromas in a patient with type I neurofibromatosis (von Recklinghausen's disease).

❑❑  What is the inheritance pattern in neurofibromatosis type I?

Autosomal dominant with a mutation on a tumor suppressor gene on chromosome 17.

❑❑  In a 20-year-old patient with a malignant peripheral nerve sheath tumor (MPNST), what should you suspect as an associated diagnosis?

Young patients with MPNST typically develop the tumor in a preexisting neurofibroma and have neurofibromatosis type I.

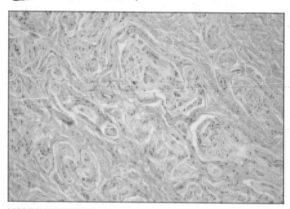

MORTON'S NEUROMA (TRAUMATIC NEUROMA)

❑❑  What is the typical location for a Morton's neuroma such as the one shown above?

This is enlargement and perineural fibrosis of an interdigital plantar nerve.

❑❑  What is the most common cause of selective type I fiber atrophy?

Myotonic dystrophy.

❑❑  What is the most common cause of type II fiber atrophy?

Corticosteroid therapy.

❏❏  **What type of muscle fiber atrophy is seen in myasthenia gravis?**

Type II.

❏❏  **What is the most common of the muscular dystrophies?**

Duchenne muscular dystrophy (DMD).

❏❏  **Where is the gene for DMD located?**

Chromosome Xp21.

❏❏  **What is the product of the DMD gene?**

Dystrophin which is a lattice-like protein for the myocyte.

❏❏  **What is the typical disease course in DMD?**

It typically becomes evident by age 5 with progressive weakness leading to wheelchair dependence and death by the third decade.  Remember, the classic pseudohypertrophy of the calf muscles occurs in association with simultaneous calf muscle weakness.

❏❏  **How does Becker's muscular dystrophy differ in its clinical course from DMD?**

It occurs later, is less severe and progresses slower than DMD.

❏❏  **What is the typical inheritance pattern in most limb-girdle dystrophies?**

Autosomal recessive.

❏❏  **What is the most common muscular dystrophy in adults?**

Myotonic muscular dystrophy (MyD).

❏❏  **Where is the gene found for MyD?**

19q13.2-13.3, inheritance is autosomal dominant.

❏❏  **What are some typical systemic signs and symptoms of MyD?**

Cataracts, hyperinsulinism, cardiomyopathy, dementia, and atrophic testes.

❏❏  **What are the most prevalent etiologic agents of parasitic-related myopathies in North America?**

Toxoplasmosis, trichinosis, and cysticercosis.

❏❏  **What is the most common parasite found in skeletal muscle?**

Trichinella spiralis.

❏❏  **How does polymyositis differ from dermatomyositis in clinical presentation?**

Polymyositis simply lacks any of the cutaneous manifestations that are seen in dermatomyositis and occurs predominantly in adults.

322    PATHOLOGY MEDICAL STUDENT PEARLS OF WISDOM

❏❏ **Which muscle groups (proximal or distal) are more markedly effected in polymyositis?**

Proximal, although the clinical weakness is generalized.

❏❏ **In addition to generalized weakness, what other clinical manifestations are seen in polymyositis?**

More than two thirds of the patients develop interstitial lung disease (30% in dermatomyositis) and there is a slight increase in incidence of development of visceral cancers.

❏❏ **What is typically the first manifestation in patients with dermatomyositis?**

95% of patients develop a skin rash of varying patterns as the first symptom of disease.

❏❏ **Can there be a vasculitic component in dermatomyositis?**

You guessed it, yes. This is seen in many of the childhood cases.

❏❏ **What would you expect to see on immunofluorescence in polymyositis versus dermatomyositis?**

Immune deposits are typically absent in polymyositis while they are typically seen in dermatomyositis (IgG and IgM).

❏❏ **Of the main inflammatory myopathies, which is characterized by a distal muscle weakness as opposed to proximal?**

Inclusion body myositis (IBM).

❏❏ **What is the typical age and presentation of a patient with IBM?**

It is more common in males in contrast to polymyositis and dermatomyositis, age 50-70. Although indolent, it is progressive and resistant to steroids. Painless, asymmetric, generalized weakness which is more prominent distally, and normal serum CK are the characteristic findings.

❏❏ **Describe the typical clinical presentation of a patient with drug-induced myositis.**

They typically present with a mild muscular weakness in the absence of pain. The serum CK is only mildly elevated and muscle biopsy demonstrates a perivascular infiltrate with numerous eosinophils and minimal or absent muscle fiber necrosis.

❏❏ **What is the characteristic histologic finding in the muscles of patients with branching enzyme deficiency (type IV glycogenosis)?**

They demonstrate deposits of polysaccharide (polyglucosan bodies) that are often found at the periphery of the myofibers.

❏❏ **A patient presents with complaints of exercise intolerance which first became manifest in childhood. A muscle biopsy shows small, subsarcolemmal vacuoles and a lack of myophosphorylase with special stains. What is your diagnosis?**

Type V glycogenosis or myophosphorylase deficiency (McArdle's disease).

❏❏ **What is the basic histologic finding in muscle biopsy specimens from patients with carnitine deficiency?**

They have increased lipid droplets in the type I myofibers and, to a lesser degree, in the type II myofibers.

❏❏ **What is the most common metabolic cause of myoglobinuria in adults?**

Carnitine palmitoyltransferase deficiency.

❏❏ **Is there a gender preference for carnitine palmitoyltransferase deficiency?**

Yes, it is much more common in men.

❏❏ **What is the term used to describe the appearance of type I myofibers histologically in a mitochondrial myopathy?**

"Ragged-red" fibers.

❏❏ **What is the characteristic clinical finding in alcoholic neuropathy?**

There is a pronounced sensory loss with sparing of the motor nerves.

❏❏ **In Duchenne muscular dystrophy, when do the symptoms become most prominent?**

At about the time the child begins to walk, it becomes evident that he is weak and frequently falls. Early, the pelvic girdle is the main muscle group involved although eventually all muscles become involved.

❏❏ **What are some of the clinical manifestations of Kearns-Sayre syndrome?**

This mitochondrial myopathy is manifested by external ophthalmoplegia, ataxia, peripheral neuropathy, retinal degeneration, increased CSF protein, short stature, and hearing impairment. The manifestations are typically apparent by age 20 and death can result secondary to cardiac conduction abnormalities.

❏❏ **What are the main clinical signs/symptoms of Batten's disease?**

Batten's disease (neuronal ceroid lipofuscinoses) is divided into four types depending on the age of onset - infantile, late infantile, juvenile, and adult. The main manifestations include mental retardation, seizure activity, and sight impairment. The pathology rests in the accumulation of lipopigments in a variety of tissues.

❏❏ **What are some of the clinical manifestations of malignant hyperthermia?**

A rapid and pronounced elevation in body temperature, tachycardia with associated arrhythmias, rhabdomyolysis, and muscle rigidity.

❏❏ **What are some drugs that have been associated with development of toxic myopathies?**

Ethanol, chloroquine, colchicine, zidovudine, steroids, and several others.

❏❏ **What is the basic mechanism behind the pathology of myasthenia gravis (MG)?**

These patients have circulating antibodies against the postsynaptic acetylcholine receptor protein (AChR) at the motor end plate. In particular, there appears to be a specificity in many cases for the AChR which contains the gamma subunit.

❏❏ **Describe the typical patient and presentation in myasthenia gravis?**

This occurs more commonly in adult females younger than 40. They typically complain of facial and extraocular muscle weakness including development of "double vision". They also suffer from increasing weakness and fatigue throughout the day.

❏❏ **What specific tumor is associated with myasthenia gravis?**

Up to 15% of patients have a thymoma and the vast majority have thymic hyperplasia.

☐☐ **How does Lambert-Eaton myasthenic syndrome (LE) differ from myasthenia gravis?**

LE is characterized by proximal muscle weakness rather than the face and eye weakness seen in MG. In addition, LE is very commonly associated with an underlying malignancy, most commonly small cell carcinoma of the lung. LE also is notable for associated autonomic dysfunction and they do not show the lack of acetylcholine receptors seen in MG, rather they release fewer vesicles at the synapse.

☐☐ **In a muscle biopsy that shows "target fibers", what is the best diagnosis?**

Chronic denervation.

☐☐ **When a muscle biopsy demonstrates grouping of the fiber types rather than the usual "checkerboard" staining pattern, what does that typically indicate?**

Denervation with reinnervation.

# BONE, SOFT TISSUE, AND JOINTS

❑❑ **What cell lines the surface of bone and is responsible for initiating mineralization?**

Osteoblast.

❑❑ **What cell is typically multinucleated and is responsible for resorption of bone?**

Osteoclast.

❑❑ **What is the connective tissue which covers the surface of the bone?**

Periosteum.

❑❑ **What is the name of the cell which is surrounded by and embedded in the bone?**

Osteocytes.

❑❑ **What are the two forms of ossification or bone development?**

1. Long bones exhibit endochondral ossification whereby a cartilaginous cap is replaced by bone.
2. Intramembranous ossification occurs in flat bones whereby there is no cartilaginous intermediary.

❑❑ **What are the two basic types of bone?**

Woven (random) and lamellar (layered).

❑❑ **Where is woven bone normally found in the adult skeleton?**

It's not. In the fetus, it is found at growth plates; however, it is pathologic in adults and formed in many conditions including fractures and infection.

❑❑ **Which is stronger, woven or lamellar bone?**

Lamellar.

❑❑ **What cell acts as one of the main mediators of the activity of osteoclasts?**

Osteoblasts. In fact, many of the cytokines responsible for regulation and stimulation of bone resorption (IL-1 and TNF) act on osteoblasts and not osteoclasts.

❑❑ **What is the inheritance pattern of achondroplasia?**

Autosomal dominant, with some 80% of cases representing new mutations.

❑❑ **What is the name of the gene which is mutated in achondroplasia?**

There is a mutation (usually arginine for glycine at position 375) in the gene that codes for FGF receptor 3. Thus, there is constant activation at the growth plate which allows for cartilage proliferation.

❑❑  **Describe the prognosis in achondroplasia.**

These patients have no significant alteration in life span.

❑❑  **What type of collagen is deficient in osteogenesis imperfecta?**

Type I collagen.

❑❑  **What is the prognosis of type II osteogenesis imperfecta?**

It is lethal in utero.

❑❑  **What are some of the other characteristic clinical manifestations in patients with type I osteogenesis imperfecta?**

They classically have blue sclerae, a combined sensorineural and conductive hearing loss, lax joints, and abnormal dentition.

❑❑  **What is the term which depicts an age-related loss in bone mass?**

Osteoporosis.

❑❑  **Does age-related bone loss occur at a greater rate in men or women?**

The greater incidence of symptomatic osteoporosis in females is likely related to a lower peak bone mass compared to men.  Both sexes exhibit a similar rate of bone loss; however, men start with greater bone density.

❑❑  **What effect does exercise have on osteoporosis?**

Exercise, particularly resistance type, helps maintain bone mass.

❑❑  **What effect does menopause have on osteoporosis?**

Following menopause, women have an accelerated loss of bone which is related to deficient estrogen. Thus, replacement of estrogen after menopause is protective against bone loss.

❑❑  **What is osteopetrosis?**

This is a congenital disease which is characterized by osteoclast dysfunction in which the bones become extremely dense, although brittle, nearly obliterating the narrow space.

❑❑  **What are the two main forms of osteopetrosis?**

There is a so-called benign form which is inherited in an autosomal dominant manner and a so-called malignant form which is inherited in an autosomal recessive fashion.

❑❑  **What is the typical course of disease in patients with the "malignant" form of osteopetrosis?**

They present at birth with significant problems related to fractures, anemia, hydrocephaly, and recurrent infections.  The dense bone literally replaces the medullary cavity forcing them to rely on extramedullary hematopoiesis resulting in profound hepatosplenomegaly.  They typically die at a young age.

❑❑  **What is the typical clinical course in patients with the benign form of osteopetrosis?**

They typically present in adolescence with multiple fractures.  They have milder degrees of anemia and some cranial nerve deficits.

**❑❑ What is the prognosis of thanatophoric dysplasia?**

This is the most common lethal form of dwarfism that shares a common general site of mutation (FGFR3) with achondroplasia; however, these patients have an underdeveloped thoracic cavity as well as multiple other bony abnormalities and die either at birth or very soon after.

**❑❑ What virus has been proposed as a possible etiologic agent of Paget's disease?**

Paramyxovirus.

**❑❑ What is the pathognomonic histologic appearance of bone in Paget's disease?**

The hallmark is a mosaic pattern of lamellar bone which may impart a "jigsaw puzzle" appearance.

**❑❑ What are the three basic phases of Paget's disease?**

In order of occurrence:

1. osteolytic
2. mixed osteoclastic-osteoblastic
3. quiescent osteosclerotic

**❑❑ Does Paget's disease typically effect a single bone or multiple bones?**

85% of cases have multiple bone involvement (polyostotic). 80% of the cases include the axial skeleton or proximal femur.

**❑❑ What is the most common clinical manifestation of Paget's disease?**

Pain.

**❑❑ What are some other signs/symptoms which occur during the course of Paget's disease?**

They can develop extensive bone overgrowth particularly in the craniofacial skeleton, pronounced secondary osteoarthritis secondary to weakened, weightbearing bones, fractures of the long bones, compression fractures, and high-output heart failure.

**❑❑ What are some of the tumor associations with Paget's disease?**

Sarcomas (including osteosarcoma) develop in up to 10% of patients that have marked polyostotic disease. Many benign conditions including giant cell tumor and giant cell reparative granuloma also occur.

**❑❑ What are some of the general categories which predispose to development of rickets (children) or osteomalacia (adults)?**

Inadequate synthesis/dietary deficiency of vitamin D, decreased absorption of vitamin D, abnormal vitamin D metabolism, end-organ resistance to active vitamin D, and phosphate depletion.

**❑❑ What are some of the morphologic changes seen in rickets?**

Frontal bossing, squared head, prominent costochondral junctions, pigeon breast deformity, lumbar lordosis, and prominent bowing of the legs.

**❑❑ What are some of the common morphologic features seen in osteomalacia (deficient vitamin D in adults)?**

Morphologically, the adults appear normal as the abnormality occurs following cessation of bone growth. These patients develop fractures as the bones are weak.

❑❑  **What is the morphologic manifestation of severe hyperparathyroidism, which is now rarely seen, but is characteristic radiographically?**

Osteitis fibrosa cystica.

❑❑  **What are some of the typical manifestations in the bone of vitamin C deficiency?**

As it is denoted by capillary fragility, there are characteristic hemorrhages in the periosteum as well as the gums and skin.  The osteoblasts appear abnormal and there is a diminished trabecular bone mass.

❑❑  **What are the changes seen in the bone secondary to vitamin A deficiency?**

This deficiency results in cessation of bony remodeling and osteoclast activity.  Subsequently, the bones are short and thick.

❑❑  **What effect does hypervitaminosis A have on the long bones of children?**

It results in premature closure of the epiphyses.

❑❑  **In general terms, how does chronic renal failure result in skeletal changes (renal osteodystrophy)?**

Phosphate retention occurs which induces secondary hyperparathyroidism. Hypocalcemia occurs secondary to decreased conversion to the active vitamin D (1,25-dihydroxyvitamin D3) in the damaged kidneys. This furthers the secondary hyperparathyroidism resulting in increased activity of osteoclasts.

❑❑  **What is a compound fracture?**

This is the fracture of a bone in which the bone breeches the skin's surface.

❑❑  **What is a comminuted fracture?**

This is a crushing or splintering fracture of the bone into multiple pieces.

❑❑  **What is the term given to describe the tissue reaction to a bony fracture by the end of seven days which is composed of an organizing hematoma and granulation tissue amidst the fractured ends of the bones?**

Soft tissue callus or procallus.

❑❑  **What are some of the causes of avascular necrosis?**

Fracture, chronic steroid use, thrombosis, vasculitis, venous hypertension, hyperuricemia, Gaucher's disease, SLE, alcoholism, and trauma.

❑❑  **How common is avascular necrosis?**

It accounts for about 10% of the joint replacement surgeries performed in the United States.

❑❑  **Which joint is most commonly effected in avascular necrosis?**

It most commonly occurs in the head of the femur in men.

❑❑  **What is the method of spread in most cases of osteomyelitis?**

Most are hematogenous and occur in the vertebra or long bones.

❑❑  **What is the most commonly recovered organism causing osteomyelitis?**

Staphylococcus aureus.

❑❑  **What particular organism is a frequent cause of osteomyelitis in patients with sickle cell disease?**

Salmonella.

❑❑  **What is the term given to describe a subperiosteal abscess which progresses, disrupts the blood supply and results in segmental bone necrosis in osteomyelitis?**

Sequesterum.

❑❑  **What is Pott's disease?**

This is tuberculous osteomyelitis of the spine.

❑❑  **What bones are most frequently effected in skeletal syphilis?**

Nose, palate, skull, and the long bones.

❑❑  **What is the typical location in the bone for chondroblastoma and giant cell tumors?**

Epiphysis of long bones.

❑❑  **What are some conditions which are associated with an increased incidence of bone tumors?**

Bone infarcts, chronic osteomyelitis, Paget's disease, radiation, metal prostheses, Li-Fraumani syndrome, and many others.

❑❑  **What is the risk of transformation of an osteoma into an osteosarcoma?**

None, this does not happen.

❑❑  **What syndrome is associated with multiple osteomas?**

Gardner's syndrome.

❑❑  **What bones are most commonly involved with osteomas?**

Skull and facial bones.

❑❑  **What tumor is most commonly seen in men in their teens and 20s, in the femur or tibia, and is characterized by nocturnal pain which is relieved by aspirin?**

Osteoid osteoma.

❑❑  **Histologically, what is the appearance of an osteoid osteoma?**

They are composed of a central nidus with surrounding haphazardly arranged interconnecting trabeculae of woven bone that has a prominent rim of osteoblasts.

❑❑  **What is the most common primary malignant tumor of bone?**

Osteosarcoma.

**□□ What is the age distribution of osteosarcoma?**

It is bimodal with the majority occurring in patients less than 20; however, there is a second peak in older adults.

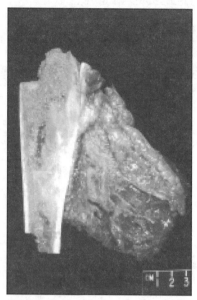

GROSS OSTEOSARCOMA

**□□ What is the most common location of osteosarcoma?**

They occur in the metaphyses of the long bones of the extremities most commonly. More than half are found in the proximal tibia/distal femur.

**□□ What is the manner of spread in metastatic osteosarcoma?**

They spread hematogenously with 1 in 5 patients presenting with pulmonary metastases.

**□□ What is the characteristic but not diagnostic radiographic finding in osteosarcoma?**

The so-called Codman triangle occurs when the periosteum is raised off the cortex creating a triangular configuration.

**□□ What is the inheritance pattern of multiple hereditary exostoses?**

Autosomal dominant.

**□□ What is the benign tumor which is characterized by an outgrowth of cortical and medullary bone with a hyaline cartilage cap?**

Osteochondroma (exostosis).

**□□ What is the intraosseous cartilaginous tumor which arises in the medullary cavity of bones in patients in their 20s-40s?**

Enchondromas.

**□□ What is the typical location in the bone of enchondromas?**

Metaphysis.

❑❑  **What is Ollier's disease?**

This is a syndrome characterized by multiple enchondromas or enchondromatosis.

❑❑  **What is the syndrome characterized by enchondromatosis in concert with hemangiomas of the soft tissue?**

Maffucci syndrome.

❑❑  **What is the favored location of origin of chondroblastoma?**

They arise in the epiphyses, particularly around the knee.

❑❑  **What is the characteristic mineralization  pattern  seen  frequently in chondroblastoma?**

The tumor cells are embedded in a hyaline matrix which, when mineralized, imparts a "chicken-wire" pattern.

❑❑  **What is the typical age and sex of a patient with chondromyxoid fibroma?**

Adolescent to young adult males.

❑❑  **What bones are typically effected by chondromyxoid fibroma?**

They tend to arise in the metaphyses of long, tubular bones.

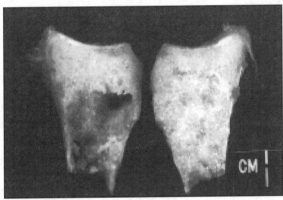

CHONDROSARCOMA

❑❑  **How does clear cell chondrosarcoma like the one depicted differ from conventional chondrosarcoma?**

Clear cell chondrosarcoma tends to arise in the epiphyses of long bones and occurs in adolescent and young adult patients.  In contrast, conventional chondrosarcoma tends to occur in patients older than 40 and tends to arise in the pelvis, shoulder, and ribs.

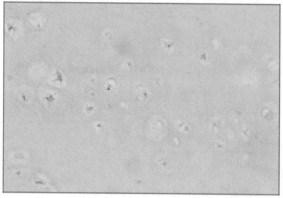

GRADE 1 CHONDROSARCOMA

❑❑  **What are two key histologic features to help differentiate between a low chondrosarcoma like this one and a high grade chondrosarcoma?**

Cellularity and mitotic activity.

❑❑  **What is the average five year survival for a conventional chondrosarcoma?**

For grade I tumors about 90%, grade II about 80%, and grade III about 40%.

❑❑  **What is the most common benign tumor of bone in patients less than 21?**

Osteochondroma.

❑❑  **What is the treatment of chondroblastoma?**

Curettage or local excision.

❑❑  **What is the most common clinical presentation of patients with chondromyxoid fibroma?**

Pain.

❑❑  **What is the treatment of choice in osteosarcoma?**

Amputation with chemotherapy.

❑❑  **Is there a gender preference in chondrosarcoma?**

Yes, they are three times more common in men.

❑❑  **What is the typical age and clinical presentation of patients with Legg-Calve-Perthes disease?**

This form of osteonecrosis occurs in children (peak age 5) and is more common in males. They classically present with a limp and associated pain. It may be bilateral and its precise etiology is unknown.

❑❑  **What are the most common sites of involvement by fibrous dysplasia?**

For the monostotic form (single bone involvement), the most frequent sites are ribs, femur, tibia, jaw, calvarium and humerus, in descending order of frequency.

For the polyostotic form (multiple bone involvement), it is the femur, skull, tibia, humerus, ribs, fibula, radius, ulna, mandible and vertebrae, in descending order of frequency.

❏❏  **Which is more common, the monostotic or polyostotic version of fibrous dysplasia?**

About 80% of cases are monostotic.

❏❏  **What is the typical histologic picture of fibrous dysplasia?**

The lesion is composed of curvilinear trabeculae of woven bone in a moderately cellular fibroblastic stroma. The trabeculae are said to mimic the appearance of Chinese letters.  Importantly, there is no osteoblastic rimming of the trabeculae.

❏❏  **What is the McCune-Albright syndrome?**

This is the combination of polyostotic fibrous dysplasia with cafe-au-lait spots and endocrinopathies.

❏❏  **What is the most common clinical presentation in patients with McCune-Albright syndrome?**

Precocious puberty and girls are effected more frequently than boys.

❏❏  **Do most fibrosarcomas and malignant fibrous histiocytomas arise de novo or are they secondary to other conditions?**

The majority are de novo; however, a small percentage do arise in areas of previous irradiation, Paget's disease, bone infarcts, or other benign bone tumors.

❏❏  **What oncogene is expressed in Ewing's sarcoma?**

c-myc.

❏❏  **What is the age, gender, and sex predilection for Ewing's sarcoma?**

80% of cases occur in patients younger than 20 and males are slightly more likely to develop it than females.  Blacks rarely develop this tumor.

❏❏  **What is the translocation and fusion gene in Ewing's sarcoma?**

t(11;22)(q24;q12) and the fusion gene is EWS-FLI1.

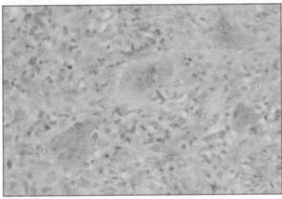

GIANT CELL TUMOR

❏❏  **What is the normal age and location of giant cell tumor of bone like the one shown above?**

They arise in patients from the third to fifth decade and typically involve the epiphyses and metaphyses.  It is more common in females.

**□□  What is the typical behavior and treatment of a giant cell tumor?**

Treatment is aggressive curettage or complete resection.  Interestingly, in spite of a bland appearance, many will recur (1/3) and some will exhibit distant spread including, most commonly, the lung.

**□□  What are some tumors that produce lytic type bone lesions when they metastasize?**

Examples include kidney, lung, colon, and melanoma.

**□□  What general type of metastatic bone lesion does prostate carcinoma produce?**

It tends to produce an osteoblastic lesion with a sclerotic appearance.

**□□  What type of osteosarcoma is characterized by an origin from the surface of the bone, is twice as common in women, arises very frequently from the distal femur, and is associated with a bland histologic appearance and excellent prognosis?**

Parosteal osteosarcoma.

**□□  What is the most common age and site of adamantinoma?**

This is a very rare tumor which typically occurs in patients in the second-fourth decade of life.  The vast majority (90%) involve the diaphysis of the tibia.

**□□  What is the most common site of aneurysmal bone cyst?**

They tend to occur in the metaphysis of the extremities, particularly the femur and proximal tibia. However, almost any bone can be involved.

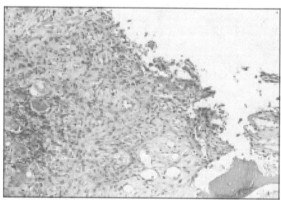

ANEURYSMAL BONE CYST

**□□  What is the typical histologic appearance of aneurysmal bone cysts?**

They are composed of multiple cysts which are devoid of endothelial lining. There may be giant cells and mitotic figures within the connective tissue cyst lining; however, the mitoses are not atypical in appearance.  There may be reactive new bone formation present.

**□□  What is the prognosis for aneurysmal bone cysts?**

They recur at a fairly high rate (approximately 20%) but recurrences may be treated by curettage and packing similar to the primary tumor.

**□□  What are some of the etiologic factors that predispose to the development of osteoarthritis?**

Aging, previous injury, excessive/repetitive use, obesity, and synovial disease.

❑❑  **What are the most common joints involved in osteoarthritis?**

Hips, knees, distal phalangeal, and vertebrae.

❑❑  **What are Heberden's nodes?**

These are nodules which are found at the base of the terminal phalanges of the fingers in patients with osteoarthritis.

❑❑  **How prevalent is osteoarthritis?**

Up to 90% of all people have evidence of some degree of osteoarthritis by age 65.

❑❑  **What are so-called "joint mice"?**

These are portions of bone and articular cartilage which get knocked loose into the joint space in patients with osteoarthritis.

❑❑  **What are the characteristic symptoms of osteoarthritis?**

Morning stiffness, pain that is aggravated with use, range of motion limitation, and crepitus.

❑❑  **What is the typical age and gender of a patient with rheumatoid arthritis (RA)?**

It is four to five times more common in women with a peak in the third to fifth decades.

❑❑  **What are the most common joints involved in rheumatoid arthritis?**

The interphalangeal joints of the fingers and metacarpophalangeal joints of the hands and feet are most commonly involved.  The involvement is bilateral and symmetric.

❑❑  **What is the characteristic deformation of the fingers which occurs in patients with long-standing RA?**

They show ulnar deviation of the fingers and dislocation of the interphalangeal joints.

❑❑  **What are the lesions seen in a quarter of patients with RA that are characterized by a subcutaneous location, central fibrinoid necrosis with a surrounding rim of palisaded histiocytes admixed with lymphocytes and plasma cells?**

Rheumatoid nodules.

❑❑  **What vascular disease can develop in patients with rheumatoid arthritis?**

They can develop a small to medium sized vessel vasculitis which is similar to polyarteritis nodosa.  They also develop obliteration of the vasa vasorum in digital arteries.

❑❑  **What is a commonly found HLA haplotype in patients with RA?**

Up to 80% of patients have HLA-DR4 or HLA-DR1 or both.

❑❑  **What is rheumatoid factor?**

This is predominantly IgM antibody to the Fc portion of autologous IgG which is generated in 80% of patients with rheumatoid arthritis.

❏❏ **What are some of the ways in which juvenile rheumatoid arthritis (JRA) is different from RA?**

Onset before age 16, oligoarthritis (less than 5 joints) is more common, large joints greater than small joints, antinuclear antibody positivity is common, absent rheumatoid nodules and rheumatoid factor.

❏❏ **What is the prognosis in JRA?**

The vast majority of patients (up to 90%) recover with only 10% manifesting pronounced joint deformities that persist.

❏❏ **What joints are most commonly effected in bacterial (septic) arthritis?**

Larger joints such as the knee, hip, ankle, and wrist are most commonly effected.

❏❏ **What are the most common etiologic agents in septic arthritis occurring in pediatric patients?**

Haemophilus influenzae and gram-negative bacilli.

❏❏ **What is the most common anatomic location of tuberculous arthritis?**

The spine.

❏❏ **Describe the typical patient with ankylosing spondyloarthritis.**

It is more common in males and typically begins in adolescence. 90% of patients have the HLA-B27 haplotype and the sacroiliac joint is most commonly involved.

❏❏ **What is Reiter's syndrome?**

Arthritis, urethritis, and conjunctivitis.

❏❏ **Describe the typical patient with Reiter's syndrome.**

It is more common in men and occurs typically in the 20s and 30s. Again, about 80% are positive for the HLA-B27 haplotype.

❏❏ **What type of arthritis is characterized by abrupt involvement of the knees and ankles, a course of about 12 months, HLA-B27 positivity, previous bowel infection with organisms such as Yersinia, and inducement of joint damage by the lipopolysaccharides of the organisms?**

Enteropathic arthritis.

❏❏ **What is the nature of the arthritis seen in Lyme disease?**

80% of patients with Lyme disease develop joint manifestations and the arthritis tends to be migratory and waxes and wanes. It typically involves large joints most commonly the knees, shoulders, and elbows.

❏❏ **What is the plasma level of urate in which, at normal body temperature and pH, urea would exceed its saturation?**

7 mg/dl.

❏❏ **What are the two pathways of purine synthesis?**

There is a de novo pathway in which purines are built from nonpurine precursor substances and a salvage pathway in which purine bases broken down from nucleic acids are saved and used for further production.

❑❑  **What is the enzyme which is involved in the salvage pathway of purine synthesis and is absent in Lesch-Nyhan syndrome?**

Hypoxanthine guanine phosphoribosyl transferase (HGPRT).

❑❑  **What is the term given to the large aggregates of urate crystals in the joints and soft tissues in gout?**

Tophi.

❑❑  **What are some of the drug treatments used in gout?**

Colchicine, probenecid, and allopurinol.

❑❑  **What is the appearance of the crystals in gout?**

They are needle-like and appear yellow under parallel polarized light.

❑❑  **What is pseudogout?**

This is calcium pyrophosphate crystal deposition disease (CPPD), occurs in patients who are older than 50, and is often asymptomatic but can produce arthritic complaints with subsequent joint damage.

❑❑  **What is the benign cyst which typically presents as a mobile subcutaneous nodule on the wrist and contains mucoid material?**

Ganglion cyst.

❑❑  **What is the most common soft tissue tumor?**

Lipoma.

❑❑  **While most lipomas are painless, which type is characterized by clinical presentation as a painful mass?**

Angiolipoma.

❑❑  **What types of liposarcomas feature the most aggressive behavior?**

Round cell and pleomorphic. The well-differentiated liposarcoma is indolent; however, when located in the retroperitoneum it presents a difficult surgical problem and can be locally aggressive over a long course.

❑❑  **Describe the typical presentation of nodular fasciitis.**

It most characteristically occurs in men on the volar aspect of the forearm with a history of a very rapidly (weeks) growing mass which sometimes elicits pain. A history of trauma is provided in a minority of cases.

❑❑  **An 18-year-old male football player presents with a very hard, painless, well-defined mass in the upper arm. He tells you that he received a significant hit during a game in that area and the area became painful and swollen very rapidly. It gradually evolved into this hard, painless mass. What is your best diagnosis?**

Myositis ossificans.

❑❑  **Describe the typical "zonation" which occurs microscopically in myositis ossificans.**

This zonation occurs within three weeks of origin of the tumor. Centrally, there is a proliferation of fibroblasts. The intermediate zone contains osteoblasts and irregular trabeculae of woven bone. The third and most peripheral zone contains mineralized trabeculae which are microscopically similar to normal cancellous bones.

❑❑  **What is another name for palmar fibromatosis?**

Dupuytren's contracture.

❑❑  **What tumor is benign yet locally aggressive and tends to arise from the anterior abdominal wall in pregnant or postpartum women?**

Abdominal desmoid (fibromatosis).

❑❑  **What benign, locally aggressive tumor tends to occur in the mesentery and/or pelvic wall in patients with a history of Gardner's syndrome?**

Intra-abdominal desmoid (fibromatosis).

❑❑  **What soft tissue sarcoma is classically characterized by a prominent herring bone pattern microscopically?**

Fibrosarcoma.

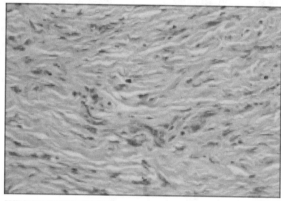

SUBCUTANEOUS NODULE

❑❑  **What is a common benign fibrohistiocytic tumor which occurs in the dermis and subcutis in middle-aged adults which has ill-defined borders but does not involve the overlying epidermis?**

Benign fibrous histiocytoma (dermatofibroma) like the one shown above.

❑❑  **What is the tumor which is essentially a malignant fibrous histiocytoma that occurs in the superficial skin?**

Atypical fibroxanthoma.

❑❑  **What is the most common subtype of malignant fibrous histiocytoma (MFH)?**

The pleomorphic-storiform type is the most common. Other types include myxoid, inflammatory, giant cell, and angiomatoid.

❑❑  **What is the prognosis in MFH?**

It is poor, the tumors are locally aggressive and metastasize at a rate of up to 50%.

❏❏  **What is the most common soft tissue sarcoma found in children and adolescents?**

Rhabdomyosarcoma.

❏❏  **What is the most common location of rhabdomyosarcoma in the pediatric population?**

Head and neck and the genitourinary tract.

❏❏  **What is the most common type of rhabdomyosarcoma?**

Embryonal.

❏❏  **What type of rhabdomyosarcoma is most commonly seen in adults?**

Pleomorphic.

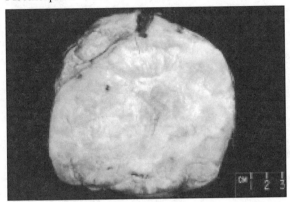

SMOOTH MUSCLE TUMOR OF UTERUS

❏❏  **The above photo represents the most common neoplasm in women and is a benign smooth muscle tumor.  What is it?**

Leiomyoma.

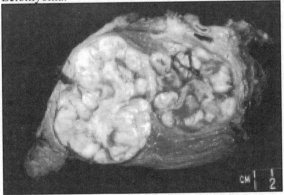

LEIOMYOSARCOMA
*(Photo courtesy of Julie Breiner, MD - University of Nebraska Medical Center)*

❏❏  **What are the most common sites of origin of leiomyosarcoma like the one shown?**

Uterus and the gastrointestinal tract.

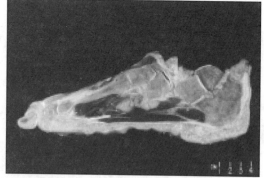
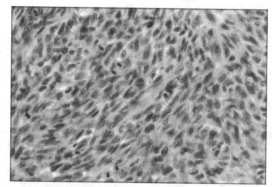

GROSS SARCOMA;                                    MICROSCOPIC SARCOMA

❑❑  **The sarcoma shown above is characterized by occurrence in young adults, 90% occurrence in the extremities (2/3 in the lower extremities), sometimes showing a biphasic histologic pattern, and tendency to spread via lymphatics.  What is your diagnosis?**

Synovial sarcoma.

❑❑  **What benign reactive lesion most commonly occurs in the ear lobe following ear piercing and has a greater incidence in African-Americans?**

Keloid (hypertrophic scar).

❑❑  **What is the most common postirradiation sarcoma?**

Pleomorphic-storiform MFH.

❑❑  **Compare the prognoses for pleomorphic storiform MFH, atypical fibroxanthoma, myxoid MFH, MFH of giant cell type, and inflammatory MFH.**

Pleomorphic-storiform MFH is high grade and associated with a poor prognosis with frequent local recurrence and high metastatic rate (mostly lungs).  MFH of giant cell type is said to behave similarly as does inflammatory MFH. Atypical fibroxanthoma has an excellent prognosis and myxoid MFH is less aggressive than the pleomorphic-storiform with metastases occurring in about 25% of the cases.

❑❑  **What is the name of the benign vascular tumor which occurs in the skin at all ages and, in infants, may spontaneously regress?**

Hemangiomas, capillary or cavernous.

❑❑  **What reactive vascular proliferation bares a resemblance to granulation tissue and classically occurs on the gums of pregnant females?**

Pyogenic granuloma.

❑❑  **What cystic lesion is typically found as a neck mass in small children and sometimes in aborted fetuses with Turner's syndrome?**

Cystic hygroma (cystic lymphangioma).

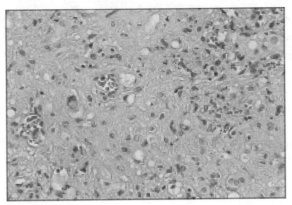

SOFT TISSUE TUMOR

❏❏  **What relatively uncommon soft tissue tumor occurs in adults, usually follows a benign course, and is characterized by multivacuolated cells which often contain red cells and represent intracytoplasmic vascular lumens?**

Epithelioid hemangioendothelioma (see above image).

❏❏  **What is the favored location of cutaneous angiosarcomas?**

They typically occur on the scalp or face of elderly patients.

❏❏  **A 32-year-old male with AIDS presents with multiple cutaneous plaques which, when biopsied, consist of a vascular spindle cell proliferation containing numerous mitoses, extravasated red cells, and intracytoplasmic PAS-positive globules in the spindle cells.  What is your diagnosis?**

Kaposi's sarcoma which is associated with human herpersvirus 8 (HHV 8).

❏❏  **A patient presents with a painful subungual lesion.  What is your best diagnosis based on history alone?**

Glomus tumor.

❏❏  **What associated condition is seen in half the patients with malignant peripheral nerve sheath tumor (MPNST)?**

Neurofibromatosis type I.

342

# SKIN

□□ **How does vitiligo differ from albinism?**

In vitiligo, there is extensive or complete loss of melanocytes resulting in hypopigmentation. In contrast, in albinism melanocytes are present in normal numbers but melanin pigment is not produced owing to a deficiency or lack of tyrosinase enzyme.

□□ **What is an ephelis?**

This is also referred to as a freckle and represents increased melanin pigment within basal keratinocytes. Melanocytes are not increased in number typically.

□□ **What is the term used to describe a benign proliferation or hyperplasia of melanocytes?**

Lentigo.

□□ **What happens when a lentigo is exposed to the sun?**

Nothing. Unlike a freckle, they do not darken when exposed to sunlight.

□□ **What type of melanocytic nevus is characterized by a proliferation of small, typical appearing melanocytes in nests which are confined to the epidermis at the dermal-epidermal junction?**

Junctional nevus.

□□ **What is the name given to a melanocytic nevus which features both an epidermal and dermal component?**

Compound melanocytic nevus.

□□ **What are some of the clinical signs/symptoms of melanoma?**

Change in size and shape of a pre-existing pigmented lesion, itching or pain in a pre-existing pigmented lesion, development of a new pigmented lesion as an adult, change in color of a pigmented lesion.

□□ **What is the best predictor of prognosis in malignant melanoma?**

The depth of skin invasion as measured from the granular cell layer.

□□ **A 65-year-old male presents with a lesion on his back that features a granular surface and appears as if it can be "peeled off". A biopsy demonstrates acanthosis and pseudohorn cysts. What is your diagnosis?**

Seborrheic keratosis.

□□ **An older patient presents with acanthosis nigricans, what should you rule out?**

An underlying adenocarcinoma.

□□ **Which is more common in acanthosis nigricans, the benign type or the malignant type?**

The benign type occurs in younger patients and accounts for about 80% of cases.

❑❑  A patient presents with a polypoid skin growth which you resect. Histologically, it is composed of normal appearing epidermis overlying a polypoid dermis with a fibrovascular core. What is your diagnosis?

Acrochordon (skin tag, fibroepithelial polyp).

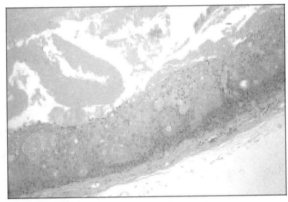

EPITHELIAL CYST

❑❑  This epithelial cyst is characterized by a squamous epithelial lining which is devoid of a granular cell layer and is filled with a homogeneous eosinophilic keratin and lipid debris. What is your best diagnosis?

Pilar or trichilemmal cyst.

❑❑  What epithelial cyst is characterized by a squamous epithelial lining with associated appendages inherent within its wall?

Dermoid cyst.

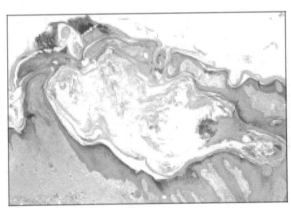

KERATOACANTHOMA

❑❑  Describe the typical patient with a keratoacanthoma like this one.

These are more common in the sun-exposed skin of white males older than 50. It involves the skin of the face and the dorsal hands most commonly.

❑❑  What is the prognosis in keratoacanthoma?

It is excellent, these lesions spontaneously regress in the majority of cases.

❏❏ **What is the most common location for an eccrine poroma?**

The palms and soles.

❏❏ **What is the most common location for a cylindroma?**

Forehead and scalp.

❏❏ **What is the most common location for a syringoma?**

Lower eyelids.

❏❏ **What is the most common location for a sebaceous carcinoma?**

They most commonly arise from the meibomian glands of the eyelid. These can be extremely aggressive both locally and systemically.

❏❏ **What are some of the treatment options in actinic (solar) keratoses?**

Curettage, cryotherapy, or topical chemotherapy (5-FU).

❏❏ **What are some of the associations in patients who develop squamous cell carcinoma?**

It is twice as common in males. There is an increased incidence in immunosuppressed patients, patients with xeroderma pigmentosum, ulcers, scars, chronic osteomyelitis and, of course, previous ultraviolet light (sunlight) damage .

❏❏ **This tumor is characterized by slow growth, origin on sun-exposed skin, an excellent prognosis and characteristic clefting between the groups of tumor cells and the surrounding stroma. What is your diagnosis?**

Basal cell carcinoma.

❏❏ **What is the form of inheritance in basal cell nevus syndrome?**

Autosomal dominant.

❏❏ **What are some of the types of xanthomas?**

Eruptive, tuberous, tendinous, plane, and xanthelasma.

❏❏ **What type of xanthoma is found in a patient with type IIA hyperlipidemia and primary biliary cirrhosis?**

Plane xanthomas.

❏❏ **An infant presents with multiple skin lesions comprising papules and nodules. A biopsy shows a diffuse dermal infiltrate of large cells with nuclear indentations and grooves. Immunoperoxidase staining is performed and demonstrates the presence of CD1a antigen. Electron microscopy shows the presence of intracellular Bierbeck granules. What is your diagnosis?**

Histiocytosis X.

❏❏ **What is the name of the condition characterized by a proliferation of CD4 positive cells (T lymphocytes) that involve the epidermis both as single cells and small groups (Pautrier microabscesses), has a "cerebriform" appearance and follows an indolent course?**

Mycosis fungoides.

❏❐ **What is this condition referred to in a patient with mycosis fungoides who develops diffuse erythroderma and circulating Sezary cells?**

Sezary syndrome.

❏❐ **What is urticaria pigmentosa?**

This is a localized cutaneous form of mastocytosis seen in children. The skin lesions are widely distributed and consist of papules and small plaques.

❏❐ **What is the general category of diseases which are characterized by impediment of normal epidermal maturation with the resultant appearance of fishlike scales?**

Icthyosis.

❏❐ **What is the inheritance pattern of icthyosis vulgaris?**

There is an acquired type in adults that is often seen in association with lymphoma or visceral malignancies. In addition, there is an autosomal dominant form.

❏❐ **What substance is deficient in patients with hereditary angioneurotic edema that results in continued activation of complement?**

C1 esterase inhibitor.

❏❐ **What is the classic, but not always present, skin appearance of the lesions associated with erythema multiforme?**

Classically, there are target lesions which are characterized by a central "blister" or epidermal necrosis with surrounding macular erythema. However, these patients get multiple types of lesions including typical macules, papules, vesicles, and bullae.

❏❐ **What are some of the conditions which are associated with erythema multiforme?**

Various infections such as herpes simplex, mycoplasma and many others; certain drugs such as penicillins, sulfonamides and others; malignancies; and collagen vascular disorders.

❏❐ **What is Stevens-Johnson syndrome?**

This is a severe febrile form of erythema multiforme which is more common in children and includes bullous eruption of the skin and mucous membranes.

❏❐ **Is there a genetic component to psoriasis?**

Yes, certain HLA types have an increased incidence. Some experts think the disease may represent incomplete penetrance of an autosomal dominant condition.

❏❐ **What condition is classically characterized by "pruritic purple polygonal papules"?**

Lichen planus.

❏❐ **Do most patients with discoid lupus erythematosus (DLE) go on to develop systemic LE?**

No.

❏❐ **What would you expect to find on immunofluorescence in DLE?**

DLE shows a granular band of positive immunofluorescence of immunoglobulin and complement along the dermal-epidermal junction ("lupus band test"). Patients with DLE typically do not demonstrate immunofluorescence in nonlesional skin while patients with SLE may show positive immunofluorescence in both lesional and nonlesional skin.

☐☐  **What is the most common form of pemphigus?**

Pemphigus vulgaris accounts for greater than 80% of cases.

☐☐  **Describe the typical bulla in pemphigus vulgaris.**

It demonstrates a suprabasal acantholytic blister leaving behind a row of basal cells sometimes referred to as "tombstones".

☐☐  **Describe the typical immunofluorescence in pemphigus vulgaris.**

IgG deposits in the intercellular areas in sites of acantholysis. This has been likened to a "fish net" pattern.

☐☐  **What is the immunofluorescence pattern in bullous pemphigoid?**

Classically, there is linear deposition of immunoglobulin and complement along the basement membrane.

☐☐  **What is the location of the bulla in bullous pemphigoid?**

It is a subepidermal, nonacantholytic bulla, in contrast to pemphigus vulgaris.

☐☐  **Describe the typical patient who develops dermatitis herpetiformis.**

It is more common in males and tends to occur in the third and fourth decade; however, this is quite variable. It has a strong association with celiac disease and, like the gastrointestinal disease, the skin manifestations respond to a gluten free diet.

☐☐  **What are some common HLA haplotypes seen in dermatitis herpetiformis?**

HLA-B8, DRW3, and A1.

☐☐  **Describe the immunofluorescence pattern seen in dermatitis herpetiformis.**

The subepidermal microabscesses are characterized by granular deposits of IgA and C3.

☐☐  **What are some conditions which are associated with subepidermal bulla formation with little or no associated inflammation?**

Epidermolysis bullosa, bullosis diabeticorum, pseudoporphyria, porphyria cutanea tarda, cell-poor bullous pemphigoid, and thermal injury.

☐☐  **What is the immunofluorescence pattern in the porphyrias?**

They demonstrate linear immunoglobulin (most commonly IgG) and C3 staining around the vessels.

☐☐  **What anaerobic bacterium may play a role in acne vulgaris?**

Propionibacterium acnes.

☐☐  **What are some of the treatments for acne vulgaris?**

Vitamin A derivatives (13-cis-retinoic acid) and tetracyclines.

❑❑  **What is the name for the lesions seen in acne vulgaris commonly referred to as "blackheads"?**

Comedons.

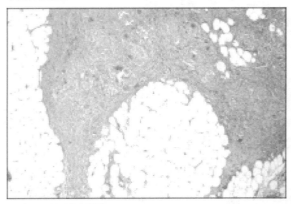

SEPTAL PANNICULITIS

❑❑  **What is the most common form of panniculitis which is shown above?**

Erythema nodosum.

❑❑  **What is the general pattern difference between erythema nodosum and erythema induratum?**

Erythema nodosum is a septal panniculitis while erythema induratum is a lobular panniculitis.

❑❑  **What is Weber-Christian disease?**

It is also referred to as relapsing febrile nodular panniculitis, occurs in children and adults, and is rare.  It is a lobular panniculitis without associated vasculitis and is characterized by plaques or nodules on the lower extremities.  Histologically, there is a granulomatous-type inflammation with neutrophils, lymphocytes, and giant cells.

❑❑  **What is the skin lesion associated with Lyme disease?**

Erythema chronicum migrans.

❑❑  **What is the causative agent of verruca vulgaris?**

Human papillomavirus (HPV).

❑❑  **What is the causative agent of molluscum contagiosum?**

A poxvirus.

❑❑  **What is the most common causative agent of impetigo?**

Coagulase-positive staphylococci or, less commonly, group A beta-hemolytic streptococci.

❑❑  **What are the most common locations for molluscum contagiosum?**

Trunk and anogenital regions.

❑❑  **What is the term given to describe the dermatophyte infection on the scalp?**

Tinea capitis.

☐☐  **What is the name given to the dermatophyte infection of the foot?**

Tinea pedis.

☐☐  **What is the causative organism of tinea versicolor?**

Malassezia furfur.

☐☐  **What is the causative agent of scabies?**

The mite Sarcoptes scabiei.

☐☐  **What are some of the etiologic associations with acne vulgaris?**

Heredity, diet, adequate cleanliness, stress, and warm climates.

☐☐  **What is the enlargement of the nose which occurs in patients with rosacea called?**

Rhinophyma.

☐☐  **What is the causative agent of tinea cruris?**

Trichophyton rubrum.

☐☐  **What is the causative agent of tinea pedis?**

Trichophyton mentagrophytes or T. rubrum.

# BIBLIOGRAPHY

Auclair, P., Ellis, G. Atypical features in salivary gland mixed tumors: their relationship to malignant transformation. Mod Pathol 1998;9;(6)652-657.

Barnhill, R.L., Busam, K.J. Textbook of Dermatopathology, New York: McGraw-Hill 1998.

Batts, K., Ludwig, J. Chronic hepatitis an update on terminology. Am J of Surg Pathol 1995 19(12):1409-1417.

Brunning, R.D., McKenna, R.W. Tumors of the bone marrow. Atlas of Tumor Pathology, Third Series, 1994.

Burger, P.C., Scheithauer, B.W. Tumors of the central nervous system. Atlas of Tumor Pathology, Third Series, 1994.

Byers, P. , Holbrook, K., Emery, A., Rimoin, D. Ehlers-Danlos syndrome in principles and practice of medical genetics, New York: Churchill Livingstone, 2nd Ed, 1990, p. 1065.

Cochand-Priollet, B., et al. Renal chromophobe cell carcinoma and oncocytoma, Arch Pathol Lab Med. 1997; 121:1081-1086.

Cotran, R., Kumar, V., Collins, T. Robbins Pathologic Basis of Disease. Philadelphia: W.B. Saunders Company, 6th Ed, 1999.

Cotran, R., Kumar, V., Robbins, S. Robbins Pathologic Basis of Disease. Philadelphia: W.B. Saunders Company, 5th Ed, 1994.

Damjanov, I. Linder, J. Anderson's Pathology. St. Louis: Mosby, 1996.

Delahunt, B., Eble, J.N. Papillary renal cell carcinoma: a clinicopathologic and immunohistochemical study of 105 tumors. Mod Pathol 1997; 10(6) 537-544.

Deugnier, Y., et al. Primary liver cancer in genetic hemochromatosis: a clinical, pathological, and pathogenetic study of 54 cases. Gastroenterology 104, 1993: 228-234.

Devaney, K., Wenig, B., Abbondanzo, S. Olfactory neuroblastoma and other round cell lesions of the sinonasal region. Mod Pathol 1998;9;(6):658-663.

Dorfman, H.D., Czerniak, B. Bone tumors. St. Louis: Mosby, 1997.

Elston, C.W., Ellis, I.O. The breast, Systemic Pathology, New York: Churchill Livingstone, 1998.

Enzinger, F.M., Weiss, S.W. Soft tissue tumors. St. Louis: Mosby, 1995.

Epstein, J. Prostate biopsy interpretation. Philadelphia: Lippincott-Raven, 2nd Ed, 1995.

Fechner, R.E., Mills, S.E. Tumors of the bones and joints, Atlas of Tumor Pathology, Third Series, 1993.

Foucar, K. Bone marrow pathology. Chicago: ASCP Press, 1995.

Fukunaga, M., Nomura, K., Matsumoto, K., Doi, K., Endo, Y., Ushigome, S. Vulval angiomyofibroblastoma. Am J Clin Pathol 1997; 107:45-51.

Hsing, A., et al. Cancer risk following primary hemochromatosis: a population-based cohort study in Denmark. Int J Cancer, 60, 1995:160-162.

Hubbert, N., Sedman, S., Schiller, J. Human papilloma virus type 16 increases the degradation of p53 in human keratinocytes, J Virol 66: 3547, 1992.

Hwang, H., Mills, S., Patterson, K., Gown, A. Expression of androgen receptors in nasopharyngeal angiofibroma: an immunohistochemical study of 24 cases. Mod Pathol 1998;11(11):1122-1126.

Ishak K. Chronic hepatitis: morphology and nomenclature. Modern Pathol 1994 7(6):690-713.

Kurman, R. J., Norris, H.J., Wilkinson, E. Tumors of the cervix, vagina, and vulva, Atlas of Tumor Pathology, Third Series, 1990.

Levinson, W., Jawetz, E. Medical microbiology & immunology, examination and board review. Stamford: Appleton & Lange, 1996.

LiVolsi, V., Merino, M., Brooks, J., Saul, S., Tomaszewski, J. Pathology - the national medical series for independent study. Philadelphia: Harwal Publishing, 3rd Ed, 1994.

Ludwig, J., Batts, K. Practical Liver Biopsy Interpretation Diagnostic Algorithms Chicago: ASCP Press, 2nd Ed, 1998.

MacSween, R., Anthony, P., Scheuer, P., Burt, A., Portmann, B. Pathology of the liver. New York: Churchill Livingstone, 1994.

Motzer, R.J., Bander, N.H., Nanus, D.M. Renal cell carcinoma. NE J of Med, 1996; 865-875

Newland J. Pathology - examination and board review. Norwalk: Appleton and Lange, 1995.

Ockner, D.M., Sayadi, H., Swanson, P.E., Ritter, J.H., Wick, M.R. Genital angiomyofibroblastoma. Am J Clin Pathol 1997; 107:36-44.

Rosai, J. Ackerman's Surgical Pathology. St. Louis: Mosby, 8th Ed, 1996.

Rosen, P.P., Oberman, H.A. Tumors of the mammary gland, Atlas of Tumor Pathology, Third Series, 1993.

Rossi, E., Simon, T., Moss, G., Sould S., Principles of transfusion medicine. Baltimore: Williams and Wilkins, 2nd Ed, 1996.

Sampson, B., Jarcho, J., Winters, G. Metastasizing mixed tumor of the parotid gland: a rare tumor with unusually rapid progression in a cardiac transplant recipient. Mod Pathol 1998;11(11):1142-1145.

Sherlock, S. Primary biliary cirrhosis: clarifying the issues. The American Journal of Medicine, 96(suppl 1A), Jan 1994: 27S-32S.

Sherris, J. Medical microbiology, an introduction to infectious diseases, New York: Elsevier, 3rd Ed, 1994.

Silverberg, S., DeLellis, R., and Frable, W. Principles and Practice of Surgical Pathology and Cytopathology. New York: Churchill Livingstone, 3rd Ed, 1997.

Silverberg, S.G., Kurman, R.J. Tumors of the uterine corpus and gestational trophoblastic disease, Atlas of Tumor Pathology, Third Series, 1991.

Sternberg, S.S. Diagnostic Surgical Pathology.  New York:  Raven Press, 2nd Ed, 1994.

Tavassoli, F.A.  Pathology of the Breast.  Norwalk:  Appleton & Lange, 1992.

Vengelen-Tyler V et al,  Technical Manual American Association of Blood Banks. (12th Ed.) Bethesda, MD. 1996.

Werness, B., Levine, A., Howley, P.  Association of human papilloma virus types 16 and 18 E6 proteins with p53.  Science 248: 76, 1990.

Young, R. & Scully, R.  Testicular Tumors. Chicago: ASCP Press, 1990.